Breast Cancer Basics and Beyond

DEDICATION

To all whose lives have been touched directly or indirectly by cancer

Ordering

Trade bookstores in the U.S. and Canada please contact:
Publishers Group West
1700 Fourth Street, Berkeley CA 94710
Phone: (800) 788-3123   Fax: (510) 528-3444

Hunter House books are available at bulk discounts for textbook course adoptions; to qualifying community, health-care, and government organizations; and for special promotions and fund-raising. For details please contact:

Special Sales Department
Hunter House Inc., PO Box 2914, Alameda CA 94501-0914
Phone: (510) 865-5282   Fax: (510) 865-4295
E-mail: ordering@hunterhouse.com

Individuals can order our books from most bookstores, by calling
(800) 266-5592, or from our website at www.hunterhouse.com

Breast Cancer Basics and Beyond

TREATMENTS, RESOURCES, SELF-HELP,
GOOD NEWS, UPDATES

Delthia Ricks, M.S.

Hunter House PUBLISHERS

Hunter House Inc., Publishers
PO Box 2914
Alameda CA 94501-0914

Library of Congress Cataloging-in-Publication Data

Ricks, Delthia.
Breast cancer basics and beyond : treatments, resources,
self-help, good news, updates / Delthia Ricks.— 1st ed.
p. cm.
Includes bibliographical references and index.
ISBN-10: 0-89793-454-7 (pbk.)
ISBN-13: 978-0-89793-454-1 (pbk.)
1. Breast—Cancer—Popular works. I. Title.
RC280.B8R535 2005
616.99'449—dc22   2005007293

Project Credits

Cover Design: Brian Dittmar Graphic Design
Book Production: Hunter House
Copy Editor: Kelley Blewster
Proofreader: Rachel E. Bernstein
Indexer: Nancy D. Peterson
Acquisitions Editor: Jeanne Brondino
Editor: Alexandra Mummery
Publishing Assistants: Antonia T. Lee, Herman Leung
Publicist: Jillian Steinberger
Foreign Rights Coordinator: Elisabeth Wohofsky
Customer Service Manager: Christina Sverdrup
Order Fulfillment: Washul Lakdhon
Administrator: Theresa Nelson
Computer Support: Peter Eichelberger
Publisher: Kiran S. Rana

Printed and Bound by Bang Printing, Brainerd, Minnesota

Manufactured in the United States of America

9 8 7 6 5 4 3 2 1   First Edition   05 06 07 08 09

Contents

❧ ❧ ❧

IMPORTANT NOTE

The material in this book is intended to provide a review of re-sources and information related to breast cancer. Every effort has been made to provide accurate and dependable informa-tion. However, professionals in the field may have differing opinions and change is always taking place. Any of the treat-ments described herein should be undertaken only under the guidance of a licensed health-care practitioner. The author, editors, and publishers cannot be held responsible for any error, omission, professional disagreement, outdated material, or ad-verse outcomes that derive from use of any of the treatments or information resources outlined in this book, either in a pro-gram of self-care or under the care of a licensed practitioner.

Foreword

❦ ❦ ❦

One out of every five patients who pass through the front entrance of our cancer center has breast cancer. As a practicing oncologist for thirty years, I have listened to many women and a few men tell their stories about the single most important event in their lives: that initial, and often shocking, moment when they were diagnosed with breast cancer. In *Breast Cancer Basics and Beyond*, Delthia Ricks' stories of breast cancer patients accurately depict reality. Her collection of moving and inspiring first-person accounts from patients, caregivers, and other people clearly separates the book from the many others that are focused on this significant health issue. The stories also add a personal touch to this scientifically accurate, evidence-based, very educational, and superbly written book.

The audience for this book is not only breast cancer patients, but also their families, all those at risk for the disease, and the medical professionals who care for patients and their families. Because of the enormous amount of helpful information and the many resources contained in this book, I recommend it to all who must confront breast cancer in one capacity or another.

That Delthia could or would write such a valuable book is no surprise to me. I have known her as an extremely talented science writer for most of my career. We became friends and colleagues in the business of sharing health-related information with the public when, in her early career, she was the health writer for the *Orlando Sentinel* and I was a young practitioner of medical oncology in the same city. Delthia never seemed reluctant to give me a call when she wanted a physician's perspective on a health topic about which she was reporting. Because of her exceptional ability to grasp the essence of the issue at hand and report it with uncanny accuracy, I always honored her request for input.

It is indeed a privilege to be asked to write a Foreword to Delthia Ricks' *Breast Cancer Basics and Beyond*. It is a book with which I am very pleased to be associated.

Clarence H. Brown III, M.D.
President and Chief Executive Officer
M.D. Anderson Cancer Center Orlando
Orlando, Florida

Introduction

❧ ❧ ❧

Within minutes after Senator John Kerry, the Democrat from Massachusetts, delivered his concession speech announcing his loss in the 2004 race for the U.S. presidency, Elizabeth Edwards, the wife of Kerry's running mate, was whisked away by Secret Service agents to Massachusetts General Hospital. During the hotly contested campaign, Mrs. Edwards had discovered a lump in one of her breasts but had waited until the outcome of the race before seeking treatment.

What happened to Elizabeth Edwards immediately after going public with her diagnosis should not have happened to anyone. In many ways, news commentators and the "talking heads" that television outlets hire for "expert" commentary essentially blamed Mrs. Edwards for being derelict in her duties when it came to cancer screening. Worse still, seasoned reporters sent wrongheaded messages to probably thousands of other women facing a breast cancer diagnosis, making them feel guilty for a wide range of reasons that were not fully grounded in fact. In the current pop-fitness culture, in which any kind of illness is viewed as personal failure, you can quickly be made to feel guilty for breaking an important health rule. Accusing fingers begin to point when you come down with a serious condition these days—surely you must have done something to seal your own fate.

Mrs. Edwards was taken to task for what was deemed a major infraction: She hadn't gotten a mammogram in the previous four years. On NBC, she was chastised before millions of television viewers. And though it wasn't stated, the implication was evident: Had Mrs. Edwards been timely about her mammograms she would have been in a far better position than she was at that moment. You really had to ask yourself why this know-it-all TV personality was upbraiding this woman so publicly. Mrs. Edwards' doctors were nowhere in

1

sight to provide technical details on what the lapse in her mammography schedule really meant. Still, Mrs. Edwards was on the hot seat, and the talk-show host found her guilty of neglect, essentially marking her as a conspirator in her own cancer.

A similar tone was taken on CNN, where, again, the mammography lapse was pointed out. No one bothered to explain that mammography is detection—not prevention. The accusatory tone of the "news" made it seem the other way around.

By highlighting the lapse, an opportunity to teach about breast cancer was missed: Given that Mrs. Edwards already had cancer, the issue shouldn't have been colored by speculation on how she got it, but how she would move forward. In other words, how do people find the strength to cope when abruptly handed a cancer diagnosis? In her case that question had special resonance. Only eight years earlier her oldest son was killed in a car crash, her husband had just lost a major election—now breast cancer. Empathy would have been much more galvanizing. But the story unfortunately doesn't end there.

Some reporters dug deeper into Mrs. Edwards' personal life and spoke of her late-in-life pregnancies, noting that she gave birth to her youngest child at age fifty. Having children later in life indeed is linked to an elevated breast cancer risk. But some reporters brazenly stated that the pregnancies had probably caused her cancer. None of the reporters had access to Mrs. Edwards' private medical records. The documents would have enabled media commentators to discuss her diagnosis in the full context of her medical history. Thank goodness for medical privacy laws; there's no telling how armchair doctors would have interpreted such sensitive material.

The final slap involved Mrs. Edwards' weight. More than one cable outlet made reference to her size, saying that obesity "causes" breast cancer. Again, no one had access to her private medical records. These assessments were simply a matter of eyeballing the lady and deciding she looked fat. In all instances, reporters and talk-show hosts alike wished Mrs. Edwards a speedy recovery, gestures that seemed obligatory and that rang desperately hollow, tacked on to reports in which the real news was her inattention to having routine mammograms and to her diet.

For anyone newly diagnosed with breast cancer it is virtually impossible to avoid the daily onslaught of medical news, especially when it involves someone famous. *Breast Cancer Basics and Beyond* is designed to help you cut through the myths, sensationalism, and scare-mongering surrounding the topic of breast cancer. It presents the basic facts about the condition framed in the words of survivors, activists, physicians, and nurses who know better than most the truth about the disease and about the strength that comes with survivorship.

The Reasons for This Book

Curiously, more than for any other form of cancer, accusations, myths, and misinformation about breast cancer have proliferated alongside the stunning advancements made in its treatment. Why this is so remains a mystery. Who hasn't heard that deodorants and antiperspirants "cause" breast cancer, or that under-wire bras might be associated with the disease? Even more puzzling are the scares that frequently crop up about breast cancer. In 2004, panic ensued when a small study associated antibiotics—some of the most commonly used pharmaceuticals—with the cancer. In response, the American Council on Science and Health listed this widely reported "link" as one of its Top Ten Unfounded Health Scares of 2004. The council blamed poor reporting in newspapers and other media outlets for raising the alarm. Of course, all of these "causes"—deodorants, bad bras, and antibiotics—belong to the category of mythology surrounding the cancer. It is misinformation such as this that I attempt to dispel in this book through testimonies from people who know the truth.

There are several other reasons I chose to write this book. As a newspaper medical writer I frequently report on breast cancer and its treatment, but the confines of newspaper writing do not allow for expansive interviews or permit me to provide readers with the kind of context they need to fully understand their condition and what to expect from the health-care system.

Additionally, I wanted to tackle the subject of risk and to put it into its proper perspective through the comments of experts who are best able to explain it. Dr. Silvana Martino, of both the John Wayne Cancer Center in Santa Monica, California, and the University of Southern California, states so eloquently that "just being female" is breast cancer's greatest risk factor. Therefore, if you have been newly diagnosed, do not assume that you did something wrong, even in a world now so obsessed with placing blame. Indeed, Dr. Martino points out, three-quarters of all cases of the disease diagnosed in the United States cannot be explained by the known risk factors.

And finally, while there are hundreds of breast cancer books on the market, this one is different because it is aimed at cutting throught the hype by having survivors of all ages and from all walks of life, people who possess intimate knowledge about breast cancer, address many of your concerns.

Quotes and Anecdotes

Throughout the book you will read firsthand accounts of survivors' experiences that run the gamut from discovering a lump or other suspicious symptom to treatment, medications, and recovery. Doctors and advocates for patients from throughout the United States were interviewed and quoted to provide a stronger grounding in what newly diagnosed patients can expect.

Many of the survivors quoted are people I have met over the years as a writer for newspapers and for an international news service. Friends, breast cancer survivors, and family members introduced me to several others. In Chapter 5, many of the women who were treated for breast cancer as a result of a genetic predisposition were members of an online breast cancer listserv and were brought to my attention by Musa Mayer, a New York–based advocate who has written extensively about the disease.

You will notice that the first and last names of physicians and advocates are used throughout the book, but only the first names and last initials of survivors are published. Steps were taken throughout the interviewing phase and writing of the book to avoid revealing too much of each individual's identity. This was to ensure a degree of privacy in the ever-expanding era of Google and other search engines. Many survivors spoke about medical privacy issues, and one woman who discussed her thoughts about genetics and breast cancer asked that not even her last initial be published. Survivors, nevertheless, were free to talk openly about their medical experiences and to convey only as much information as they felt comfortable revealing.

There is much to learn from those who have been treated for breast cancer. The testimonies of these survivors depict both the emotional tug-of-war and the strength that comes from surmounting one of the biggest—and most threatening—obstacles life can throw in your path.

How to Use This Book

The twelve chapters are designed to answer many of the questions that may arise throughout your odyssey from cancer discovery to cancer recovery. The book will walk you through the steps involved in getting a diagnosis and will introduce you to medical terminology and procedures. It invites you to keep a journal chronicling both practical matters regarding your care and your thoughts and feelings about the journey. It also attempts to answer a few questions about insurance and legal issues to give you a somewhat stronger footing as you enter the world of the health-care system, a parallel universe with its own language and protocols.

If you want to conduct your own research about breast cancer, you may want to make note of some of the pointers outlined in the Appendix at the back of the book, which offers guidelines on tracking down the most credible sources of medical information. If you cannot find something in the chapters themselves, turn to the Resources section at the end of the book, which contains information on a wide range of topics. There, you can find the telephone numbers, postal addresses, and e-mail and web addresses for cancer centers, support groups, listservs, and even sources to help you find a wig if you are facing chemotherapy or a prosthesis if you have had a mastectomy.

Certainly, a single volume cannot provide all of the answers, but in *Breast Cancer Basics and Beyond*, with the words of medical professionals and "survivor experts" woven throughout the text, you will at least learn that many have traveled this path before you. You will discover that during no part of this journey are you ever alone.

Chapter *1*

Diagnosis

I wanted it to be a lie. I sat down and stared out the window
and imagined that if I sat very still all of this would just go
away. But of course that didn't happen.

— *Diahann Carroll, actress*

When word of the diagnosis comes, however it comes—face to face
with your doctor or from a nurse over the phone—life splits instan-
taneously into distinct parts: the time before breast cancer and the
time afterward. There's no moving backward in time. A breast cancer
diagnosis brings the meaning of mortality front and center. Life from
the point of diagnosis onward, survivors say, is viewed through a different lens.

From a medical viewpoint your diagnosis is a sequential process
that very likely may have begun with you. You may have noticed a
telltale sign such as a lump, a discharge, or a reddening or deeper discoloration of the skin. But as is often the case, the symptom may
have been invisible and painless, revealed to you and your physicians
only after a routine test, such as a mammogram or ultrasound.

Naturally, reactions vary to the prospects of breast cancer. No
two people respond identically. You may react calmly to the news or
respond with a sense of shock, disbelief, sadness, rage—or some in-
describable combination. The diagnostic process may mark your

first encounters with myriad medical tests and the likelihood of surgery.

Mindful of all these possibilities, this book is intended as a resource for anyone who has been told that she—or he—will be treated for early breast cancer (which involves a tumor that has not spread to a distant site). Your cancer may have been discovered at any one of several stages, from the very earliest point in a tumor's evolution to a stage in which it has invaded deeply in the breast. Your adjoining lymph nodes, in the armpit, may show evidence of the cancer or may be free of the disease. Whatever the case, this book has been written to help you.

In this chapter you'll meet people who recount the moment when they found a lump or were told of a suspicious shadow on a mammogram. Later in the chapter you'll learn what doctors think about the role of mammography and other imaging procedures. The purpose of the biopsy is discussed, as is the range of emotional responses that occurs with the conveyance of unfavorable health news.

But take a deep breath. No treatment decisions have to be made within a week or so after diagnosis, even if you are facing care for invasive breast cancer. The key to emerging from the jolt of the diagnosis is to understand where in this medical odyssey you've been and where along its paths you have yet to go.

Noticing a Lump or Other Symptom

Finding a mass, the symptom most often associated with breast cancer, is a sobering discovery. You may have noticed the abnormality during a routine self-examination. Your doctor may have found it during a physical, or your spouse or partner may have come upon it during lovemaking. Palpable growths are not the only way breast cancer makes its presence known. Symptoms of the disease are numerous and insidious.

Your lesion may have been discovered on a mammogram and may be far too small to palpate. Or it may have developed in a nearby lymph node, producing a nodule in the armpit. Some people notice a dimpling in the breast, pronounced changes in skin texture, a discharge, or an eczema-like rash affecting a nipple.

While breast cancer usually develops silently and produces no discomfort, some patients do report episodes of breast pain preceding their diagnosis. Certain forms of the disease have very conspicuous and striking symptoms. Paget's disease, a very rare form of breast cancer, can cause a crusting and scaling around the nipple. Inflammatory breast cancer can trigger an intense reddening on the chest. Some patients who have been diagnosed with inflammatory breast cancer report itchiness and swelling among their symptoms, which they initially mistook as the prelude to their menstrual cycle. Paget's disease and inflammatory breast cancer will be discussed in greater detail in Chapter 4, "Types of Breast Cancer."

Most who seek medical attention do so after discovering a suspicious lump. Forty-five-year-old Lynne J. discovered one while showering.

> I had been really busy. I'd noticed a couple of times while taking off my bra that my left nipple seemed to point a little off center. I somehow thought my bra was too tight and I needed to buy new bras. One day in the shower, while soaping up, I felt a hard, gravelly lump in my left breast. I made the immediate connection with my nipple's appearance and knew that the lump shouldn't be there, and it was probably bad news.
>
> I was traveling at the time. For days, I kept touching my breast to see if the lump was still there. It always was. When I got home, I called the doctor's office right away, but at first I let them talk me into an appointment far in the future for a "checkup." My fear of having this lump confirmed as breast cancer had to battle my fear of not having it looked at and treated. I finally called back and got an earlier appointment.

Lula F., a nurse for more than four decades, noticed an abnormality only after she developed an itchiness that wouldn't stop. What seems unusual now, she says in retrospect, is that the itch seemed to come on suddenly, as though it were a bug bite.

> My tumor was about an inch in diameter. It was at the base of my breast, just where my bra sits. I discovered it when it

started itching quite a bit, and automatically I started scratching and scratching. When I looked to see what was causing
the itch, that's when I noticed the lump. That's what takes
your breath away, when you first discover it, and you think,
"Where did that come from, it wasn't there before." I was
sixty-one. This was on a Saturday. All evening I kept touching
it. It was stationary. It was not moveable. That's when I
thought, "Oh, no, this is serious."

On Monday, as soon as I thought his office was open, I
went to see my doctor. I explained that I had found a lump, so
they ordered a mammogram. My doctor did a needle biopsy
that day. That weekend I was scheduled to go to San Diego
with my daughter. I didn't say anything to her about it. When
we got back, she heard the message as I was listening to my
answering machine. She started asking questions: "What's
so urgent that you have to call your doctor right away?"
That's when I told her about the lump, and it was no longer a
secret. She said if she had known about the lump, we would
not have gone to San Diego.

Gayle-Marie A., who gave birth for the first time at age forty-
two, also noticed a lump but assumed it was associated with breast-
feeding, despite having weaned her son a year earlier.

I kept thinking it would go away. I had always heard that if
you breast-feed your baby you won't get breast cancer. So
every time I noticed it, I thought it had something to do with
being a new mom. I ignored it. It was a lump, yes, but I never
knew about breast engorgement or what that was like until I
had a baby. That's why I thought the lump had something to
do with all of those things you experience as a mom. It was
only after I asked other mothers at the day-care center if they
also had a lump after they had finished breast-feeding that I
realized it wasn't normal. No one else had gotten anything
like that. That's when I went to the doctor and they found out
it was cancer.

Sometimes the initial sign that breast cancer is present eludes
everybody—doctor and patient. Pat G., thirty-six, had a nagging
pain that bothered her when she walked or sat. She describes it as an

achy feeling that would not go away. The persistent discomfort was something she and her doctor at first assumed was an orthopedic problem.

> I had a pain in my hip; that's why I went to an orthopedic doctor. He gave me medication for it, but the pain didn't go away. He didn't take a bone scan or anything like that. Then about two weeks later a red area showed up on my chest, and I went to a different doctor. This doctor immediately recognized it as the "burn." That's what we call the redness that develops on your chest when you have inflammatory breast cancer.
>
> I was lucky because the doctor recognized inflammatory breast cancer when he saw it. I know it takes a long time for some people to get a diagnosis for this kind of breast cancer because it isn't easy to diagnose.

Barbara G. experienced no symptoms whatsoever. Her diagnosis came after undergoing a routine mammogram.

> There were no symptoms. No lump. Nothing. I felt fine. I was in perfect health. So it was very difficult hearing him tell me I had something life-threatening. I couldn't believe it. You're never prepared for this moment. I thought, "There's something wrong here—he's got it all wrong." I was almost forty-four. I had no family history of breast cancer. So how could this happen? That's what I was thinking.

Yvonne M., fifty-one, found she was facing cancer after an annual mammogram, a test she never thought would find evidence of cancer.

> I had just gotten my yearly mammogram. I was very proactive about getting them, really consistent. It had been ten months since the last one. And I guess I never expected to have breast cancer—well, because it didn't run in my family. But the people giving me the mammogram seemed to have some concern. The same day I got the mammogram, they did the biopsy. I was thinking the lump they saw was from drinking coffee, because I had heard that coffee can cause cysts and all kinds of other breast problems. It was February

when I went in for the exam, and the doctor didn't call me for a week. My friends at work kept telling me it was probably nothing. But he called and said, "We just got your results, and it's not a death sentence—but it is cancer."

Geraldine M., sixty-four, also didn't notice any symptoms and discovered her lesion inadvertently. Apparently, a well-developed mass was growing in her right breast. It had been detected a few months earlier during a routine mammogram. No one at her doctor's office bothered to tell her about the need for further diagnostic testing.

I went in there for a sprained ankle and came out with an Ace bandage and breast cancer. That shouldn't have happened to a dog, but it happened to me and the Lord has kept me here to tell the story. It seems that somebody forgot to give me a call. They had filed away my chart with the breast cancer information in it. But as far as a symptom is concerned, I'd have to say it was the sprained ankle. Divine Providence put that broom handle on the back steps and made me fall. I'm told it was a pretty big tumor. But I didn't know it was there. I didn't feel a thing. They saw it on the mammogram.

Arriving at a Diagnosis

If your mass was not discovered on a mammogram, generally your doctor's first step after physically examining a lump or other symptom is to put in an order for a specific set of images, called a diagnostic mammogram. This series of films will include two images of each breast. Additional images of the area involving the mass are also taken. Mammograms provide information about the position and size of the abnormality.

Studies conducted by the Centers for Disease Control and Prevention demonstrate that among women who undergo routine screening, a mammogram generally detects tumors 1.7 years before they can be felt by hand. Mammograms also spot the tiniest of lesions, including the malignant growths known as ductal carcinoma in situ (DCIS). These growths are composed of abnormal cells in

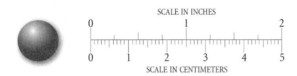

SCALE IN INCHES

SCALE IN CENTIMETERS

Average-size lump found by getting yearly
mammograms when past films can be compared:
0.43 inches or 1.1 cm

Average-size lump found by first mammogram:
0.59 inches or 1.5 cm

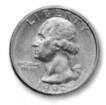

Average-size lump found by women doing regular BSE:
0.81 inches or 2.1 cm

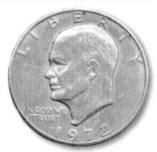

Average-size lump found by accident:
1.40 inches or 3.6 cm

Figure 1. *The size of tumors found by mammography and breast self-exam.*
(Reprinted with permission from the Susan G. Komen Breast Cancer Foundation)

the lining of a milk duct. And while they can grow to a size that you or your doctor might be able to feel as a lump, for many women these clusters are so small that it takes mammography to bring them into view. See Figure 1 to see the average tumor size found using different detection methods.

Dr. Lloyd B. Greig, a gynecologist at Cedars-Sinai Medical Center in Los Angeles, says that to obtain the best possible images a breast must be compressed to flatten it somewhat during a mammogram. To do this, a technician must position the breast on the machine's lower metal platform. The upper one, which is made of see-through plastic, is then eased downward to compress the breast, allowing the image to be taken. Although women have remarked that some technicians can be too aggressive with compression, Dr. Greig says few patients have complained of severe pain after the procedure. "The compression is necessary to get the full diagnostic value of the mammogram," he explains. "If this weren't done, then an abnormality could be missed. Fortunately, it doesn't take much time, just a few seconds. So that's a few seconds of discomfort for taking the right steps. A diagnostic mammogram is a very important part of getting the right information about the abnormality."

For most patients, Dr. Greig continues, the initial visits to a physician will be to a primary care doctor—a family practitioner, internist, or gynecologist—who will not only help you understand early suspicions but also get you started on the path to additional testing. Some women, he says, find it easier to pose questions and voice fears to someone they've known for many years. "We are familiar with the patients," he says. "We've known them, sometimes for many, many years. So we can answer a lot of their questions. This is a very difficult time, and we know that it is important for patients to feel as comfortable as possible—and as confident as possible—as they face their next steps."

Among these initial steps, he tells patients, is the need for the taking of a complete medical history, during which the following series of questions is asked:

❖ Is there a history of breast cancer in your family?

❖ What about other forms of cancer?

❖ Have you noticed a discharge or anything else unusual about either breast?

A complete physical examination also is required. Such simple steps are pivotal, Dr. Greig says, as patients make progress toward obtaining a definitive diagnosis.

At Cedars Sinai, he and other gynecologists work closely with specialists in the medical center's breast-care center, where all types of breast conditions are diagnosed. A vast number of growths detected on mammograms turn out to be benign, according to Dr. Greig. And even when an abnormality turns out to be cancer, a mammogram—an X ray—cannot determine whether a tumor has spread to a distant site, such as the bones, liver, or lungs. Laboratory tests as well as additional imaging procedures, such as a ductogram, ultrasound, or MRI, may be needed to better understand your lesion.

A mammogram provides a picture only of the breast's interior and often does not easily distinguish between tumors and other types of growths that can develop in breast tissue. The radiologist who reads your mammogram will be the first physician to view the contours of the mass and to evaluate where it is situated in the breast. The radiologist, however, does not have the final word on whether the abnormality seen on the mammogram is malignant. Any suspicions must be confirmed by laboratory testing.

> **A Primer on Prevalence**
>
> According to the American Cancer Society, an estimated 211,000 cases of invasive breast cancer are diagnosed annually in the United States. More than three-quarters of those cases occur in women age fifty or older. Women who have been consistently screened from age forty onward tend to have smaller cancers at the time of diagnosis.

In the process of diagnosis, each advancing step either confirms or rejects suspicions from the previous step. The linchpin in the diagnostic process is the biopsy, a test in which a small amount of tissue is removed from the breast to be closely examined in the laboratory.

What Cancer Specialists Think about Mammography

Doctors involved in virtually all aspects of your care will want to know the results of your mammogram as well as the findings from the tests that follow. The mammogram, therefore, is of importance not only to the radiologist. Viewing the mammogram also ultimately helps direct the surgical oncologist in how best to operate to remove the cancer. With such a detailed image of the breast's interior, the surgeon essentially has a map, and thus in many cases is enabled to perform a more precise, breast-sparing operation.

Dr. Lisa Newman, director of the Breast Care Center at the University of Michigan's Comprehensive Cancer Center in Ann Arbor, says the mammogram is critical as patients embark upon each of the steps involved in a breast cancer diagnosis. She says, "When breast cancer is suspected we do not want to leave any stone unturned. The workup is intense, and I think patients appreciate that fact. The mammogram is very important in the overall scheme of things."

Dr. Newman, also a former assistant professor of surgical oncology at the M.D. Anderson Cancer Center in Houston, adds that the numerous procedures patients undergo during the course of having a breast abnormality diagnosed may seem daunting. However, most patients ultimately are pleased about the thoroughness of the medical procedures.

As one of the initial diagnostic steps, the mammogram is the physician's first view of what may be developing within the breast, explains Dr. Freya Schnabel, chief of the breast-surgery section at New York-Presbyterian Hospital/Columbia University Medical Center in New York City. Having a mammogram in hand eliminates what largely was left to guesswork a generation ago. She says, "There is no guesswork, speculation, or 'what ifs' when it comes to diagnosing breast cancer—not anymore. The reason why so many of our patients fare so well these days is because we work very hard to get the right diagnosis, and we have the technology to do it."

Mammogram Findings

A mammogram is a low-dose X-ray procedure that is used for the screening of healthy women and for the diagnosis of breast disorders, which include breast cancer and benign conditions.

Currently, the average tumor size found through this technology for women who've had consistent mammograms is about 0.43 inches. The best machines are able to detect growths that are even smaller. Again, one of the key benefits of mammography is detecting tumors that are too small to feel by touch (palpate).

Some centers use digital mammography, a new technology in which X-ray film is replaced by detectors that convert X rays into electronic signals. The detectors are comparable to those found in digital cameras. Doctors say the digital images can be seen on a computer screen or examined like an ordinary mammogram when the image is printed on a special film. The benefit of this technology is that it produces sharper images of breast abnormalities.

Very few centers have these machines, and the Food and Drug Administration, which oversees medical devices, offers no listing of medical facilities that have them. The FDA advises women interested in digital mammography to contact the manufacturers to find which medical centers in their area may offer this evolving technique. Makers of digital mammography equipment include G.E. Medical Systems, Fischer Imaging, and Lorad/Hologic.

Even though conventional mammography is widely cited for its role in detecting tumors, it remains an imperfect tool. The accuracy of a mammogram depends on the age and type of equipment, the skill of the technician operating the machine, the skill and experience of the radiologist reading the film, and the density of the breast tissue being imaged. Experts from the American Cancer Society have strong recommendations about the use of mammography. They say, "It is important for women to have their mammograms at a facility where breast imaging is regarded as a specialty, an area of concentration, and where interpretation of mammograms is a significant proportion of the imaging they do."

If you are not being treated at a major medical center you may want to ask if the mammography equipment is up-to-date and accredited by the American College of Radiology and the FDA.

Lourdes R., fifty-four, had been getting regular mammograms since age forty. In retrospect she believes the mammography program that offered services free of charge gave her a false sense of assurance. She was stunned when she found a growth in her left breast on her own that later proved to be a tumor. When doctors at the teaching hospital where she was diagnosed examined her previous mammograms, they found their quality to be very poor. Lourdes does not speak English; here, her daughter Magdalena translated and commented about the problem.

> When the doctor looked at the X-ray pictures he told her he couldn't tell when the tumor started and that he should have been able to see it on her mammogram from last year. He said those were the worst mammograms he had ever seen.
>
> My mother was so upset. She was crying and crying because she thought she'd been doing the right thing. But she says there was no way for her to tell if the people were taking a good mammogram picture or a bad mammogram picture. There are a lot of ladies who live around here who get mammograms all the time at this place. I think this can happen to them, just like it did to my mom.

Greta L. recalls dismissing a gut-level feeling that a mammogram was not being properly performed.

> Two years before I was diagnosed, I was still in my forties and on a mammography screening schedule of every two years. When I went in for my mammogram, there was a new tech doing the test. I noticed that she didn't compress my breast much. I almost said something but then decided, What the heck. It's easier and less painful this way—who am I to ask for more pain? Two years later, when I found the lump and it was noted as "highly suspicious" in the subsequent mammogram, I must admit I thought back to that last mammogram. If I had told them there wasn't sufficient pressure to see any-

thing, would they have found the lump earlier? It's just one of those "what ifs" I've had to let go of.

Getting the Best Possible Mammogram

There are some things you can do to ensure that there are no problems with the results of your film. On the day of a mammogram, make certain you do not wear antiperspirant or talcum powder. Aluminum is a constituent of underarm deodorants and on a mammogram may be easily confused with the tiny microcalcifications suspected to be precancers. Talc likewise gives a misreading of microcalcifications. If you have had mammograms performed in the past at a different center, have those X rays sent to the physicians involved in your diagnosis. The old films can help the radiologist better evaluate your current mammogram.

Traditionally, mammography has had its greatest benefits in women fifty and older. Breast tissue becomes less dense with age, so the X ray is more likely to bring early tumor growth sharply into view. Dr. Newman, of the University of Michigan, notes that as women age, fatty tissue is more likely to pervade the breast. Tumors, she says, show up white on a mammogram, in sharp contrast to the grayish color of fat.

Your radiologist may want more than one mammogram to confirm or clarify what was seen in earlier images. Additional breast X rays may be needed to reach a diagnosis. Yet being called back for additional mammograms sometimes frightens patients. A few may even find it a bother. Jean G., sixty-three, felt that returning to her physician's office for an additional mammogram would interrupt her travel plans with her husband to Florida. When someone called from her doctor's office to ask her to come in for a second mammogram, she asked if it could wait a couple of weeks. She was told no.

What the radiologist saw in the first screening was confirmed by the second: a tiny tumor too small for Jean or her doctor to find. The Florida trip was postponed. A biopsy proved what doctors had suspected from both mammograms: a small cancer developing in a milk duct.

Mammography and Younger Women

Women under age forty are not routinely screened by mammography, though women from age twenty onward are encouraged by the American Cancer Society and the National Cancer Institute to conduct a monthly breast self-examination (BSE). Health agencies do not recommend routine mammograms for younger women because of the infrequency of breast cancer among women in their twenties and thirties. An estimated 77 percent of breast cancer cases occur in women fifty and older. For women in their twenties, the disease is extraordinarily rare.

Dr. Newman says there are several issues involving mammography and younger women: "Mammography has become very sophisticated, and it is very good at evaluating the breast tissue of most women, but not that of younger women. If you are young and have fairly dense breasts, then that can obscure the appearance of a cancer. On a mammogram, tumors appear whitish, and so does the dense glandular tissue of younger women. Although mammography has become much better over the years, there are still some cancers that are not apparent mammographically."

There are several reasons why younger women are not routinely offered mammograms. Some reasons are medical, others are economic.

> ❖ Routine screening, which is used to identify early tumors in older women, has not proven to have the same medical usefulness in younger women. Moreover, the procedure would produce a lopsided cost/benefit ratio for bottom-line-

---

Understanding the Odds

One of the most prevalent misunderstandings about breast cancer susceptibility is the statistic 1 in 8. It is often used to refer to all women. Experts have found that risk differs dramatically by age. The odds are as follows:

– In women age thirty and younger the disease is extremely rare, accounting for 1.5 percent of all reported cases of breast cancer.

– The chance at age forty is 1 in 217.

– At age fifty, it's 1 in 50.

– At age eighty-five, it's 1 in 8.

conscious health insurers. For the amount of money spent on screening, too few tumors would be detected. If doctors were to order additional screening techniques, costs could soar even higher with still no likelihood of catching more cancers earlier.

❖ In younger women the milk production glands are denser, producing an opaque image on a mammogram. Tiny tumors—DCIS—that mammography identifies so well in older women also appear opaque and can be difficult to find in those who are young.

❖ Mammography is considered very safe, but some experts say it is not a zero-risk procedure. These experts contend that younger women have more rapidly dividing healthy cells, and therefore the cumulative risk of periodic X-ray exposure could prove greater over time.[1] For that reason, healthy women under thirty-five, and certainly women just in their twenties, should not be screened. However, mammography has been used routinely for years to screen women as young as twenty-five who have an elevated genetic risk for the disease. A majority of doctors have long insisted that risk is not increased as a result of the exposure, although most now are turning to MRI screening for this population (see Chapter 5).

> ## Men and Mammography
>
> Men who are being examined for a breast abnormality undergo diagnostic mammography just as women do. The core concern involving men with breast cancer is that tumors often are found at a much later stage. This difference can make breast cancer in men quite challenging to treat. Breast cancer manifests in men just as it does in many women, and a lump usually is the telltale sign. But because men do not undergo routine screening—and mammograms are not even part of their annual physicals—tumors may very well evade the attention of patients and doctors alike until they've advanced to significant size. Breast cancer strikes an estimated thirty-four hundred men annually in the United States. Men also account for 1 percent of the forty thousand deaths each year from the disease.

Dr. Newman adds that none of these caveats should serve as excuses to avoid ordering mammograms for younger women who have symptoms. While tissue density contributes to poorer mammogram quality among women in their twenties or thirties, a diagnosis can be delayed unless doctors continue to hunt down the cause of the complaint.

Conscientious physicians, Dr. Newman says, probably will also order other procedures. Concerns about white-appearing glandular tissue and the whiteness of a tumor are not issues with other forms of imaging.

Some Cancers Are Not Easily X-Rayed

Regardless of age, women with inflammatory breast cancer comprise a group for whom mammography often is of little value. This form of breast cancer is very aggressive and can produce symptoms that some people may not at first associate with the disease, such as changes in skin coloration and texture. Itchiness is also a symptom some patients experience initially, leading them to think they may be experiencing an allergic reaction to certain fabrics or to their laundry detergent. As mentioned earlier in this chapter, warmth and redness—the "burn"—are signs of inflammatory breast cancer, but so are pitting of the skin, dimpling, and swelling. The affected breast can enlarge significantly as a result of fluid buildup. Mammography is of limited use in the examination of this rare cancer's unique symptoms.

Additional Imaging Choices

Besides mammography, doctors can order several other procedures as part of the diagnostic process.

ULTRASOUND

Ultrasound, also known as sonography, produces an image of the breast's internal structures by way of high-frequency sound waves. It is the same technology used to bring a developing fetus into view during pregnancy. The problem with ultrasound as a tool in routine breast screenings is its inability to produce an image of the tiny lesions that are too small to detect by hand; only mammography is capable of producing a sharp image of such tiny abnormalities.

Despite that shortcoming, ultrasound offers numerous other benefits. It is an important aid in the diagnosis of dense breast tissue. Ultrasound also helps distinguish between breast tumors and benign, fluid-filled cysts. An increasing number of studies also demonstrate that ultrasound can detect some deep-seated tumors missed by mammography.

MRI

Magnetic resonance imaging—MRI—is another way of viewing internal breast structures. An MRI may be ordered as part of the diagnostic process, particularly for younger women and those with breast implants. An MRI is an imaging technique that uses magnetic fields and radio waves to produce computer images of internal structures. No X rays or radiation are involved. Tissue density is not a problem with an MRI as it is with mammography, and the procedure does not require compression, which is a welcome benefit for many patients. Another advantage of MRI is its ability to spot some very tiny lesions.

A breast MRI is obtained with specialized equipment that captures images of both breasts simultaneously. It can help doctors determine the approximate depth of the abnormality within the tissue. But while MRI technology has many favorable points, it is not without drawbacks. The technique does not always distinguish between tumors and the benign lesions called fibroadenomas. Cost is another concern. An MRI can run in excess of a thousand dollars, up to fifteen times more than the cost of a mammogram.

As part of the MRI procedure, images are taken in multiple directions (front to back; side to side; top to bottom) to give physicians extensive and highly detailed views of both breasts. To obtain the images, the patient must lie on her stomach on a large moveable platform. The breasts are exposed through an opening. Once the patient is positioned correctly the technician will advance her into the magnet. Dozens of images can be obtained during the time she is in there, which can run up to an hour.

Additional evidence of the usefulness of MRIs can be found in the growing number of physicians researching it as a tool to screen healthy younger women at high risk of breast cancer because they carry one of the known breast cancer genes. Medical scientists from the United States and Europe reported at a recent meeting of the American Society of Clinical Oncology (ASCO) in 2003 that MRI is becoming increasingly helpful in screening younger high-risk patients. These women must undergo frequent screening similar to the schedules of older women, whose risk increases with age. Using MRI in the younger high-risk population avoids excessive radiation exposure.

Although these researchers cite the benefits of MRI screening for younger women, they have not ruled out the importance of mammography. When a suspicious mass is detected by way of an MRI, physicians probably will also want to confirm the finding with a mammogram. It is important to note that while ultrasound and MRI may be used in the diagnostic process and in special-circumstance screening, neither method has been recommended as an alternative to mammography in routine physicals.

DUCTOGRAM

Dr. Greig of Cedars-Sinai points out that a ductogram (also known as galactography or ductogalactography) is sometimes used to obtain a keener view of a breast's milk ducts. Ductograms are a type of mammography but take more time to perform—up to an hour—and require the use of a contrast medium. The medium is injected into the breast to make a duct show up sharper on the image. The technique can be useful as doctors gather evidence on an abnormal discharge or an intraductal papilloma, which is a wartlike formation that can develop within a duct. Intraductal papillomas are a common cause of nipple discharge. The contrast medium is injected from a cannula (a small tube used for such injections) into the suspected duct. A mammogram is then taken, focusing on the area highlighted by the contrast medium.

The Activist's View of Mammography

Advocates for breast cancer patients have long argued that something more precise and free of radiation exposure is needed for tumor detection and routine screening—regardless of a patient's age or gender. Too many breast cancers, they point out, are still diagnosed far too late. In fact, by the time the smallest tumors detectable through mammography are found, the lesions have been developing for at least eight to ten years.

A technique known as *ductal lavage* is a minimally invasive method of collecting a relatively large sample of cells from milk ducts, cells that provides doctors with biological information on a patient's level of risk. The test, which is FDA approved, is reserved for women already considered at high risk and is not made available to women undergoing routine screening.

> ## Ductal Lavage: Screening for Risk Without X Rays
>
> Ductal lavage is a relatively new way to collect and identify abnormal cells in the breasts' milk ducts, a technique that provides doctors with answers about a woman's level of breast cancer risk. The technique is minimally invasive and allows doctors to collect a sample directly from the site where a majority of breast cancers originate. Although approved by the FDA, currently this screening method is only for those deemed at high risk and is not designed to replace mammography. When used as part of a comprehensive work-up, however, the procedure works especially well, helping clinicians confirm results from other diagnostic procedures.

Doctors say it is most effective when used as one component in comprehensive testing. Ductal lavage is not intended as a replacement for mammography.

As an advocate for patients, Fran Visco, president of the National Breast Cancer Coalition, contends that more precise methods of breast cancer detection are needed—tests that focus on biological markers, such as proteins and other cancer-specific molecules. Tests such as those could pinpoint the presence of precancerous conditions years before tumor growth begins. The idea isn't as radical as it may seem initially. Studies are under way worldwide to identify such markers. Mammography, she emphasizes, could never match the accuracy of precision-driven biological tests.

> Mammography is woefully inadequate as a screening tool, and even as a diagnostic device we feel that it has very definite limitations. We would like to see, and would much prefer, something that is minimally invasive or, better yet, a blood test that is inexpensive and capable of detecting breast cancer very early. That is what is most important.
>
> We need to develop strong biomarkers and prognostics that will tell us which normal cells will turn into cancer and which ones will metastasize. Mammography does not detect all breast cancers. That's the problem. It's a major problem.
>
> Mammography is not effective in younger women, it doesn't detect tumors in all older women, and it can't distinguish well among the various kinds of breast cancer. Almost every woman with breast cancer has a different disease, but you can't tell that from imaging a breast. But having said all of that, mammography is the best we have right now.

Delays in Being Tested

An estimated forty-three million people in the United States are without health-care insurance, and their ranks continue to grow. This lack of basic coverage is one of the primary impediments to the early detection and diagnosis of all forms of cancer. The U.S. is one of the few industrialized countries where serious illness can become a red-alert financial situation that can lead to a family's economic ruin and a patient's poor prognosis.

Studies have found that women without health-care insurance, or those who have inadequate health coverage, are 30 percent to 50 percent more likely to die from breast cancer than those with sufficient coverage. Money—or the lack of it—can have a profound impact on a cancer prognosis. If you have been "downsized" and your job "outsourced," it is very likely that your health coverage is gone as well.

If you have found a suspicious mass or other symptom that could be suggestive of breast cancer, please heed these words: *Do not ignore the condition.* It probably will not go away and very well might get worse.

The American Cancer Society has guidelines focusing on the early detection of breast cancer. The society actively supports programs in every state to help low-income and uninsured women obtain access to mammography and other forms of diagnostic testing. If you do not have health insurance but need medical assistance, you can obtain it through the National Breast and Cervical Cancer Early Detection Program. The program is sponsored by the U.S. Centers for Disease Control and Prevention (CDC) and is administered individually within states. Through the early-detection program, you may even qualify for low- or no-cost treatment. However, states differ on how much they will pay. To find information about the program in your state, call the following toll-free number at the CDC and follow the prompts on the automated telephone line: (888) 842-6355.

Inadequate health insurance, or a total lack of health insurance, are two causes of delayed breast cancer diagnosis.

Overlooked Populations

Activists cite numerous factors that delay a breast cancer diagnosis. Among them are physical disability and mental illness. Women with these conditions often are not aggressively sought for routine screening, which means by the time a cancer is found it can be at an advanced stage. Studies by the CDC and other leading research groups confirm that disabled women are less likely to receive routine mammograms. Additionally, activists point to the issue of problematic mammography equipment in some medical centers, particularly smaller ones, which make it virtually impossible for women who cannot stand to undergo the procedure. Many mammography machines can be adjusted to accommodate a patient who cannot stand, but the patient has to be helped to a chair or stool. G.E. Medical Systems and Trex Medical Corp. manufacture special mammography machines found in leading teaching hospitals that allow a patient to stay in a wheelchair.

Survivors say there are several others. Women who don't speak English or Spanish have trouble explaining their symptoms to health-care providers. And on occasion, some women report being taken less than seriously when they have found a lump that isn't apparent to others.

Persistence when Faced with a Long Delay

Maryanne B., a mother of four, discovered she had breast cancer only after a significant delay and after advocating strongly for appropriate testing. At age thirty-eight she detected an unusual crescent-shaped mass at the bottom of her left breast. It was a growth that neither her doctor nor her husband could palpate. It took a full calendar year to convince her doctor she needed a mammogram, and even the mammogram couldn't bring the tumor into view.

> I found the lump at the time my sister-in-law had breast cancer and was very sick. Breast cancer was on everybody's mind so I didn't want to seem too paranoid about it, but I did want somebody to tell me what it was.
>
> You always hear about getting a lump checked right away. But this didn't feel the way I thought a lump should feel. I thought a lump should have a roundish shape. This was shaped like a *U*.
>
> I told my husband that something was wrong. I said, "You've got to feel this thing." But when he tried to find it, he couldn't. He said, "Maryanne, you're just looking for problems." But I wasn't. I knew it was there.

Maryanne's doctor told her that lumps come and go and that as far as he was concerned, her lump had long since disappeared. Maryanne would not budge from her belief that something was awry. Her doctor, on the other hand, was steadfast in his belief that Maryanne's imagination had gotten the best of her. He told her to give the situation some time. She waited to see if he was right. The lump, nevertheless, persisted. In January of the following year she insisted on a mammogram.

> I had to demand a mammogram. I had to say, "I want a mammogram. Give me a mammogram." This was really frustrating. He kept commenting on the [large] size of my breasts. I know that; that wasn't the problem. But it got to where even I thought I was imagining things because when I got the mammogram, nothing showed up. They were giving me a clean bill of health.

By October, now well over a year since she'd first found the lump, Maryanne began to feel a bizarre sensation, which she equates to what she felt while breast-feeding her children. The lump, which her doctor insisted was not there, a belief confirmed by a mammogram, was now producing physical symptoms.

Convinced, finally, that she knew her body better than her family doctor did, Maryanne went to a different clinic at St. Vincent's Medical Center in Los Angeles, not far from her home. There, doctors ordered another mammogram, and also a breast ultrasound. The second mammogram also produced negative results.

The ultrasound, however, revealed a two-centimeter mass growing in a lower quadrant of the breast. A biopsy concluded that the tumor was malignant, confirming the fear Maryanne had harbored all along.

Understanding the Biopsy

Mammograms and other types of technology used to obtain a picture of a breast abnormality are important to doctors, but imaging alone doesn't tell them definitively whether the lump is cancerous or benign. The biopsy, a procedure in which a sample of tissue is removed from the breast and sent to a pathology laboratory for examination, makes that determination. Pathologists conduct a wide range of cellular, hormonal, and genetic tests on the tissue. Details in the pathologist's written report will form the foundation of your doctor's treatment recommendations. Without a biopsy, you will never know whether you have cancer.

For many patients, breast biopsies will rule out cancer. In the United States more than 500,000 biopsies are performed for breast conditions annually. With an estimated 211,000 cases of invasive breast cancer and another 50,000 of localized malignancies that are contained in milk ducts (DCIS), clearly thousands of biopsies are performed for breast abnormalities that turn out to be benign.

The following section describes the various ways in which tissue samples are collected for biopsies. Chapter 4 contains a more extensive description of how biopsy results are interpreted, what they mean, and how a pathologist's report of laboratory findings can ultimately affect your care. When a biopsy is positive for breast cancer, your physicians will also want to know whether your lymph nodes are affected. They will conduct specific tests to make that determination.

Tissue samples are a vital medical record equal in importance to the written reports that doctors enter into your chart. The specimens contain a permanent record of your cancer and thus are important for a variety of reasons. Future illness is one example. If breast cancer occurs years later in a close family member—a daughter, sister, mother, or aunt—the tissue specimens would be available for genetic comparison.

Many advocates for patients emphasize that you should request in writing that the hospital keep your biopsy samples for as long as possible—indefinitely if at all possible. Cancer survivors have found that some hospitals have policies allowing samples to be maintained for only a few years. Without the samples, your oncologist may run into obstacles years down the road if your cancer recurs and there is a need to compare a newer tissue sample to the earlier one.

Types of Biopsies

Biopsies can be surgical or nonsurgical, but the aim, regardless of how they are performed, is to obtain tissue samples of the lesion. Once removed, the specimen is sent to the hospital pathology laboratory for microscopic and molecular examination. The object is to find out whether malignant cells are present.

Most physicians prefer needle (nonsurgical) biopsies and tend to order surgical biopsies only when the abnormality is more difficult to reach or when a larger sample size is needed. Dozens of studies in recent years have compared needle and surgical biopsies. Needle techniques are less invasive than surgical ones, and there are several ways in which each of the procedures can be performed. The technique that is ultimately chosen for a specific patient's biopsy is based on a number of variables, such as the size of the mass and its location. You may want to discuss the merits of the various biopsy techniques with your physicians.

NONSURGICAL BIOPSIES

Nonsurgical biopsies include both the fine-needle aspiration and core-needle techniques. The needles come in a variety of sizes and are chosen based on several criteria, mainly the size and location of the growth being tested. Needle biopsies often involve the simultaneous use of imaging technology, which enable doctors to view the specimen's removal as the procedure is performed.

SURGICAL BIOPSIES

These types of biopsies include incisional and excisional techniques. An incisional biopsy may be the doctor's first choice when only a portion of the mass is needed for study. During this procedure a small incision is made, usually directly over the growth, and a sample of the lesion is removed. An excisional biopsy involves removing the entire mass along with the rim of the healthy tissue that surrounds it. For many patients, this serves as their lumpectomy and the complete surgical treatment of their cancer. Excisional biopsies are also performed when preliminary tests strongly suggest the presence of a benign growth known as a fibroadenoma. In either case, a local anesthetic is injected into the breast to blunt pain. Your doctor may choose to administer an additional medication to induce drowsiness during the procedure. Even though this biopsy can serve as a lumpectomy for cancer, it is performed on an outpatient basis.

Lymph Node Biopsy

Also known as axillary lymph node dissection, lymph node biopsy is another type of surgical biopsy. It can be performed soon after a biopsy produces positive breast cancer results, or at the time of a lumpectomy or mastectomy. The procedure is performed under general anesthesia. Now that you know a little bit about the distinctions between the various types of biopsy techniques, you may want to grasp a few more details.

Core-Needle Biopsy

Of the two needle procedures, the core-needle technique is the one most commonly performed. In a core-needle biopsy, a spring-loaded hollow needle is used to remove tissue samples. An average needle size is about the diameter of a toothpick. Generally, only local anesthesia is necessary. Core needles can range from size 14-gauge to 18-gauge (compared with the 27-gauge needle used in fine-needle aspiration). Smaller gauge numbers in biopsy needles are equated with larger needles, and vice versa.

When the lump in the breast can be easily felt, a core-needle biopsy can be performed in the physician's office. If the abnormality is deep-seated or is so small that it is seen only on a mammogram, then the procedure must be performed with the aid of imaging equipment. Doctors can use either stereotactic mammography or ultrasound imaging to guide needle placement. Stereotactic mammography involves X-ray imaging and the use of a computer to map the coordinates of the abnormality for precise placement of the needle.

Given the needle's diameter you may wonder whether it can retrieve a sample sufficient enough to examine. A study conducted by Dr. Darrell Smith, director of mammography at Brigham and Women's Hospital in Boston, compared core-needle biopsies to surgical procedures and found no difference in effectiveness between the two methods.[2] Needles, his study confirmed, were comparable to the surgical knife. Reporting his study in the *Journal of the American Medical Association*, Smith also found that women who underwent a core-needle biopsy tolerated it well.

Fine-Needle Aspiration

With fine-needle aspiration biopsy (FNA or FNAB), doctors use a needle whose diameter is approximately equivalent to that of a sewing needle. The needle is under vacuum pressure, which is the force that enables it to aspirate (draw by suction) cells from the growth. When all types of biopsy techniques are taken into consideration, the fine-needle procedure is the least invasive. Again, only local anesthetic is required.

FNA can be performed in several ways. Some doctors who feel confident about the position of the lump, based on what has been seen in earlier images, perform the procedure without the aid of imaging equipment. This choice is usually made when the abnormality is located near the surface of the breast. FNA also can be performed under the mammogram-guidance technique called stereotactic needle biopsy.

Surgical Biopsies

Surgical biopsies are more invasive than those performed with needles, but surgical biopsies are still used regularly. An incisional biopsy might be performed to reach a lesion otherwise difficult to approach with a needle, or it may be needed after a needle biopsy in order to obtain a more complete specimen. The incisional technique may also be recommended because the mass is close to the breast's surface and is easy to reach. Again, reasons for using each technique vary.

To obtain a tissue sample in an incisional biopsy, the surgeon makes a cut above the mass, having located its position on the mammogram. Local anesthesia is applied to the breast to relieve pain. The small piece of the lesion that is obtained is then used to make slides for microscopic analysis and tumor marker tests, which help determine whether the cancer has spread. Finally, even though surgical biopsies, whether incisional or excisional, are called "surgery," they can be performed on an outpatient basis in an ambulatory-care center.

In some cases, after tissue is confirmed as malignant, a surgical biopsy may be necessary to determine if cancer has spread to local lymph nodes. This procedure involves removing a small pad of fat under the arm adjacent to the affected breast. Anywhere from ten to twenty lymph nodes can be contained in the specimen. The nodes are then examined in the pathology laboratory. This type of biopsy is formally known as an axillary lymph node dissection. In Chapter 7 there is a description of an increasingly used procedure called a sentinel node biopsy.

Wire Localization

Wire localization may be used for a hard-to-reach abnormality, especially a tiny microcalcification in a duct that is brought into view through mammography.

After the patient has been given a local anesthetic, a radiologist guides a thin, hollow needle to the site, then inserts a wire through the needle. The needle is removed and the wire left in place. The wire marks the spot of the tiny lesion. The patient is then wheeled into surgery. A surgeon removes the abnormality, which is sent to the pathology department for analysis. Although wire localization is an available option, most biopsies are performed surgically or through one of the needle techniques.

Sharon M., a high school art teacher and divorced mother of two sons in college, recalls the sense of dread she felt on the day of her biopsy. She drove herself to the procedure and kept her fingers crossed that everything would turn out fine. Her doctors already suspected cancer based on her mammograms. She hoped the biopsy would prove them wrong.

> The doctor told me he would do a core-needle biopsy. I had no idea what that meant, and I kept asking how he'd get enough tissue to do all of the tests he said would be done. He explained the particulars about the biopsy, and it didn't sound too frightening.
>
> Still, the very idea of this needle being stuck inside me didn't seem like a walk in the park, either. But there was classical music playing while the biopsy was being done, and he worked very quickly. I kept praying that there would be good news in the end, but of course there wasn't.

Getting the News

When a biopsy comes back positive for breast cancer, it is only natural that emotions well up, and at least for a while they will probably overwhelm you. A wide range of sentiments surface when word of the diagnosis comes. A growing array of studies show that being confronted with life-altering news ranks high among the causes of clinical depression and anxiety. And the emotional impact of learning about a cancer diagnosis is as strong as that which floods the spirit upon learning about the death of a loved one.

It is normal to break down and cry when you hear of a breast cancer diagnosis; it is okay to lose it. The late Diane Sackett Nannery, an advocate and writer from Long Island, discussed her feelings about receiving a breast cancer diagnosis in several interviews for this book as well as for a series of articles I wrote for a health website. Diane said when she first found out about her diagnosis she was overwhelmed by shock, sadness, and an inability to focus her thoughts. Diane died of breast cancer in November 2003, after a long and valiant fight that lasted for more than a decade.

During her interviews she talked of the diagnosis (and a later recurrence) as having a transforming effect. "I didn't understand the Diane Nannery who was newly diagnosed," she said. "My sides hurt from holding myself so tightly and not letting go. I was shaking. The feeling is crippling. Your mind races when you're first diagnosed. People are talking to you, but it's like your head is underwater because nothing they say seems to make sense." Diane eventually turned her grief into a positive force of energy. She conceived the first U.S. postage stamp honoring women with breast cancer.

The sense of being engulfed in unknowns—especially the unknown of what lies ahead—intensifies the fear, denial, anger, and myriad other responses patients have when they receive a breast cancer diagnosis. As a leader in the pioneering field of psycho-oncology at Memorial Sloan-Kettering Cancer Center in New York City, Dr. Mary Jane Massie is a psychiatrist who specializes in mental health issues facing breast cancer patients. She has observed and analyzed the emotional reactions that occur among those who have received unfavorable health news.

Dr. Massie acknowledges that receiving word of a breast cancer diagnosis can have a profound impact on a patient's emotional stability. For some newly diagnosed breast cancer patients, the thought of mastectomy compounds the anxiety brought on by the cancer diagnosis itself. Still, the reactions to the news vary from patient to patient. Some may experience more than one response. It is possible, Dr. Massie says, to be sad, angry, and grief-stricken all at once.

The following list, in alphabetical order, covers the reactions cited most often by the breast cancer survivors interviewed for this book when they learned of their diagnosis.

ANGER

Anger can have good points as well as bad. It may help you realize that you are in a red-alert health situation that must be dealt with quickly. But anger may also trigger you to dislike or distrust the people who have handed you the verdict. You may think, What a horrid doctor to tell me such terrible news, or, How dare that laboratory insist that such a tiny tissue specimen revealed the presence of cancer. You are so angry you could explode.

The trouble with anger is that it can be projected in all directions. You can project it toward anyone who crosses your path: your friends, husband, children, the grocery checker—anybody. No one is missing the point that you're pissed. Anger, unfortunately, has a way of backfiring. Rest assured, if you continue tossing hand grenades, you're likely to get several more tossed back at you—breast cancer or no breast cancer. Many breast cancer survivors cite the benefits of joining a support group because it is very helpful to explore the issues causing your anger with people who are also enraged—and saddened—by the same medical condition.

CAN'T REMEMBER A THING

You heard the news when the biopsy came back with a diagnosis of breast cancer. Or did you? Your doctor said come back next Wednesday for additional tests, or was that two weeks from Thursday? Just as the activist Diane Sackett Nannery found that her mind raced upon hearing the news, and that the words of people around her seemed not to make sense, others have recalled a similar reaction, saying they could hear people talking but what they said went in one ear and out the other. One woman remarked that after receiving news of her diagnosis she walked around the hospital parking lot for over an hour, searching for her car, only to realize that a friend had dropped her off and was planning to meet her on the opposite side of the building.

DENIAL

Denial can be a very powerful response, potent enough to let you forget about cancer in the short term. Denial may also lead you to believe the doctor doesn't have the right chart, that someone else's diagnosis is being reported to you. As Barbara G. stated earlier in this chapter, she initially felt her doctor had gotten the wrong information. "There's something wrong here," she told herself. "He's got it all wrong."

If your sense of denial is so strong that it interferes with treatment, then it is vital that you discuss these issues with your doctor or someone who can help you move toward acceptance. There are other ways of channeling your disbelief. If you think the diagnosis is wrong and the results of your tests to date are a lie, then you'd better get to work on obtaining a second opinion. That way, you'll hear the results from more than one source. Later in the book, labs that specialize in reanalyzing specimens and offering second opinions are discussed. The sooner you get to work on shedding your denial, doctors say, the better.

DETACHMENT

Could it be that you're on the moon looking down watching all of these interesting medical procedures happen to someone else? Being detached allows you to accept the news as if it were a minor problem that is easily fixed. "Breast cancer?" someone who's detached might ask. "No problem." The bizarre thing about detachment is that it allows you to accept what you hear without the denial, forgetfulness, or anger associated with other reactions to the news. Detachment, however, may suddenly wear off, leaving you with the stark realization that you have been diagnosed with breast cancer, that you're scheduled for a mastectomy, and that you'll have to tell your boss you won't be coming to work for a while.

FEAR

Fear can envelop you like a straightjacket—and it can keep you from telling family and friends about your diagnosis because you're uncertain how they'll react. You may be afraid they'll distance themselves from you or treat you like a leper. Fear may also drive a need to seek offbeat therapies. That, of course, can leave you vulnerable to hucksters pushing weird concoctions and other potentially dangerous remedies.

Helen C., a college professor, says her only direct knowledge of breast cancer was her grandmother's case more than thirty years ago. Even though Helen found helpful websites allowing her to better understand treatment choices, fear snuffed out her ability to remain rational—at least temporarily. "I couldn't stop thinking about the mutilating surgery and the pain and the agony my grandmother went through, and our inability to help her." Helen was afraid that something similar would happen to her—despite knowing better. "I had to get a grip because I was becoming fearful of things that weren't part of my reality."

GUILT AND BLAME

It may be impossible at first to convince yourself that you did not cause yourself to develop breast cancer. This sense of guilt can become so consuming that you are occupied by it constantly. Guilt naturally leads to blame as you search your mind for the exact thing you did to cause your cancer. You may blame your diet, the fact that you didn't exercise for thirty minutes a day, or whatever the reason du jour happens to be. You may even blame the amount of stress in your life. This mindset also can lead to blaming others: "My husband/mother/boss/lover/children have caused me so much stress that I got breast cancer." Guilt and blame must be released because the reality is so simple: Breast cancer is an extraordinarily complex disease. You can't give yourself breast cancer, and no one can give it to you.

SADNESS AND GRIEF

Many people—men and women—interviewed for this book said

they cried and were deeply depressed upon learning about their life-changing diagnosis. But they also said they felt better having done so. Sadness is, of course, an entirely normal reaction to a cancer diagnosis. As noted in the opening of the book, a breast cancer diagnosis brings the meaning of mortality front and center. Due to that fact alone, survivors say they saw life through a different lens from that moment forward.

Making Sense of It All

At major cancer centers in the United States, where psychiatrists specialize in helping women cope with the emotional aspects of breast cancer, patients often are counseled to take some time to absorb the news. At Memorial Sloan-Kettering Cancer Center, Dr. Massie tells patients they don't have to make decisions right away. Instead, patients are encouraged to collect themselves as a way to adjust to their new reality. Dr. Massie says she has long recognized that patients must pass through several phases of emotional struggle before they reach acceptance of their diagnosis. Some reach a degree of acceptance faster than others. But acceptance generally overtakes confusion and denial in short order, she emphasizes, because the will to survive inevitably kicks in, becoming for most people a powerful and unstoppable force.

On occasion, some patients need help from her to find their fighting spirit. Dark moods and thoughts of death, Dr. Massie believes, are natural, even when the prognosis is bright. She says, "The very first thing the newly diagnosed ask is whether they're going to die. They also want to know if they're facing something very painful physically and whether they will be disfigured. They want to know how the people who depend on them will manage while they're coping with serious illness. Many ask if they have the strength and fortitude to go through the therapy."

Such questions, Dr. Massie says, are fairly common. But to help her patients, she has to probe a little deeper to find out what they really think and know about the disease they are confronting. Most of the women she sees at Memorial are very knowledgeable about breast cancer and the procedures involved in treating it. A few are less so. "First I wait to see where they are emotionally and what they know about breast cancer," she says. "I've found that what some women know about breast cancer is wrong. There are a lot of myths out there. I try to help them through that and to understand how treatment of the disease has changed so dramatically."

The key, Dr. Massie and other experts emphasize, is in finding support. Support can come from family, friends, a lover, religion, a breast cancer support group, and even through conversations with professionals such as her.

For some patients, though, the diagnosis seems to come as a face-to-face meeting with a specter that has long stalked them. Catherine B. recalls being numbed by the news of her diagnosis. Her mother was diagnosed with breast cancer in 1972, and breast cancer continued to occur throughout her family. A cousin on her mother's side of the family, a nun, developed the disease, as did another cousin on her father's side, in Ireland. As is the case with a growing number of women, word of Catherine's illness came not as a result of seeking care for an overt symptom, but as the surprising outcome of a routine mammogram.

> It all happened pretty fast. I had gone to the doctor and had gotten a mammogram, but I was called back because they told me they wanted to have another one taken because there was a suspicious spot. When I got there, they told me they also wanted an ultrasound. This time they also saw calcium spots. So they told me I'd have to go for a biopsy. When that came back, they told me one of the spots had cancer.

That wasn't the end of Catherine's ordeal. After she was admitted to the hospital and was in the operating room being prepared for a lumpectomy, her surgeon handed her additional news.

> He said they found another spot with cancer in the opposite breast, and that rather than have me go home and then come back he could take care of both of them that day. What could I say? That was the first I had heard of the second cancer.

Catherine's physician gave her no indication prior to the day of surgery that a second malignancy was suspected based on the findings of the mammogram and her biopsy. But now, several years past the double lumpectomy, her mammograms have shown no signs of cancer.

Catherine's stoic response to the news is in sharp contrast to Fran D.'s reaction when she learned that she had breast cancer. Fran has been a breast cancer survivor for nearly a decade. She remembers as if it were yesterday the day she received the news of her biopsy report. Fran's doctor calmly reported evidence of breast cancer and three affected lymph nodes.

> I would like to say that I was braced for it, because I knew something was up. After all, I had found the lump and had gone in to have it checked. But you're never really braced for bad news, even when you expect it. You've heard that old saying, forty days and forty nights? That's how long I cried, forty days and forty nights. I couldn't stop crying. I was forty-nine at the time and had been divorced for about six months. I kept thinking, Why are all of these horrible things happening to me?

✼ ✼ ✼

A cancer diagnosis is, without question, devastating news. But as you will see in the coming pages, some survivors find that their diagnosis helps to lead them to new friendships. Others adopt a mindset that refuses to let breast cancer dominate their lives. And one woman, you'll find as you read on, discovered that even though she was diagnosed with breast cancer, her funny bone remained completely unscathed.

Chapter *2*

A Postdiagnosis Checklist

> There was no other way to approach it. I had to look this
> situation in the face and take control of it, otherwise it would
> control me—and I certainly didn't want that to happen.
>
> — *Wendy Chioji, television news anchor and*
> *breast cancer survivor*

Certainly after you have absorbed the news of your diagnosis you
justifiably may ask who is in charge of your care. Is it your primary
care physician? Should it be the oncologist who treated a friend or
relative for breast cancer in the past? Who can guide you at what
may seem to be a bewildering time?

This chapter is designed to help you answer that question and to
help you marshal your two important teams: your team of supporters, people who will be there for you and help you cope; and your
team of medical professionals, who will provide your treatment.

As television anchorwoman Wendy Chioji emphasizes, it is important to be surrounded by supportive people and to become
knowledgeable about the medical condition you're facing. The Orlando, Florida, journalist says she went into this critical juncture of
her life with an attitude of "just take control." Having sufficient
knowledge about your condition, Chioji says, will help you shed
some of your fears about the disease while at the same time allowing
fuller participation in your treatment and follow-up care.

As part of helping you become a well-informed patient, this chapter also explores where to seek credible medical information. In time, you may have questions about chemotherapy, radiation, medications, support groups, cancer clinical trials, medical studies, wigs, or breast prostheses. Where do you turn to find such information? A logical answer is the Internet. But as a physician-expert explains, you won't simply want to log on to Google and plug in the words *breast cancer*. There are methods that should guide an effective Internet search about the disease and help you find the exact information you need.

A Brief Checklist of What to Do Now

❖ Gather a support team of relatives and friends.

❖ Choose the medical and surgical oncologists who will be involved in your care. If you have no clue about where to turn for such information, several tips are offered in this chapter in the section "Choosing Your Health-Care Team." You do not have to leap into treatment as soon as you get the diagnosis, so take some time to be thorough.

❖ Become informed about the other professionals who will take part in your treatment. Oncology nurses will assist you throughout your treatment and will likely prove invaluable as they explain medical procedures and steps involved in your care. You may also meet with a medical social worker, technicians, and probably even a relaxation or music therapist. Complementary and alternative approaches to stress reduction are increasingly becoming integrated into conventional cancer care.

❖ Start and maintain a diary or journal, which need be nothing more than a notebook. Use it to write down *everything*. You'll need a handy record of necessities, such as your insurance information and your doctors' names and phone numbers. Try also to chronicle some of your thoughts on these pages. Consider your journal a record of your life during this very trying and important phase. Spelling out your thoughts and concerns can help you cope. Write about anything that comes to mind—anything you deem noteworthy. Your diary or journal is also a good place to jot down questions as they come to mind, which can later be answered by your doctors, friends, or fellow cancer patients.

❖ Consider joining a support group of others with breast cancer and participating in a breast cancer "listserv" group on the Internet.

❖ Don't be afraid to seek out the help of psychiatric experts if you think you need such assistance.

❖ Have a firm grip on what type of adjuvant treatment or treatments you may be facing. The term *adjuvant treatment* refers to chemotherapy, radiation, and hormone therapies that are prescribed to ensure that breast cancer does not return.

❖ Become fully informed about your disease.

Don't Be Afraid of the "C" Word

There was a time in the not-too-distant past when the words *breast cancer* were not mentioned in polite company. People who survived it, rather than being proud of their accomplishment, tried to forget their ordeal. Embarrassment and shame were feelings many women attached to their medical condition. Although times have changed, some people are still apprehensive about telling others about their diagnosis. Some cite the sorrow and worry close friends and relatives might feel. Still others are concerned about how young children might respond to the news.

Research has shown that sharing the news of a cancer diagnosis with those who are close to you helps open the channels of communication immediately.

Julie H., forty-four, who was treated twice for early breast cancer—once in each breast, five years apart—believes that getting family and friends involved in her care was as important as assembling an excellent team of physicians.

> I was definitely afraid to mention the "C" word the first time around. I didn't tell my husband about my diagnosis for three days. I think a week had passed before I told my mom and sisters. It's hard to describe. I thought they would perceive me differently and treat me differently, that I would be perceived as fragile, about to draw my last breath. But I'll tell you, when I finally got up the courage to say the word *cancer,* that's when I found out how much everybody cared. You call it a support team. I call them my guardian angels. Even my son, Jake, who was only four, was doing everything he could to help his mommy. The second time was different. My husband, Brian, was in the waiting room, and he knew the minute I walked out of the doctor's office. We didn't even have to say anything to each other. We just sat in the car in the parking lot and held each other's hands and cried.

What if You're Alone?

Elaine H. found out she had breast cancer about a year after she retired from a thirty-five-year career as a public school teacher. Elaine has no children, she lives alone, and both parents are dead. She lives in California and has a disabled sister who lives in Arizona. After her mastectomy, Elaine was prepared to go it alone, marshaling the strength that had carried her through other crises in her life. For her, assembling relatives as a team of supporters was not possible.

> I never married, never had children. A cousin did come to visit after I was home. I found there were wonderful resources available through social services at the cancer center. That's how I got to and from my appointments. They sent a van. Also, I qualify now as a senior so I was able to get into the Meals on Wheels program, which is run by the local senior center. There were support groups at the cancer center but I didn't take part in those.

Even though Elaine was alone she was not lonely. She was surrounded by friends and acquaintances who invited themselves to be part of her experience.

> I do want to point out that the pastor of my church stopped by often, and neighbors dropped by. Some of the neighbors I had never seen before, but they heard I was getting cancer treatments, so they came to visit. One or another of them came the entire time I was on chemo, and never missed a day.

The surprise, she says, was how the visits continued throughout the duration of her treatment. Her cancer helped her meet people who had been neighbors for years. Neither had bothered to knock on the other's door.

> Who organized this? I had no idea then; I have no idea now— and I never solicited any of it. A lady came one afternoon with a beautiful mahogany box and said it was a special present. This was a Monday. I'll never forget that because she said she saw it on Saturday when she was out shopping and bought it because she thought I'd like it. I had never seen the woman in my life. I now know she lives two blocks away. But that particular Monday was my first time ever seeing her.

Other surprises were yet to come.

> You want to know what was in the box? Tea. It was a tea box with a brass lock and key. I love tea. How could she have possibly known this? If that's what you mean by a support team, that was my support team, and I was very—no, let me phrase this correctly—I was extremely grateful for it.

Taking Elaine's example, the definition of a support team depends on your willingness to accept the kindness of friends, relatives—and relative strangers.

If your life is not overflowing with people, there probably isn't a need to artificially force some into your world as a result of being diagnosed with breast cancer. But at the same time it may be a good idea when neighbors come knocking to open the door. They may be carrying the seeds of new friendships and bearing a box of your favorite teas.

Seeking Support while Telling the World

Some newly diagnosed patients want people to know about their diagnosis right away. Telling someone—anyone—is important. Writer Jami Bernard, in a *MAMM* magazine essay, comically explained how she quickly gathered a support group of friends while trumpeting to the world that she had breast cancer:

> The minute I was diagnosed I called all of my friends, who rushed me appropriate medical supplies—bottles of wine and bars of chocolate. Had I announced a hangnail they would have done the same, because that's the formula we've worked with for all crises, small and large.
>
> I suppose I could have sat alone at home and contemplated the universe, enjoying a quiet moment before all hell broke loose. But that's not my style. I come from a long line of blabbermouths who never learned to scuba dive because you can't chat while the oxygen's on. Plus, I'm a writer. Within months, I had told the readers of the New York *Daily News* (where I work) all about my prognosis, side effects and general mood. They had seen a picture of me posing bald under a white-and-gold Lurex turban. At the support group when we discussed how it felt to get up the courage to tell someone, the facilitator passed right over me. "You," she said, "we know about."[1]

What Support Can Do

According to the Susan G. Komen Breast Cancer Foundation, an advocacy organization, support from those around you can have physical benefits. It can

1. reduce stress
2. reduce side effects from treatment
3. boost your immune system
4. reduce the risk of recurrence
5. lengthen your life

Choosing Your Health-Care Team

Critical to the care you receive as a breast cancer patient is the team of professionals surrounding you. Many women enter the cancer-care system through the physician who ordered the mammogram, often their gynecologist or family practitioner. Once the radiologist who reads the mammogram finds something suspicious, the scope of your treatment inevitably advances to a different and more highly specialized medical arena.

Many primary care physicians work with a network of specialists and probably can recommend an oncologist and breast surgeon. But you will want to be sure about certain criteria before you refer to your specialists as "my doctors."

Foremost, you'll want your doctors to be board-certified. That means the doctor will have completed a three- to four-year residency program in his or her specialty and passed a rigorous examination. The consensus among doctors interviewed for this book, most of whom treat breast cancer exclusively, is that patients should seek care at a major teaching institution or cancer center. A teaching hospital is one in which up-and-coming physicians are trained. Also, these centers are often the sites where major medical studies are conducted, and doctors who practice there very likely may be in the vanguard of new and more effective therapies.

Dr. Clarence Brown, president and CEO of the M.D. Anderson Cancer Center in Orlando, Florida, has some strong beliefs about the hierarchy of the breast cancer patient's health-care team. While specialists such as the oncologist, surgeon, radiation oncologist, and oncology nurses are crucial to treatment, Dr. Brown believes one member of the health-care team counts even more. He says, "Certainly the key person on the team is the patient herself, and she needs some control over things as she enters the health-care system. There is no question that she has to be at the center of it all, at the helm. Equally important, she needs to be treated at a center where doctors specialize in breast cancer. All of the major cancer centers have now put together these teams."

Special teams can be found coast to coast, often in breast-care centers like the one at Cedars-Sinai Medical Center in Los Angeles, mentioned by Dr. Lloyd Greig in Chapter 1, or the breast-care center at the University of Michigan in Ann Arbor, headed by Dr. Lisa Newman.

Other breast-care teams include those at the Avon Foundation Breast Center at Johns Hopkins University in Baltimore and the Breast Center at Vanderbilt University in Nashville, Tennessee. Special programs at these institutions bring survivors and the newly diagnosed together in one-on-one meetings. The hope is to better help the newly diagnosed by introducing them to people who have already gone through diagnosis, treatment, and recovery.

Although breast-care centers may seem to be separate entities, they have all of the clinical, research, and social-service resources of the major cancer centers with which they are affiliated. However, physicians at breast-care centers treat benign conditions as well as cancer.

Nurse practitioner Lynette Lee Pack-May, R.N., coordinator of the Carol M. Baldwin Breast Care Center at Stony Brook University Hospital, on Long Island, has found that patients prefer the center's special focus. "When a patient has a diagnosis of breast cancer," she says, "one of the major advantages of a breast center is that everything for the patient is available in one setting. They'll need to see a medical oncologist, a radiologist, and probably a surgeon. These doctors are here for them and they specialize in breast cancer. We are independent, but we are still part of the larger cancer center."

Just as the physicians at breast-care centers are specialists in breast cancer, so too are the nurse practitioners. Ms. Pack-May finds that she must function in multiple roles to help meet the needs of patients, addressing their concerns as well as answering technical questions about the disease. She says, "I function in a dual role. I am a nurse practitioner and a nurse administrator. I more or less have the opportunity to interact with the patients at the clinical level and the administrative end. I can both advocate for the patients and talk to them about clinical concerns. Patients have a lot of anxiety about breast cancer. The anxiety is something many of them really struggle with. It is very difficult. But they are free to call me when they have concerns about their diagnosis."

Differences exist from one center to another in how these special teams function. Even when a cancer center doesn't have a breast-care center it will usually have an interdisciplinary group of specialists who focus only on breast conditions, both benign and cancerous. Patients treated in such settings have access to a wide array of services, which can include psychosocial support and nutritional and genetic counseling. At all of the nation's federally designated comprehensive cancer centers, a special emphasis is placed on breast cancer through the use of either an affiliated breast-care center or an interdisciplinary team.

As you begin your search for physicians, it may be a good idea to start at a leading teaching hospital or cancer center. These are the types of facilities where you will most likely find a breast-care focus.

Can I "Shop" for a Doctor?

The key to successful cancer therapy is feeling comfortable with your doctors and being able to ask them questions. In short, you want to choose physicians who want to be on your team and want to help you through one of the most difficult periods in your life.

If for any reason you are uncomfortable with the doctor you have—for example, if he or she fails to answer your questions properly, or seems too aloof or uninterested—find someone else. There are several ways of finding physicians when the recommendations of your primary care doctor don't meet your expectations. But have some idea in mind of what you're looking for when seeking a doctor. You're not looking for a therapist, a hand-holder, or a fortune-teller. You're looking for a highly skilled physician with an excellent track record who treats breast cancer.

In her book *Working with Your Doctor: Getting the Healthcare You Deserve*, author Nancy Keene recommends carefully defining your health-care needs before going out to find a physician. In fact, before shopping for a doctor, she advises, it is important to figure out whether you want a frank discussion about your medical condition with your physician and also whether you expect to communicate openly about it. She writes, "Finding a doctor you can really work with means seeking out someone compatible. If you want a lot of information—and all your questions answered—you need a doctor who can't be easily threatened, who takes time with you, and who loves to teach and share his/her reasoning process. Some people actually prefer the old style paternalistic doctor, though, who takes care of you [and who] shields you from information that might be upsetting. Personally I think that's a bit risky."[2]

Don't be afraid to ask around when trying to find physicians. Breast cancer support-group leaders can get you in touch with survivors who can tell you about specialists who have treated them. Support groups are sponsored by hospitals, by breast-care and cancer centers, and by the major patient-advocacy organizations. If there is a telephone help line in your area operated by an advocacy group, volunteers usually have names of doctors recommended by breast cancer survivors.

Additionally, all of the major cancer centers maintain websites, and some, like that of M.D. Anderson Cancer Center, Orlando, headed by Dr. Brown, carry pictures and biographies of cancer specialists on staff. This site not only has details about the physicians' specialties but also tells you where the doctors attended medical school. Internet assistance such as this is invaluable. It can introduce you to physicians and help you better understand how they can be of assistance to you.

The American Medical Association offers people seeking cancer doctors a Physician Select program that allows people to search its database via the Internet by logging on to www.ama-assn.org. There, you can search for oncologists or surgical oncologists by city, state, or ZIP code. The American Society of Clinical Oncology (ASCO) has

---

The Doctor-Patient Relationship

What to seek...

1. From your physician: You'll want a doctor sincerely interested in patient-oriented care.

2. From yourself: You'll want to exercise your most effective communication skills.

3. From your physician: You'll want someone who does not mind if you come to appointments with a list of questions—and who will answer them in lay terminology.

4. From yourself: You'll want to tap into your reservoir of fortitude and let your doctor know you'll need steady and sound advice as you journey into the world of cancer care.

a similar search program on its website, www.asco.org. The database contains names of cancer doctors in all states and a host of cities, large and small. ASCO lists only the names of its members, but bear in mind that some of the nation's top cancer specialists are ASCO members.

Having Trouble Assembling a Medical Team?

Some patients, because of the type of medical insurance they have, particularly those in health maintenance organizations, have no control over their choice of doctors. Deborah B., who belongs to an HMO in California, insists there are ways of getting around doctors assigned to you within a health plan. She asked for the names of doctors in various cancer-related specialties at her HMO and interviewed them by phone. She felt compelled to interview the doctors after the first one to whom she was assigned proved unacceptable.

> They more or less tell you who you'll see at this appointment or that appointment and what laboratory work will be done on a specific day. So the first of these doctors I meet is the surgical oncologist, and he's a real creep.
>
> He very quickly told me how the operation would go. Then he starts telling me how many lumpectomies he does every year at that hospital and how many he usually does at the other hospital and how routine a lumpectomy is.
>
> Then, his cell phone goes off and he starts talking to somebody about his kid's soccer game. I was staggered. Here I am sitting there with a life-threatening cancer, and he's talking about soccer. He wasn't the least bit interested in my case. I got rid of him pronto.

Which Doctor Will I See First?

Your medical needs dictate the order in which you encounter each medical specialist involved in your care. Your first cancer specialist may be a surgical oncologist, the person who will remove your tumor. But the surgical oncologist may suggest another order. If you have a particularly large tumor, the surgeon may recommend chemo first, which means a medical oncologist will be the first physician involved in your care.

The process of induction chemotherapy reverses the traditional order of treatment in breast cancer care, with chemotherapy first, followed by surgery. Tumor-shrinking chemotherapy is administered to reduce the mass and destroy any cancer cells that might have migrated away from the original site. Surgery is performed after the chemotherapy regimen. There are several other situations in which chemotherapy may come before surgery. Here are some quick facts:

❖ Some breast cancers, usually because of their large size or diffuse nature, are conventionally treated with drug therapy as a first round of treatment before surgery.

❖ Inflammatory breast cancer is treated with tumor-shrinking chemotherapy as a first step.

❖ Clinical trials at several major cancer centers are testing the effectiveness of induction chemotherapy compared with standard treatment. You could, if you so choose and your doctors agree, become a participant in one of these trials.

Here are some of the health-care professionals you can expect to take part in the treatment of breast cancer:

Medical oncologist A physician who specializes in cancer treatment and who administers anticancer medications.

Surgical oncologist A doctor who performs a variety of cancer-related operations, such as lumpectomies, mastectomies, and surgical biopsies.

Oncology nurse A nurse with special training in caring for people with cancer. This practitioner's diverse roles touch on all aspects of direct patient care and patient education, and can range from administering chemotherapy and explaining the nature of the medications that are used in your treatment to helping you understand how breast cancer surgery is performed.

Radiologist A key physician on the breast cancer team because she or he is the doctor who first diagnosed the breast cancer based on a reading of a mammogram. A radiologist is also involved in a variety of other functions in your care, particularly the imaging involved in your biopsy.

Anesthesiologist A doctor who administers drugs or gases to put you to sleep before surgery.

Radiation oncologist A doctor who supervises radiation therapy, the directed-beam treatments administered to destroy any remaining cancer cells after surgery.

Pathologist A physician who examines tissue removed in a biopsy to determine if it is malignant. The pathologist subjects the samples to numerous tests, including those that examine cancerous tissue at the genetic level.

Plastic surgeon A physician who specializes in rehabilitative and cosmetic surgery. These doctors perform breast reconstruction operations.

Other health-care professionals who may very well participate in your care include the technicians involved in performing ultrasound, taking X rays, and drawing blood. If you undergo radiation therapy after surgery, you will encounter a radiation therapy technologist. This health-care professional is specially trained to help the radiation oncologist administer external beam therapy.

What Can I Expect at a Cancer Center?

Cancer centers are not just places where treatment occurs. Many have become academic powerhouses where both clinical and basic scientific research are conducted. It is possible to find physicians involved in studies that seek answers to questions about new treatment strategies as well as those investigating the molecular roots of various forms of the disease.

There are many advantages to being treated at a cancer center. There is often an interdisciplinary approach taken at these facilities that allows doctors across multiple specialties to discuss your case. You also may have access to advanced therapies years before they become available to the public at large. You may have access to conventional approaches used in innovative ways. Breast centers have adopted these same approaches, so you won't miss out when being treated at one of those institutions.

When treated at either a breast center or a cancer center, you do not have to travel to distant outposts for laboratory work. The labs, radiation treatment facilities, and outpatient chemotherapy facilities are all located at the center.

You might also find it interesting to note that cancer centers offer the types of social services designed to meet the specific needs of people with cancer. If you do not have a support team of relatives and friends and therefore need help with transportation, as mentioned earlier in this chapter by Elaine H., such an issue would not be considered unusual by the center's social workers; nor would a need for companionship if you are alone. There are ways of addressing a multitude of concerns you probably never thought of as important until you were handed a cancer diagnosis. Given the many decades that experts at cancer centers have studied the needs of cancer patients, it is no accident that certain types of services have evolved.

You may need special counseling because of the emotional struggle often associated with a cancer diagnosis. You may want to join a support group but have no idea how to go about doing so, or even where to find such meetings. You ultimately might have questions about buying wigs. Cancer centers have answers to all of those questions.

What Is a Comprehensive Cancer Center?

The term *comprehensive cancer center* was used earlier in this chapter without much explanation as to what it means. You may have heard the term in other contexts and wondered about its definition. Simply put, the term *comprehensive cancer center* refers to a designation awarded by the National Cancer Institute in Bethesda, Maryland, the nation's leading cancer research and funding center. The NCI bestows the designation on institutions that meet rigorous criteria.

In 2005 there were thirty-eight NCI-designated comprehensive centers. To qualify, the institution must have at least one cancer research program in each of three prime areas: basic clinical research, basic science research, and prevention and population-based studies. The NCI requires a high degree of collaboration among researchers from each of these domains. All of the comprehensive cancer centers are listed in the Resources section at the end of the book.

A few names of comprehensive cancer centers are probably immediately recognized because they have worldwide renown: Memorial Sloan-Kettering Cancer Center in New York City; the M.D. Anderson Cancer Center in Houston (the Orlando, Florida, center is an affiliate); the Mayo Clinic in Rochester, Minnesota; the City of Hope National Medical Center in Duarte, California; Dana Farber Cancer Institute in Boston; and the Fred Hutchinson Cancer Research Center in Seattle.

The NCI has two other designations: *clinical cancer center* and *cancer center*. NCI-designated clinical cancer centers meet most of the rigorous criteria required of comprehensive centers. There were fifteen NCI-designated clinical cancer centers in 2005. Among them are the Siteman Cancer Center at Washington University School of Medicine in St. Louis, Missouri; the Eppley Cancer Center at the University of Nebraska in Omaha; and the OHSU Cancer Institute at the Oregon Health and Science University in Portland.

The NCI's final designation, cancer center, focuses on areas of basic research. Patients are not treated at these facilities. Questions underlying many of the molecular mysteries of cancer are investigated at some of these centers while matters of cancer prevention are pursued in others. There are eight centers in this category, including Cold Spring Harbor Laboratory on Long Island, in New York; the Salk Institute in La Jolla, California; and the Massachusetts Institute of Technology's center in Cambridge.

Finally, you do not have to be treated at one of the NCI-designated comprehensive cancer centers or clinical cancer centers to receive cutting-edge care. There are cancer centers at top hospitals and medical centers throughout the United States that are not on such limited lists. Keep in mind that doctors who treat cancer are among the most highly trained and devoted physicians in medicine. You may find it interesting to note that some of the most elite academic medical centers in the country do not have an NCI designation—in either category.

Institutions that provide top rate cancer care and also have strong research programs include the Winship Cancer Institute at Emory University in Atlanta; the University of Oklahoma's cancer center in Oklahoma City, which is part of that institution's health sciences division; and Stanford University's cancer center in Palo Alto, California. Of course, numerous others abound.

At Stanford there are a number of top cancer specialists and researchers who have even contributed to Nobel Prize–winning discoveries about the molecular underpinnings of cancer. Additional excellent cancer centers are listed in Resources.

Health Insurance and the High Cost of Medical Care

Marie T., a youthful-looking fifty-eight-year-old, believes that almost as troubling as being told she had breast cancer was trying to figure out how to pay the doctor bills. Marie lost her position as a manager for a large clothing retailer a few months before her breast cancer diagnosis. The company was bought by a conglomerate that had no position for Marie or many of her colleagues in the restructured corporation.

Marie did not attempt to maintain health insurance coverage from her employer because she was also insured by her husband's medical plan. But with its high deductibles and list of restrictions, Marie found that the spotty coverage helped turn a major medical disorder into a major financial headache.

> Not all insurance is good insurance. I can only say I wish I knew then what I know now. We both thought before I was diagnosed that his policy would be enough. Both of us were very healthy. But a lot of things weren't covered. The

deductibles were very high and the coverage for prescriptions wasn't very good. Worrying about insurance at a time like that made everything much more difficult.

Marie says the insurance coverage she once had from her employer was superior to that of her husband's company. But neither she nor her husband expected a serious medical condition when she lost her job. And neither had a health savings account (HSA), which is offered through some employers to be tapped for medical expenses not covered by insurance.

Given the complexity of insurance and the rapidity with which bills arrive as you begin your journey through the health-care system, it is probably a good idea soon after diagnosis to acquaint yourself with your health insurance policy and develop an understanding about what it covers. If that seems too complex a task at the moment, ask someone to help you understand it. You might want to delegate that chore to a member of your personal support team. Ask that person to boil down the rules for you. If you're all alone, perhaps a call to the insurer might be in order.

The National Coalition for Cancer Survivorship has an excellent website to assist with a variety of issues concerning cancer (www.canceradvocacy.org). The coalition is especially informative about health-care insurance. Among the coalition's pointers is to read your policy's fine print. If you don't, you might miss benefits that are covered. The website says, "Read your policy carefully to gain an understanding of what will and will not be covered, how to get all the benefits to which you are entitled, and to work within the insurer's systems to manage bills you receive. Not all insurers send out complete policies to their clients. If you do not have a complete policy, contact your insurer and ask for it; you have a legal right to the complete document. You'll want to pay particular attention to obtaining the forms you will need to use if you will be seeking reimbursement."[3]

Certainly, if you are sixty-five or older and qualify for Medicare, or if you have comprehensive benefits from a private insurer, some of the financial issues associated with a major illness may not be a concern, such as whether the costs of certain laboratory testing will be paid. But even then you are not entirely home free. You've got to keep track of your medical visits—and the bills.

On occasion, you may have to investigate why you have been sent a bill from a provider you have never seen. With plans such as those of the Kaiser Permanente system in California, Texas, Maryland, and elsewhere, virtually all of your services, plus reduced medication costs, are covered by your premium. But some social services may be extra, so you if you have a Kaiser plan or a similar one, you may want to inquire about out-of-pocket costs.

Consumer advocates emphasize that the rules of insurers can be daunting, whether your coverage is from a private or government plan. If you become interested in a clinical trial at some point during your treatment, many private insurers will not provide coverage. These companies cite the experimental nature of the trials, which of course is no reflection on the treatment's merit but is very much in keeping with some insurers' efforts to avoid risk. Medicare, on the other hand, which provides medical coverage for older Americans, now pays for costs associated with clinical trial participation.

Figuring out how to pay for treatment when you are unemployed or uninsured can be a nightmare. Medicaid is the program for those with financial need. It is run cooperatively by the federal government and individual states. Eligibility rules differ from state to state. To find out more about Medicare or Medicaid, log on to the website for the Centers for Medicare and Medicaid Services, www.cms.hhs.gov. If you do not have a computer, ask a representative in the social-services department of your treatment center to help you better understand the programs.

For those covered by private insurance, the National Coalition for Cancer Survivorship offers other basic pointers on coping with insurance issues and insurance companies. The coalition warns that health-care providers sometimes send "enormous bills" reflecting costs before an insurer has paid. According to the coalition, you "need not pay anything until the insurer has paid." Moreover, you should contact the provider's billing office to make certain the insurer has been billed. The site also offers other good advice: "If a claim is denied, and you have reason to believe the claim should be covered, contact your insurer and ask for a detailed written response. Take notes during any phone conversations—[write down] the insurance company representative's name, title, phone [extension] and comments as well as time of day and date. If need be, seek additional information to support your claim, such as a letter from a physician explaining the need for the treatment, and re-submit the claim. If the claim continues to be denied, it may be wise to ask your attorney to explore the matter with the insurer."[4]

If insurance issues become particularly troublesome, if you've been denied coverage to which you are entitled, or if you believe other serious violations have occurred, you can contact your state insurance commissioner. Some states offer a toll-free line to their commissioner's offices.

COBRA

The Consolidated Omnibus Budget Reconciliation Act of 1986 allows you to continue your employer's health-care insurance if you leave your job (voluntarily or involuntarily) or if your hours are reduced. Your employer, however, no longer foots any of the costs.

Advantages under COBRA regulations include continuation of comprehensive coverage, possibly allowing you to be treated by physicians you prefer under a medical plan you have always used. However, insurance coverage through COBRA is available by law only for specified periods. The maximum is eighteen months, but under certain circumstances coverage can be extended for as long as thirty-six months. COBRA coverage begins when your employment ends or when your hours are reduced. A human-resources officer at your place of employment can help you understand your specific plan and COBRA rules.

Insurers can discontinue your coverage under COBRA when premiums are not paid on time. You also can lose your benefits if the employer ceases to maintain the group plan that carries your coverage. Not all forms of employment are covered under COBRA regulations. Workers in certain types of jobs (e.g., positions with the federal government) have a similar plan and do not qualify for COBRA coverage.

Disability Insurance

Although many patients being treated for early breast cancer can continue working, others, because of chemotherapy, find it best not to do so. Disability insurance that you have paid for through payroll deductions or through a personal contract generally activates after a specified waiting period. Check your policy to make certain that it can be activated for cancer therapy. Another option: If doctors determine that your cancer is advanced, you may be eligible for Social Security–Disability Insurance, which pays a monthly benefit to people unable to work. You can find further information about Social Security Disability Insurance at the program's website, www.ssa.gov, or by calling the Social Security Administration at (800) 772-1213.

For Those Who Lack Adequate Insurance

For patients with less-than-adequate insurance coverage, medical bills can become overwhelming. A loss of employment, as was Marie's case, can only worsen the situation. As you peruse your policy before treatment, you may want to think about how you might go about paying for aspects of your care that are not covered. Marie and her husband ultimately chose to refinance their house to consolidate bills. Home equity loans have helped other patients. But if you are not a homeowner and are without any form of health-care insurance, you may have to rely on your ingenuity.

Here are a few tips you might want to keep in the back of your mind. Most states offer pharmacy assistance programs for people sixty-five and older, as well as for those who are disabled and eligible for Medicare benefits. A few states, such as Maine, Maryland, and Vermont, offer assistance to residents of any age who cannot afford to pay for prescriptions. Another avenue for those on Medicare, the drug benefit signed into law by Congress in 2003 and effective January 1, 2006, was designed to lower patients' skyrocketing drug costs and is considered the centerpiece of the Medicare Modernization Act.

While some advocacy organizations have praised federal efforts to offer discounts to all Medicare recipients, they still question whether the measure favors pharmaceutical companies more than it helps patients. The measure stipulates that medications cannot be purchased in bulk by the government, a move that would automatically substantially lower costs to consumers. The American Association of Retired Persons (AARP) has promised to keep an eye on drug prices and to hold legislators accountable should consumer costs rise appreciably despite the discounts given to Medicare recipients.

Qualifying for Free Medical Care

Medical centers that receive money from Congress through the Hill-Burton Program have agreed to provide free services for a specified number of patients. The number of patients varies from one facility to another, and not all cities have facilities that participate in the Hill-Burton Program. To find out if there are any facilities near you, call this toll-free number: (800) 638-0742. If you are a Maryland resident, call (800) 492-0359.

With respect to chemotherapy, oncologists began lobbying Congress in 2005 because the Medicare Modernization Act also called for a $500 million reduction in how much the government would provide for cancer care. The reduction comes despite a 34 percent increase ($66.60 in 2004 to $89.20 in 2006) in the monthly amount Medicare charges recipients. The American Society of Clinical Oncology (ASCO) charged that such cuts jeopardize cancer treatment. ASCO doctors have vowed to fight cuts in funds for cancer treatment and to maintain a presence on Capitol Hill to ensure their voice is heard.

If you're neither elderly nor disabled, and do not have teams of activists and doctors lobbying on your behalf in Washington, you'll need other options. One possibility is to seek assistance through the Pharmaceutical Research and Manufacturers Association (PhRMA), a consortium of forty-eight major pharmaceutical companies that manufacture and sell medications in the United States and abroad. If you can demonstrate a need, you may qualify for free medications. You can learn more about the association by logging on to www.pharma.org. There you will find the names of participating companies that provide medications to physicians whose patients cannot afford to purchase them. You also can inquire about PhRMA in the social-services department of your medical/ cancer/breast center. Social workers should be familiar with the program. If they are not, ask them to log on to the site and print the information for you.

Pursuing assistance through the Pharmaceutical Research and Manufacturers Association is one path to ease the cost burden—but it may not work. In addition to PhRMA, many pharmaceutical companies offer "patient-assistance programs," which provide free medications. The rules are tough because the qualifying populations for these programs are usually at—or substantially below—the federal poverty level. Patient-assistance programs are offered by some of the best-known pharmaceutical companies in the world. AstraZeneca, makers of tamoxifen, the most widely prescribed breast cancer drug around the globe, has such a program.

Generally, rules for patient assistance stipulate that you must be uninsured and ineligible for your state's Medicaid program. Pharmaceutical giant Merck sponsors a patient-assistance program, also aimed at the uninsured and those with a particularly low annual income. But if your income is more than the specified cutoffs ($18,000 or less for individuals; $24,000 or less for couples; $35,000 or less for a family of four), your doctor can request an exception when there is a special circumstance. A list of patient-assistance programs is included in Resources, at the end of the book.

Drug Discounts for Middle-Income Patients

If you meet certain income requirements—somewhat less stringent than those for free medications—or rank among the uninsured, you may qualify for drug discounts sponsored by pharmaceutical companies. Pfizer, the world's largest drug maker, allows discounts on its products. Knowing this, of course, is helpful only if you're prescribed

Pfizer medications. But when you're trying to optimize your options, it's always best to have a long list from which to choose.

The Pfizer program, which began in August 2004, cut prices by an average of 37 percent for families earning up to $45,000 a year. Anyone earning more but who is without health-care insurance can qualify for discounts of 15 percent on Pfizer drugs. The company's price slashing was hailed by New York Senator Hillary Rodham Clinton, a longtime advocate for the uninsured. She said one of the lesser-known health-care disparities has been the steeper out-of-pocket medication costs paid by those without health-care insurance. People with higher incomes and adequate insurance traditionally have had lower prescription-drug bills because of the amount offset by coverage.

Additionally, you can enroll in private supplemental prescription-drug programs to help lower costs. These are not insurance plans but do allow discounts at many larger chain pharmacies. The programs have been widely advertised on television and the radio. Some are helpful; others leave a lot to be desired. Discounts are possible because companies sponsoring the cards are able to pool the buying power of the program's enrollees. You pay the program an annual fee, which can range anywhere from $20 to $100, and that in turn makes you eligible for discounts on your prescriptions. The cards can be used for any prescribed medication.

For example, if during chemotherapy you're prescribed the antinausea drug Zofran (ondansatron), you may want to shop for the best price, using your card. Zofran isn't cheap. It runs between $530 and $607 for a thirty-day supply, depending on the pharmacy filling the prescription and the region of the country where you live. Consumer advocates say it may be a good idea to enroll in more than one prescription discount plan. If one card doesn't lower the price substantially enough, perhaps another will.

One such discounter is the Omni Choice Prescription Drug Plan, which advertises discounts ranging from 15 percent to 65 percent on name-brand and generic medications. Although deep discounts are advertised, don't expect them for all drugs. Also, be aware of the company's fine print, which doesn't differ much from that of similar card sponsors. "Please note," its caveat says, "not every prescription claim will receive a discount."[5] That being the case, remember the earlier advice: Having more than one card is probably the smartest move.

The Canadian Connection

A final option to help lower your medication costs is attempting to purchase drugs over the Internet from Canada. It is a choice that has proved both rewarding and increasingly difficult, as more Americans have turned to their northern neighbor in search of lower prices—and trillion-dollar pharmaceutical companies have tried to stop them. U.S. pharmaceutical giants, alarmed by the flood of American prescriptions crossing the border, have instituted a series of moves to block purchases. Some conglomerates have placed limits on the number of medications sold to Canadian pharmacies, which has meant some Canadian outlets have fewer medications available for sale.

In 2004, the FDA entered the fray, confiscating packages of medications in Canada that had been destined for U.S. households. Such aggression was a prime example of one of the more abhorrent moves initiated by the government in cooperation with pharmaceutical companies.

Most U.S. chain pharmacies sell drugs over the Internet, which is very convenient. Major chains offer discounts and honor many of the drug-discount cards mentioned earlier. But beware of Internet medication wholesalers whose names you do not recognize. The drugs may be less expensive, but they might also be dangerous knockoffs, possibly made in a growing prescription-drug underground emanating from India.

A Good Book and a Hot Cup of Joe (or Tea)

After being diagnosed, it is essential that you become as knowledgable as possible about breast cancer. The Appendix at the back of the book contains helpful advice on how to obtain current information on breast cancer as well as find support via the Internet. While the Internet is one way to become informed about breast cancer, good old-fashioned printed and bound material—like the book you now hold in your hands—still gets the job done. Ask your doctors, support-group leader, or a breast cancer survivor to recommend reading material. You'll find a list of Recommended Reading at the end of the book with several editions you might want to add to your library on breast cancer.

Other sources of information include videotapes, available through some physicians; articles in newspaper archives; medical textbooks; and pamphlets from medical centers and nationally renowned advocacy organizations.

MAMM, a magazine devoted to information about breast cancer, can be particularly enlightening. You can find subscription information at the magazine's website, www.mamm.com. While you're there, check out some of the archived articles that cover a wide range of issues confronting patients and survivors. Among the articles archived on the site are those focusing on Nicki Marsh, a New York woman who was diagnosed with the disease at age twenty-six. The magazine covered a year in Nicki's life.

More Info on Info

Other highly useful resources include telephone help lines, particularly the one operated by the National Cancer Institute, which can be reached by dialing (800) 4-CANCER (800-422-6237). There, trained volunteers can provide information about virtually any aspect of the disease. It operates during business hours: 9:00 A.M. to 5:00 P.M., Monday through Friday.

The advocacy group Y-Me National Breast Cancer Organization operates a twenty-four-hour hotline staffed by breast cancer survivors. It can be reached toll free by dialing (800) 221-2141 (English) or (800) 986-9505 (Spanish).

Bev Parker, who was diagnosed twice with breast cancer, is director of Y-Me's hotline, the only twenty-four-hour telephone service devoted to the disease. She believes it is an invaluable experience for the newly diagnosed to chat with someone who has already been through diagnosis, treatment, and recovery. "No question about it," she says. "One of the best things in the world is being able to talk to someone who has already been there, who knows what you're going through, who can provide some tips about navigating the medical maze, and who can help you understand that you are not alone."

Chapter 3

Facts, Fiction, and Urban Legends

> If chemotherapy doesn't make you sick, then it's
> not working.
>
> — A *myth passed by word of mouth and over the Internet*

Just about everybody knows a little bit about virtually every common medical condition. Take a stroll down Broadway in Manhattan or along Lombard in San Francisco and ask any three people what causes heart attacks and you'll probably hear fairly reasonable explanations outlining the Cholesterol Theory of cardiovascular disease. Lung cancer? A no-brainer. Your astute experts-on-the-street will fire back: smoking. Ulcers? Your smart respondents would say stomach ulcers are caused by the wily bacterium *Helicobacter pylori*. Well, maybe only one out of three will get that one.

My examples underscore the pervasiveness of medical information. It's inescapable. People are better educated about common medical conditions now than they were a generation ago. Medical information comes at you from all directions, all day, every day. You find it reported prominently in newspapers and magazines, on television and radio, and over the Internet. Why? Because people have an insatiable desire to learn about the human condition in health and disease. Breast cancer is no exception. As the leading cause of cancer in women, the subject is frequently in a media spotlight.

Even as women affected by breast cancer increasingly seek out highly technical information about the condition, myths and misconceptions surprisingly persist. Arguably, there are more myths about breast cancer than there are about any other malignancy, and there may even be more than there are about possibly any other type of medical condition. It is a matter so mystifying that even the experts are at a loss for words.

Many of these myths are widely reported in the media as fact. Who hasn't heard, for instance, that soy prevents breast cancer? It is a "fact" that has been widely reported for years. The belief is so potent that in the first few years of this century, sales of soy-based foods rose 44 percent over purchases in the 1990s, posting nearly four billion dollars in annual sales for manufacturers.[1]

Despite these impressive sales, there never has been a large-scale, long-term, randomized, placebo-controlled study examining the effectiveness of soy when consumed in foods or supplements to prevent a breast cancer recurrence or stave off the disease in those at high risk. Nurse practitioner Lynette Lee Pack-May of the Carol M. Baldwin Breast Care Center in New York says the truth about soy is that it is a matter under intense debate. Women who have breast cancer or who are at risk for the disorder should thoroughly discuss the soy issue with their physicians.

So, if you're feeling guilty about not having properly protected your health because you didn't eat any soy energy bars or gulp down gallons of soy milk, stop. The purpose of this chapter is to help you eliminate any guilt about your cancer based on the preponderance of poorly interpreted scientific data, myths, and other half-baked notions currently in global circulation.

This chapter opens with an analysis of breast cancer facts and fictions, a subject that is important to explore because of the question it raises: How is it possible for myths about a major form of cancer to persist? From there, an examination of "urban legends" is taken into account. That term was chosen because some beliefs—though based on at least some scientific research—have taken on lives of their own quite apart from the medical findings.

The soy issue is one, but there are several others that you will probably recognize very quickly.

These beliefs, born of studies widely promoted in the news media, often are reported without much explanatory context. Example: Researchers have suggested that broccoli can help prevent breast cancer. What does that mean for someone who may have regularly eaten it and yet now has the disease? And even if broccoli *is* the cancer-fighter that people say it is, how much would you have had to consume to be protected? Should you have consumed it daily, twice daily? By the cup, bowl, or plateful? No one really has that answer.

Similarly, legends have grown about antibiotics, the consistency of earwax (women with sticky wax supposedly are more prone to the cancer), and the proximity of homes to power lines. This chapter is to help you sift fact from fiction. It ends with a discussion on cancer clusters, which have evoked powerful fears that have swept communities, galvanizing some to seek unusual causes. Scientists, government health officials, and major advocacy groups generally dismiss the possibility of cancer clusters for common forms of the disease. We'll examine why.

Myths and Misconceptions

Breast cancer myths have become so deeply woven into the fabric of popular beliefs that patients frequently ask their oncologists about them, thinking they are inquiring about a fact pertinent to their survival. Often, they quickly discover their concern is a misconception. But before we get too deeply into this discussion, keep in mind that there are no "dumb" questions from patients, doctors say, and they invite the newly diagnosed to continue to ask whatever concerns come to mind. Doing so is a way, say doctors, to snuff out harmful myths.

Fiction about breast cancer runs the gamut. Some patients believe the disease is invariably fatal. Others among the newly diagnosed carry a deep and abiding belief that if the disease doesn't kill them, then the treatments certainly will. To this day, some breast cancer patients are convinced their diagnosis promises treatments that will scar them for life, exactly the way radiation and destructive surgeries marred friends or relatives in the distant past.

As president of the National Breast Cancer Foundation in Washington, patient advocate Fran Visco has found that myths are obstacles that need thorough vetting from popular culture. She says, "A lot of women have some very unfortunate ideas about the disease and what causes it. We can only hope that as more women take advantage of the many resources that are available out there, these unfortunate ideas will disappear. One of our biggest problems is that some of these ideas seem to have taken on lives of their own."

Some experts believe many of the myths that have surfaced about breast cancer arose because of the near secrecy in which previous generations endured the condition. Breast cancer was not a disease discussed openly. While medical and surgical advances have occurred at an ever-quickening pace, antiquated views have been much slower to exit.

Stories of devastating medical experiences are handed down in family folklore, or passed along as "advice" to friends or relatives facing surgery and radiation. You may recall Helen C., from Chapter 1, a college professor who said that even though she knew better, she couldn't help thinking about the mutilating surgery and scars on her grandmother's chest caused by radiation treatments in the 1960s. At some primal level, Helen felt that disfiguring surgery and radiation burns would become her fate as well.

Hanging on to beliefs about medical practices rooted in a deep and misty past can only get in the way of your own treatment and recovery, experts say. But while obsolete medical treatments triggered fears in Helen, other women harbor fears that their cancer may have been caused by common products. Bras, deodorants, coffee, and seat belts are a few that draw a spotlight. Word has actually circulated that each of these items can cause breast cancer.

Breast cancer myths can be divided into three categories: (a) myths centered on the cause of the disease; (b) myths focused on risk; and (c) myths involving diagnostics and treatments, including medications, radiation, and surgery. During interviews for this book, physicians, nurses, breast cancer patients, and survivors were asked to convey some of the "important" misinformation about breast cancer heard on the street. The following is a roundup of their most notable responses.

Fiction Versus Fact

MYTHS ABOUT THE CAUSES OF BREAST CANCER

Fiction: *Bras, especially underwire bras, cause breast cancer.*
Fact: There is no evidence that bras even remotely promote the development of cancer, even though a small study several years ago suggested such a possibility. The rumor mill caught wind of the research, causing the tall tale about bras to grow ever stronger. It is a myth that refuses to die.

Fiction: *Deodorants and antiperspirants cause breast cancer.*
Fact: This myth, for which there is no validation, has appeared as a warning on unscrupulous "medical information" websites and has turned up as a subject of discussion in Internet chat rooms. There are no scientific data supporting this notion.

Fiction: *Drinking coffee causes breast cancer. The idea behind this myth grows out of the link between coffee (and other caffeine-containing foods and beverages) and fibrocystic breast changes.*
Fact: While some doctors still tell women to lessen their consumption of caffeine-containing foods and beverages to prevent fibrocystic changes, there are no links among fibrocystic changes, consumption of coffee, tea, or chocolate, and breast cancer. Women with fibrocystic breast changes (once called fibrocystic breast disease) usually experience thickened areas or lumpiness in one or both breasts. This sometimes painful condition is known to worsen near the time of a woman's menstrual period and can be exacerbated by the consumption of caffeine-containing foods and drinks, but women with fibrocystic changes are not at an increased risk for developing breast cancer. Furthermore, lumpiness is natural and has nothing to do with disease.

Fiction: *Seat belts cause breast cancer. This unusual idea reasons that seat belts that cross the chest limit blood supply and encourage the growth of tumors.*

Fact: The truth here is plain and simple: Seat belts do not cause breast cancer, but they do save lives in the event of an auto accident.

Fiction: *Injury to the breasts, such as being hit by a baseball or falling from a bicycle, can cause breast cancer. The idea behind this one is that injured tissue never fully recovers normal function.*

Fact: Breast tissue recovers, and many women who have been injured in falls and other accidents have gone on to successfully nurse infants, a key indication that all is working well internally.

Fiction: *Having breast-fed your baby on only one side heightens the breast cancer risk on the other.*

Fact: This fiction, offered by a breast cancer survivor from an affluent Northern California community, suggests that myths know no socioeconomic barriers. There is no scientific evidence whatsoever suggesting that breast-feeding on only one side would make someone vulnerable to cancer.

Fiction: *Emotional stress causes breast cancer.*

Fact: This belief suggests that leading a stress-filled life causes the body to produce a flood of stress hormones that transform cells and trigger the processes leading to malignancy. It springs from the ill-informed notion that you can bring on your own breast cancer. There is no evidence that leading a stressful life causes breast cancer.

MYTHS ABOUT BREAST CANCER RISK

Fiction: *Women with LCIS (lobular carcinoma in situ) definitely develop breast cancer.*

Fact: As will be explained in greater detail later in this chapter, LCIS is recognized as an abnormal pattern of cellular growth, which serves as a marker for elevated breast cancer risk. Having LCIS does not automatically mean that you will develop breast cancer. The condition was recently renamed lobular neoplasia to better define the abnormal appearance of the cells when viewed under a microscope. Data from the National Cancer Institute indicate that women with LCIS have a 25 percent chance of developing breast cancer.

Fiction: *Younger women do not develop breast cancer.*
Fact: While the majority of women who develop the disease are postmenopausal, younger women are more likely to develop aggressive forms of the disease. An estimated eleven thousand women under forty develop breast cancer annually.

Fiction: *Older women do not develop breast cancer and are at lower risk than younger women. (This is the flip side of the preceding myth.)*
Fact: Nothing could be farther from the truth. Older women, as will be discussed at length later in the book, are at heightened risk because the likelihood of developing breast cancer increases with age.

Fiction: *Men do not get breast cancer.*
Fact: Not true. Even though breast cancer is not common in men, they do develop the condition. Studies have shown that some occupations, such as those involving work on high-voltage cables, put some men at higher risk for the disease. As mentioned earlier, men often feel particularly depressed about breast cancer. They say it seems as if they have developed a "woman's disease."

Fiction: *Women with small breasts do not develop breast cancer.*
Fact: Small, medium, or large, breast cancer is an equal-opportunity disease.

Fiction: *Only women with a family history of the disease are at risk of developing breast cancer.*
Fact: Not true. Most women who develop breast cancer have no known hereditary link to the cancer.

Fiction: *Breast cancer in a family may skip a generation. This myth circulated in a family in which a mother developed the disease, but whose daughters thought they were safe. The only previous case of the*

cancer involved a maternal great-grandmother. As it turned out, two
daughters eventually developed breast cancer.
Fact: There is no medical pattern by which you can guess your family risk.

MYTHS ABOUT TREATMENT AND DIAGNOSTICS

Fiction: *Once you've had a mastectomy, breast cancer will not come back.*
Fact: Up to 10 percent of patients who have had a mastectomy experience a recurrence in the remaining scar tissue.

Fiction: *Mammograms protect you from developing breast cancer.*
Fact: Mammography is not a treatment modality. It is aimed at detection.

Fiction: *Mammograms cause breast cancer.*
Fact: Doctors who treat breast cancer patients say they have heard this one countless times from women who wonder whether their preventive health measures backfired and caused their cancer. Medical evidence repeatedly shows that mammograms do not cause the disease.

Fiction: *The treatments for breast cancer are worse than the disease.*
Fact: This myth grows out of some of the observed side effects in cancer patients. People with cancer become nauseated, can lose their hair, and are fatigued. While cancer therapy can be daunting, for a majority of patients there is a silver lining behind what may seem to be arduous rounds of medical therapy. The treatments end, vigor returns, and hair grows back.

Fiction: *Breast cancer surgery causes the disease to spread.*
Fact: Surgery can prevent the disease from spreading. When detected in an early stage, the tumor and the surrounding margin of tissue that may contain cancerous cells can be removed. A study reported in the *Journal of the American Medical Association* revealed that women in the rural South were most likely to believe that when exposed to "air" during surgery, cancer spreads. So it is likely that

this myth about surgery is more prevalent in some regions than in others.

Fiction: *Radiation therapy will result in burns and scars on the chest. This fiction stems from a time when radiation was less targeted than it is now.*

Fact: Dry skin can occur in the treatment area, but the notion of scarring burns is an old myth that has yet to lose steam. The truth is that beam radiation is mathematically calibrated and finely tuned to the specific area where the tumor grew. It is not a helter-skelter therapy.

Tapping the Roots of Urban Legends

Urban legends about breast cancer often begin with an element of truth but somehow, after being passed around for a while, start assuming new levels of meaning and importance. Legends become popular because their link to science seems to confirm their legitimacy. Often some legends take hold after scientists have found provocative evidence from only a few small studies, generally statistical ones that show an association but not a definitive cause-and-effect link. These notions then become so deeply ingrained that on occasion even doctors may believe they are the final word on an issue.

One of the best examples deals with hormone replacement therapy (HRT) and heart disease. For years doctors and the news media told women that HRT prevented heart disease based on epidemiological (statistical) studies that showed an association between HRT and a lower risk of cardiac ailments. However, when the "prospective data" (results from studies involving thousands of patients) were tabulated, researchers reported quite the opposite. HRT did not prevent heart disease—it helped cause it.

Waiting for the results from a prospective trial may take a decade or longer. But it is important to know what kind of a study generated any medical information being trumpeted loudly in the news. That way you can have some idea whether stronger or more definitive data are to come at some point in the future.

Breast cancer legends have loomed large not because of bad science, but because of good science that was poorly interpreted. From poor interpretations, legends have grown and beliefs have taken root. Legends about breast cancer largely center on two key areas: prevention and risks. Example: "If you take this or that supplement or eat this or that food, you won't get breast cancer, based on scientific data." Or, "The scientific literature indicates that you're at high risk for breast cancer if you took antibiotics, have this or that kind of earwax, or lived near power lines." Whenever you hear or read statements like these, bear in mind that breast cancer is an extraordinarily complex disease and many of the questions about prevention and risk remain unanswered.

Single-Food Saviors? A Look at Broccoli

As early as the mid-1980s scientists recognized that broccoli and its cruciferous cousins, cabbage and Brussels sprouts, contained an anticancer compound known as sulforaphane. Sulforaphane is important because it boosts the body's production of a class of proteins known as phase-II enzymes. These enzymes are capable of reducing the activity of cancer-causing chemicals in the body.

Broccoli would be good for you even if it did not contain sulforaphane. The vegetable is rich in vitamins and fiber. For years, doctors and nutritionists have urged people to include it as part of a healthy diet. But to urge people to eat broccoli as a way to prevent breast cancer, as many media outlets have done over the years, constitutes practicing medicine without complete data. While broccoli can't hurt and it might help, isn't it also likely that some people might feel greatly let down when they find they've developed breast cancer despite having consumed bushels of broccoli?

Cathy R., a mother of two adult daughters, says she began eating broccoli "at least four or five times a week," a plan she incorporated into a healthy, low-fat, low-carb diet. Cathy followed this dietary program that emphasized broccoli for more than a decade. This, she says, was part of a broader lifestyle regimen that included exercise, getting plenty of sleep, and drinking lots of water. But in

2003, she was diagnosed with breast cancer, which was discovered during a routine physical.

> I am lucky to have had such good doctors who helped me through this. I'm not mad at anybody. I still eat a lot of broccoli. I still do aerobics. But I do these things for me because I enjoy them, not because they're supposed to stop something bad from happening. Bad things happen.
>
> I come from a breast cancer family. My mom had it. My sister was diagnosed two years before I was. My aunt—my mom's sister—had it and then got ovarian cancer. She passed away three years ago. My perspective on things is probably different from that of most other people.

In Chapter 5, which explores breast cancer risk factors, the genetic basis of breast cancer is examined. In that discussion doctors underscore that 75 percent of breast cancer cases cannot be explained by the known risk factors.

What most media reports don't say about broccoli is that there have never been any clinical trials of people consuming the vegetable, using controlled preparation methods, and possibly consuming only broccoli grown under certain conditions. When several epidemiologists were asked how such a clinical trial would be conducted, they all agreed that it would take years—possibly a decade or longer—to determine how well the vegetable would serve as a breast cancer preventive.

At a meeting of the American Chemical Society in 2002, a University of Chicago study confirmed the anticancer properties of sulforaphane. Using nature as their model, Dr. Jerry Kosmeder and colleagues synthesized the compound in their lab. Dr. Kosmeder, the lead investigator, reported that in pill form the broccoli compound could be taken as easily as a vitamin tablet.[2] However, there have been no large-scale tests of the broccoli compound in pill form that have shown evidence of breast cancer prevention in a double-blind, randomized, placebo-controlled clinical trial—the gold standard of scientific testing.

What about Soy?

Soy products, as mentioned earlier, are another group of foods pushed heavily by the media as a breast cancer preventive, based on "scientific evidence." How the lowly soybean became increasingly pivotal in the global commodities market is a saga that is half fairy tale, half marketing wonder. In 1999 the FDA approved a claim that soy lowers cholesterol, a statement that could from then on be written on labels of certain soy products. Petitions to make similar claims about cancer prevention have been requested but not yet approved.

Besides the traditional soy-based foods, such as tofu and edamame (very young soybeans, eaten steamed), soy has been processed into a dizzying array of snack-food products, liquefied into "milk," dried into nuts, frothed into shakes, and formulated into supplements. Few people have missed the message about the health benefits connected to consuming soy foods or supplements. Much of the increase in sales of soy products can be attributed to women consuming it as part of a healthy diet, as well as to lessen the bothersome effects of menopause—and to prevent breast cancer.

The issue of soy as a preventive arose from studies that strongly suggested that women of Asian descent have rates of breast cancer that are substantially lower than those of their North American counterparts. These studies are largely epidemiological, which means they show a statistical association between soy consumption and lower rates of breast cancer in countries such as China and Japan. What these kinds of studies cannot prove is a direct cause-and-effect relationship between soy and lower breast cancer rates. It is plausible that a direct link may never be found.

You might also want to consider this possibility: It is very likely that soy may not be acting alone to guard against breast cancer in Asian women, as some scientists have suggested. Soy could be working synergistically—in concert—with other potent nutrients that are also more common in Asian diets. Fish is one such possibility. Like the compounds in soy, chemicals in fish have antioxidant qualities capable of quelling free radicals. (Free radicals are rogue oxygen molecules that have been implicated in cancer and other health problems.) And there is yet another thought: It is also very likely that foods may play a minor role when compared with the genetics of Asians, who simply may be less prone to breast cancer than women in the West.

Finally, because soy is a dietary staple in Asian countries, exposure for many people begins while they are in the womb, not in midlife, when hot flashes flare and vaginal dryness begins. Some studies have suggested that it is soy consumption early in life, particularly during adolescence, that is most important. Chemicals in soy may affect the growth of cells in the breasts, causing them to become more differentiated. The more differentiated cells are, scientists say, the less likely it is they will undergo the proliferative processes associated with cancer.

Thus, it is important that scientists examine more closely the difference between soy exposure that begins early in life and soy consumption that starts much later.

THE CHEMISTRY OF SOY

Soybeans contain chemicals known as isoflavones, which act as weak estrogens in the body. The estrogenic effect is the reason why soy supplements and foods have become popular among women suffering menopausal symptoms. Following reports in 2002 that hormone replacement therapy—HRT—elevates the risks of breast cancer and cardiovascular disease, women turned in greater number to soy products as substitutes for hormone pills.

Some groups of scientists believe that the isoflavones contained in soy not only act as weak estrogens, but are also endowed with the ability to act as *anti*estrogens in the body, which is very good news if it is confirmed that soy is active and safe in that capacity in humans. However, the dual nature of isoflavones is still under study, and conclusive results on the estrogenic and antiestrogenic potential of these compounds has yet to be fully elucidated.

Theories about breast cancer risk reduction attributed to soy consumption have not been lost on the public. Elaine W., a talented television personality in the Northeast, was diagnosed with LCIS, lobular carcinoma in situ, which, despite its ominous-sounding name, is not breast cancer but is a marker for increased breast cancer risk. Patients with LCIS must be closely monitored because their abnormal breast pathology makes them more vulnerable to breast cancer than women in the general population. Aware of the research suggesting that certain foods can function as weak estrogens, offering protection against menopausal symptoms and possibly guarding against breast cancer, Elaine considered adding soy and flaxseeds, another phytoestrogen (plant-based estrogen), to her diet. But first she read voraciously on the subject, and she contacted scientists at the Princess Margaret Hospital in Toronto, where medical investigators have conducted studies on soy and flaxseeds and their roles in thwarting hot flashes, night sweats, and other nagging symptoms. After she'd been consuming soy foods and flaxseeds daily for a while, she received an unfavorable lab report about her LCIS (though fortunately it was not cancer). Her physician immediately suspected that her increased intake of phytoestrogens had led to the changes. Elaine explains that she did not know that soy and flaxseed products could potentially worsen her condition:

> I was interested in finding something for perimenopausal symptoms because I can't take HRT, and from what I read about isoflavones I understood they also brought down the risk of breast cancer. But I may have overdone it. Princess Margaret Hospital had a recipe on the web for flaxseed muffins. I prepared and ate some. I was eating soy, too. I think my problem was that I ate too much soy. When I mentioned my increased phytoestrogen intake to a physician, she said, "Why are you doing that?"

SOY CONSUMPTION AFTER A BREAST CANCER DIAGNOSIS

For women diagnosed with estrogen-dependent breast cancer (the type of the disease that is driven by the hormone estrogen), clinicians suggest exercising caution about soy consumption. They emphasize that soy and other plant-based estrogens should only be cautiously added to the diet, if added at all. Legumes are the food sources particularly known to carry these chemicals. Among food sources of plant-based estrogens, soybeans are the richest source.

Nurse practitioner Pack-May says the best advice she can offer anyone with breast cancer who is considering adding significant amounts of soy to her diet is to first consult with experts. "Soy is a very controversial issue," she says. "When a woman has a diagnosis of breast cancer, the amount of soy she takes in should be limited. Soy by itself is not harmful. But we know that it can interfere with certain medications [such as tamoxifen]. It is an antagonist when it is taken during active treatments."

Again, because isoflavones act as weak estrogens, the suspicion is that these compounds can compete with tamoxifen and may even prevent the drug from latching on to its cellular targets. In a summary of scientific studies that looked into the effects of isoflavones in women being treated for breast cancer, experts at the Linus Pauling Institute of Oregon State University also underscored a need to proceed with caution when it comes to soy:

> The safety of high intakes of soy isoflavones and other phytoestrogens is an area of considerable debate among scientists and clinicians. The effects of high intakes of soy isoflavones on breast cancer survival and breast cancer recurrence in humans have not been studied. The results of cell culture and animal studies are conflicting, but some have found that soy isoflavones can stimulate the growth of estrogen-receptor-positive (ER+) breast cancer cells....
>
> Very limited data from clinical trials suggests that increased consumption of soy isoflavones (38 to 45 milligrams per day) can have estrogenic effects in human breast tissue. Given available data, some experts think that women with a history of breast cancer, particularly ER+ breast cancer, should not increase their consumption of phytoestrogens, including isoflavones. However, other experts argue that there is not enough evidence to discourage breast cancer survivors from consuming soy foods in moderation.[3]

Antibiotics and Breast Cancer

The link between antibiotics and breast cancer is relatively new, but it has generated waves of concern in Internet chat rooms. In one list-serv for breast cancer survivors, a concerned woman wrote that she took antibiotics during childhood for recurrent ear infections. "I must have taken dozens of pills. I wonder if that's what caused my cancer?"

The reasoning behind the link between breast cancer and antibiotics centers on a large statistical study by top scientists who found provocative but nevertheless inconclusive information. The team of researchers from the Group Health Cooperative's Center for Health Studies in Seattle reported in a February 2004 issue of the *Journal of the American Medical Association (JAMA)* that women who had used antibiotics for many years ran a higher than usual risk of breast cancer. The greater the usage, the higher the risk turned out to be.[4]

Still, the study left many questions unanswered . Do antibiotics actually cause the disease? Or is there something as yet to be discovered about immune suppression that more readily leads to infection, forcing the need for antibiotics? Could that same immune suppression also leave someone more vulnerable to cancer? Scientists have yet to produce additional studies to answer those questions.

The research reported in JAMA was the second to suggest a link between antibiotics and breast cancer. The first study to make such an association was conducted by Finnish scientists who reported their findings in 2000.

In the 2004 study reported by the Americans, researchers examined the medical records of 10,000 women in the state of Washington. Scientists counted 2,266 cases of breast cancer. Those who'd had more than twenty-five antibiotic prescriptions during a seventeen-year period had double the risk of developing the disease.

As frightening as the results of the study may seem, the jury is still out on whether the women's cancers can be definitively tied to their use of antibiotics. On the whole, the antibiotics ranged over many classes and were chemically different from each other. That raises the question of how drugs so different from one another can all carry the same cancer-causing capability. There is as yet no answer to that question. Doctors involved in the study advised women not to stop taking antibiotics when they are prescribed for infections.

Earwax Consistency and Breast Cancer Risk

An unusual line of research that initially began in the 1980s has looked into the consistency of earwax as a possible breast cancer risk. The dark, gooey wax typically found in people in the United States differs from the type generally found in Asians. Their wax, according to people who've compared the two types, is usually gray, dry, and flaky. From those differences, scientists made an association between rates of breast cancer based on earwax type.

Studies of earwax in the United States took inspiration from similar studies in Japan where scientists over the years have found that women with the highest rates of breast cancer tended to have the wet and sticky, brown-colored wax. Those who tended not to develop the disease were more likely to have the dry, flaky version.

The idea behind these studies suggests that the gene in charge of earwax production may also affect breast cancer risk. The reasoning? Earwax glands are related to the apocrine system, which includes the glands that secrete fluid in the breast. Scientists hypothesize, but as yet have been unable to confirm, that the gene for the wet, sticky wax could one day prove to be a marker for the disease. More work, however, has yet to be conducted before anyone's earwax type can be positively linked to the development of breast cancer.

Power Lines and Electromagnetic Energy

Associating power lines with various types of cancer also dates back to the 1980s, when scientists first announced several dramatic findings linking electromagnetic energy and cases of cancer in residents who lived near the lines. Researchers measured the distance from large electrical towers that carry power over great distances to the homes of people who developed cancer and found increased rates of malignant disease in those who lived closest to the energy source.

Among the cancers first linked to power lines were childhood malignancies, mostly brain tumors and leukemia. In time, many other types of cancer were reported to have a relationship to electro-magnetic energy, associations often made by people who lived near the giant power-carrying towers and who claimed that cancers were occurring in clusters. In addition, as time wore on, there was a trend toward linking different sources of electromagnetic energy to cancers, not just the fields that flowed from power lines.

An electromagnetic field—EMF—is an area of energy caused by the flow of electrical current. You can't see or feel an EMF, but if you're reading this passage by way of lamplight then there is an EMF very close to you. The giant towers carrying power from one town to the next are another EMF source, but there are others that are much more common in day-to-day life, such as the wiring behind the walls in your home or office and electrical appliances of all sizes, ranging from your refrigerator to the alarm clock at your beside. EMFs also flow from your computer, electric hairdryer, and TV, whenever they're turned on. It is difficult to escape EMFs, even if you decide to move to the mountains of Montana and live in a cabin free of electricity. Earth is surrounded by the Vann-Allen belt, from which electromagnetic energy constantly flows.

Still, the issue of EMF exposure and cancer has become one of the most controversial—and emotional. It has continued for nearly a quarter century, though reports of cancer clusters related to electro-magnetic fields have declined somewhat in recent years.

EMFS AND THE LONG ISLAND BREAST CANCER STUDY

On Long Island, where the breast cancer rate exceeds the national average, activists and scientists questioned whether exposure to EMFs could explain the elevated rate at which the cancer was occurring. For years, women living in Long Island's affluent suburbs were puzzled about why they were at greater risk for breast cancer than women elsewhere. (Similar patterns of elevated risk had been reported in other affluent suburbs, particularly those in the San Francisco area, in Connecticut, and near Chicago).

Scientists at the National Cancer Institute and the State University of New York at Stony Brook also questioned whether EMFs were at the root of the cancers. They began an investigation, one of several, exploring possible environmental links to breast cancer on Long Island. The EMF study involved 576 women who had been newly diagnosed with breast cancer between August 1, 1996, and June 20, 1997. Scientists compared the confirmed cases with 585 "controls," women who did not have the disease.[5]

The research project took scientists into the homes of all of the women. Participants were asked, for example, where in their homes they spent the most time, how long they slept at night, and how close their beds were to electrical wiring behind the walls. Electrical current was measured in the homes. No stone was left unturned in efforts to explore the smallest details involving possible EMF over-exposure.

Questioning was extensive because scientists had hypothesized that exposure to extremely low-frequency magnetic fields—but not electric ones—may increase breast cancer risk by affecting melatonin production. Magnetic fields were considered to be of greater concern because magnetic energy cannot be easily blocked. Electrical-field energy, on the other hand, can be.

Melatonin is a hormone produced by the pineal gland, located at the base of the brain, during darkness, such as at night, while you sleep. Melatonin, as it turns out, also has a "light-switch" relationship with estrogen. In darkness, when melatonin is flowing, it switches off estrogen. Melatonin is believed to be at its peak between 2:00 A.M. and 4:00 A.M. Scientists further hypothesized that exposure to light well into the night could increase breast cancer risk because estrogen flow would not be extinguished.

To the surprise of study participants and the scientists who conducted the study, results, which were finalized in 2002, showed no difference in the EMF exposure of women who had breast cancer and those who did not. Therefore scientists had to conclude that EMFs were not an underlying cause of the unusually high number of breast cancer cases on Long Island. Scientists instead pointed to the usual suspects: age (because breast cancer risk increases with age), family and personal history of the disease, and other demographics.

Cancer Clusters: Common or Rare?

Generally, doctors and scientists take a cautious view of reports about cancer clusters, an attitude sometimes viewed as dismissive in communities where clusters are being reported. On the whole, reports of true clusters are rare, but they have been found, sometimes in industries where an unsuspected carcinogen leads to a rare form of cancer among workers.

Does the guarded attitude scientists take toward reports of clusters mean they don't believe clustering exists? No. Both the National Cancer Institute and the Centers for Disease Control and Prevention are very interested in looking into reports that carry strong evidence of clustering, especially when something inexplicable appears to be involved, such as a large number of rare cancers.

Here are some of the National Cancer Institute's key points on cancer clusters:

❖ Cancer clusters may be suspected when people report that several family members, friends, neighbors, or coworkers have been diagnosed with the same or related cancers.

❖ Some amount of clustering may occur simply by chance.

❖ Epidemiologists (scientists who study the frequency, distribution, causes, and control of diseases in populations) investigate suspected clusters [for government agencies such as the NCI and CDC].

❖ Concerned individuals [should] report a suspected cancer cluster to their local health department or state cancer registry.[6]

Central to an investigation of possible clustering, experts at the NCI say, is determining whether the cancers being reported as part of a cluster are primary (original cancers) or ones that have spread from another organ. This is important because epidemiologists consider only primary cancers (such as the newly diagnosed breast cancer cases on Long Island) when they investigate a possible cluster.

❧ ❧ ❧

Finally, many people have long suspected environmental links to breast cancer. And even though reports of clusters and studies like the EMF research on Long Island have failed to turn up positive clues, that doesn't mean researchers have abandoned all efforts. Science sometimes proceeds down dozens of blind alleys before that one tantalizing piece of evidence surfaces to prove an association.

Sleuthing for environmental links to any common form of cancer has its difficulties. Many of the risk factors are already known and may very well explain what appears to be clustered cases of the disease. With respect to the Long Island cases, scientists ultimately attributed them to several well known risks, such as age and personal history. Also, attempting to track down new, provable risk factors linked to an environmental cause can take many years—possibly a decade or longer. This kind of science can cost millions and involve thousands of people volunteering to be tested. The conclusion to Chapter 6 briefly discusses a research project, the Sister Study, that will take the extended time necessary to search for such clues. It is a major scientific effort that asks a simple question: whether there are unique environmental links to breast cancer.

Chapter 4

Types of Breast Cancer

Women who have had breast cancer comprise the largest
proportion of cancer survivors in the United States.

— *American Society of Clinical Oncology*

Rule number one when writing a book: Don't be repetitious—don't
continue to mention the same fact or facts until your readers feel as
if they're being beaten by them. But while it has been mentioned
earlier, it probably is worth saying again: Breast cancer is an extraordinarily complex disease—so complex that countless scientific questions about it remain to be answered. Indeed, the term "breast
cancer" is merely a general description for a variety of malignant
conditions that can arise in the breast.

Your doctors may refer to your cancer as ductal carcinoma in
situ. This type of lesion generally is not palpable; typically only a
mammogram is powerful enough to bring it into view. You may have
been told that you have an infiltrating ductal carcinoma, an infiltrating lobular carcinoma, or any one of the rare forms: inflammatory breast cancer, cystosarcoma phylloides, or Paget's disease.

Details about the tumor are contained in your pathology report,
the document produced after pathologists finish studying your
biopsy specimens. You may get one pathology report or you may get
two—maybe even three. The others are usually based on additional

89

laboratory testing, especially after surgery, when the tumor is sent to pathologists for further study. Even if you receive multiple reports, consider them episodes of a larger story. The first one, of course, sets in motion the type of care you'll receive.

This chapter is aimed at examining the breast in health and disease, and at exploring the dynamics of cancer. A stronger grasp on both will help lay a better foundation for understanding your pathology findings. Late in the chapter, the pros and cons of second opinions are also explored. You may be among those skeptical patients who want to know if the doctors at your hospital have gotten the diagnosis right.

When You First Receive Your Pathology Report

You will probably embrace one of two frames of mind with respect to your pathology report: Either you will want to know the details or you won't—at least not right away. But there will be no escaping it, no hiding your head in the sand. That's because when your physician tells you of your diagnosis and your need for surgery, the basis for her or his explanation is drawn from the details contained in the pathology report.

Activists for those with breast cancer say there is an undeniable trend, signified by the growing number of the newly diagnosed who want to know as much as possible about the challenges they are facing. They want medical facts and working knowledge of what essentially amounts to human anatomy and molecular biology. For instance, officials at the Chicago headquarters of the Y-Me National Breast Cancer Organization have noticed that callers phoning its hotline are largely from the ranks of the newly diagnosed, and many of these people are calling to ask why they're facing certain therapies based on the complex findings from their tissue samples. Many are phoning with tough, technical questions.

Patients want to know about the importance of tumor margins; they want to know what it means to be estrogen-receptor positive (or negative). They inquire about the significance of the HER-2 oncogene. Basically, they want a fuller understanding of the information contained within their pathology reports.

Bev Parker, director of information services at Y-Me, has found that the tendency to seek a fuller understanding of breast cancer and the technical aspects of the condition is very helpful to many of the newly diagnosed. The organization has put together a replica of a pathology report on its website, to better aid patients in understanding the complex language and the types of information doctors seek in a biopsy.

Volunteers who answer calls at Y-Me are trained to give definitions and add context to the physicians' explanations, but not to offer medical advice. Bev counts herself among the hotline's earliest callers. She was a newly diagnosed breast cancer patient two decades ago when she phoned to get a better grasp of what her doctors had told her. She made the call long before she ever sought employment at Y-Me.

> The initial diagnosis is the real shocker. I am one who wants to know as much as I can even though I know breast cancer can't be prevented and can't always be cured. To me, it is empowering to know as much as possible. It was nineteen years ago that I called the hotline after I was diagnosed, and I have always regretted not getting the name of the volunteer I talked to.
>
> There are a lot of people who are like me. They say they never expected to get breast cancer, and when they were diagnosed they felt they needed an advanced degree to understand what they had. That's why so many women these days start surfing the Internet.
>
> Breast cancer is very complicated. It's not a simple illness. It's not, like, oh, I've got the flu. But not everyone is eager to learn about it right after they've been diagnosed. And for some people it's not a good time to learn things when they're worried. So there is this balance that most people have to reach.

Bev's predecessor at Y-Me, Judy Perotti, who authored some of the organization's literature on breast cancer, says the urge to seek a better understanding of the pathology report is part of a trend that has been growing for many years. She continues, "I say this with the caveat that not everyone wants to have a very detailed level of understanding; some women really just don't want to know. But we've recognized for some time that women, for the most part, are not passively accepting things. They really want to know about the details of breast cancer and what their options are, and what they themselves can do. While many health professionals take the time to discuss the details of their patients' pathology reports, studies also show that cancer patients absorb only a fraction of what is told to them at the time of diagnosis."

Dr. Lamar McGinnis, a past president of the American Cancer Society, remarked during a national news briefing on cancer that patients need methods to reinforce what their doctors have told them. The cancer society responded to that need by publishing treatment guidelines in English and Spanish for more than a dozen forms of cancer. According to Dr. McGinnis, when a patient is being told of a cancer diagnosis in a one-on-one meeting with a health-care provider, the patient retains only 20 percent of the information conveyed. With a family member present, he says, the retention rate reaches 50 percent. Learning about cancer is such a paralyzing event for patients and their families that few explanations register.

Some patients I interviewed remarked that the pathology report would have been simpler to understand had they possessed more knowledge about their own anatomy or had a better handle on the terminology their doctors used.

Linda G., forty-nine, says she absorbed fairly well the main points of the discussion with her physician. The big point, of course, was a diagnosis of breast cancer. Developing an understanding of the pathology report's finer details could come later.

> I just needed a little time for it to register. I mean really register. I needed some time for it to sink in. I talked to my doctor, talked to the nurse. Then a couple of weeks later I called the National Cancer Institute. There's a call-in line; the number was on the back of one of the brochures the nurse gave me. People at the NCI answer questions, and I wanted to get a

better sense of what the term *estrogen-receptor positive* meant.

Rosalyn W., who was diagnosed in 2001, says she wished she had paid more attention during high school biology, even though she attended high school in the 1960s:

> Staying awake would have helped. I vaguely remember the teacher spending time on anatomy. I remember dissecting frogs. That was a long time ago; it's hard to remember back that far. The only word that really stuck at the time my doctor was explaining it was *invasive*. I didn't need a medical dictionary for that. *Invasive* was the thing that hit like a ton of bricks.
>
> I didn't have any trouble with the word *carcinoma,* either. That's why we were all gathered in the oncology department. I called a friend of mine from work who went through her own breast cancer ordeal. She helped a lot, and I'll always be grateful. I just wanted to know what to expect.

Lee N., fifty-seven, says she went home and started searching for information on the Internet. She also bought a book with illustrations.

> I bought *Dr. Susan Love's Breast Book*. I kept it by my bed, took it to appointments, read it on the train, read it when I was getting chemo, read it just to read it. It's dog-eared and dirty. It was dry reading but really helped fill in the blanks.

Physiology of the Healthy Breast

To get a sense of what happens when the diagnosis is cancer, it may be a good idea to first understand a few facts about the physiology of the healthy breast. Certain internal structures are more likely to be targets of the disease than others. Some cancers begin in the breast's milk ducts; some begin in the lobules (see below for explanations of these terms). Still other forms of the cancer invade the nipple and areola (the area of darker skin encircling the nipple). A devastating form of the disease courses through the lymphatic system, causing redness, warmth, and swelling. Many benign breast conditions have early symptoms similar to those of cancer, usually a palpable lump, which can show up as a suspicious spot on a mammogram or produce inflammation, pain, warmth, and swelling, all the results of an infection (see Figure 2 below and the legend on the facing page).

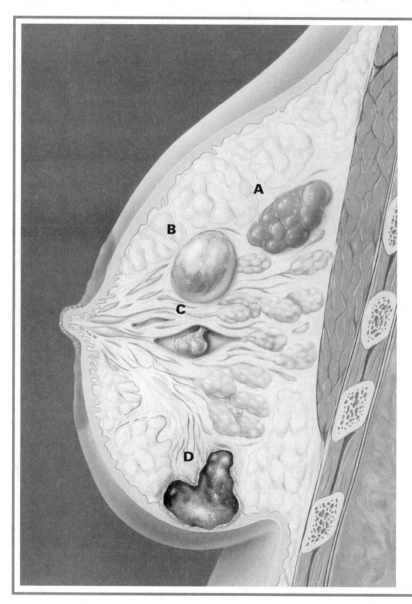

On the inside, a breast is an intricate network. The lobules are the milk-producing glands that connect to the branches of ducts through which milk flows. The ducts narrow to an end point in the nipple. These interdependent units comprise the milk-producing

---

Figure 2. Diseases of the breast. *Pictured from top down are four different kinds of masses that can develop in the breast. All are located under the breast's insulating fat tissue and in the ductal system.*

First and uppermost mass [A]: *Invasive ductal carcinoma, which is shown developing near the chest wall. When felt as a lump it is hard, unyielding, and notable for its irregular surface. Some patients say their lumps have a coarse or gravelly feel. Doctors always order a biopsy of masses that are felt. Occasionally, malignant tumors can have a smooth border, so it is vital to proceed through all diagnostic steps. Invasive ductal carcinomas are the most common form of breast cancer.*

Second mass [B]: *An oval-shaped fibroadenoma, which is generally felt as a smooth, firm lump. Fibroadenomas are benign and can grow to be fairly large. They are commonly diagnosed in young women. Doctors often can quickly distinguish between a malignant tumor and a fibroadenoma simply by feeling the mass because unlike a malignant tumor, a fibroadenoma moves around easily in breast tissue. These masses are also easily distinguished from breast cysts during a needle biopsy because cysts, which are also moveable, produce fluid in the needle whereas fibroadenomas do not. Fibroadenomas are removed surgically.*

Third mass [C]: *Intraductal papilloma, a benign, wartlike lump that often grows behind the areola (the darker area of skin around the nipple). Some women become aware of the mass when there is a sticky but clear discharge. In some cases the discharge is tinged with blood. For some women the growths develop in both breasts. Intraductal papillomas are removed surgically.*

Fourth mass [D]: *A breast abcess, which can become pus-filled as the body tries to destroy invading microbes. Such infections can involve the ducts and deeper breast tissue and cause tenderness in the lymph nodes under the arm. Both the breast and chest can become inflamed and painful. Abcesses can occur when bacteria enter through the nipple, especially if it is chafed during breast feeding. The masses can grow to be fairly large and involve large areas of breast tissue. Antibiotics are prescribed; surgery is rare but is sometimes needed to drain the abcess.*

(Credit: John Bavosi / Photo Researchers, Inc.)

system, the bulk of which is made up of ducts. Other important structures include ligaments and muscles.

The innermost network of glands and ducts is insulated in a protective layer of fat, and the entire structure is aided by a copious blood supply via the internal mammary arteries. Additionally, lymphatic vessels run through each breast, connecting to lymph nodes, small, oval-shaped structures. Lymph nodes filter infectious bacteria and cancer cells that flow into the lymphatic system, making them a major component of the body's disease-fighting immune system. There are lymph nodes in the armpits—the axillary lymph nodes—as well as some near the breastbone and others above the collarbone, the supraclavicular nodes. Breast tissue, anatomists have discovered, is widespread, extending throughout the chest wall.

Immortal Cells

Cancers, in general, are made up of various kinds of aberrant cells that have lost all ability to abide by nature's rules. These cells are hell-bent on being out of control. They misbehave because they are driven by miscues from their DNA—that is, genetic instructions that are scripted in garbled codes. Even under the general term *breast cancer* there are wide varieties of genetic mechanisms promoting the growth of cancer cells that, in turn, affect the course of the disease.

Yet for all of their differences in origin, growth rates, and prognosis, cancers—no matter where in the body they originate—have something in common: All cancers come from cells that once were normal. Once they've been transformed by irreversible assaults to their DNA, these cells can no longer go through an ordinary life cycle and die. They are by their very nature "immortalized"; they possess the capability, under certain laboratory conditions, to live forever.

The rate at which cancer cells divide is known as their doubling time—that is, how long a single cell takes to divide into two cells, resulting in a doubling of the number of cells that make up the tumor. Doubling time differs from one cancer to another. A fast-growing cancer can double its number of cells within a week to four weeks. A slow-growing cancer may take as long as six months to double.

The doubling time never stops. Two cells become four, four become eight, eight become sixteen, sixteen cells double to thirty-two, and so on. The doubling process continues until, after a period of many months or years, the aberrant cells form what is detected as a lump—technically called a tumor, a malignancy, or a lesion. All these terms are interchangeable, and they all mean cancer. The range in doubling times for various forms of breast cancer can be anywhere from 23 to 209 days.

Once a tumor reaches about one centimeter in diameter (about half an inch) and can be seen easily on an X ray, it may have proceeded through thirty doubling times and contain about a billion cells. The typical breast cancer that is imaged through mammography at this stage has been growing for eight to ten years.

Tumor biologists Cornelis Van Noorden, Linda Meade-Tollin, and Fred Bosman, writing in *The American Scientist*, report that cancers lack "the strictly controlled system of 'checks and balances' that govern the activities of normal cells." As a result, the bizarre mass of cells known as a tumor can have a profound impact on a patient's life. They write, "A diagnosis of cancer marks an abrupt change in the life of the patient. Yet the events that lead a cell to become cancerous take place gradually, sometimes over periods that can take ten years. During this lengthy evolution, cells undergoing cancerous transformation accumulate genetic abnormalities, one important consequence of which is that cellular growth becomes deregulated."[1]

These biologists also say it is not the primary tumor that makes

> ## What Is Cancer?
>
> The term *cancer* refers to many malignant conditions—more than two hundred distinct disorders altogether, each deriving its name from the organ or tissue in which it originates. Breast cancer originates in breast tissue. If it metastasizes—spreads to other parts of the body—it is still breast cancer even though the malignant cells now are found in the spine, liver, or lungs. The cells retain a distinct signature that lets pathologists know the source of the disease. When breast cancer establishes itself in distant sites, it then is known as metastatic breast cancer.

a cancer dangerous, but whether the primary tumor bears a strong likelihood of spread. All cancers are not equal. Some have greater potential for spread than others. The word *metastasis* refers to the migration of a cancer from one region of the body to another. Why cancer cells possess such wanderlust remains one of the deepest mysteries of tumor biology. It is an issue with which biologists continue to struggle. No one knows exactly why tumor cells stray.

But just as doubling times differ from one cancer to another, so does the potential for metastasis. Even within specific types of cancer, such as breast cancer, some tumors, by virtue of their genetic makeup, have a greater propensity toward metastasis than others.

The various genetic subtleties pathologists look for in tissue samples, which can reveal a cancer's potential for spread, will be discussed later in this chapter. Metastasis is the very activity cancer specialists hope to prevent by treating a malignancy early, quickly, and thoroughly. Yet for you to fully grasp the fact that cancers differ from one another in many ways, it is important to also understand, at least on a very basic level, *how* they differ. Any form of cancer, be it breast, kidney, colon, lung, or pancreatic, is grouped into broad categories that primarily define the tissue type. Cancers known as *sarcomas* originate in the muscles, bones, nerves, and tendons. Cancers known as *carcinomas* arise in what is known as the epithelium, tissues that cover or line internal organs, particularly tissues involved in secretion. Breast cancers, for the most part, are carcinomas. Breast tissue secretes milk.

Types of Breast Cancer (and Related Breast Abnormalities)

Of the 211,000 cases of breast cancer diagnosed annually in the United States, more than 80 percent are tumors that originate in the milk ducts. These are known as *ductal carcinomas*. The majority of these cancers are invasive, meaning they have broken through the membrane of the duct and have infiltrated the surrounding breast tissue. For most women with a positive diagnosis this is what doctors usually refer to when they say you have breast cancer. A lesser percentage of breast cancers develop in the lobules (milk-producing glands); accordingly, they are known as *lobular carcinomas*.

Breast cancer manifests in a variety of cell patterns, which will be duly noted when applicable on your pathology report. The names of these patterns come from the way tumor cells appear under a microscope. There may or may not be a predominance of any single type, and the tumor might very well be made up of a mix of cell patterns. Some cancers are composed of cells that are shaped like tubes and are therefore called *tubular*. Others tumor cell types include *medullary*, which derives its name from the fact the cells have a coloration similar to that of the brain's medulla. *Mucinous* cell types are so defined because they secrete mucus. *Papillary* is another type; its name derives from an appearance of little daisy-petal-like protrusions seen in milk ducts. Smaller papillary tumor cells are called *micropapillary*. For the most part these patterns are seen as variants in ductal carcinomas.

In this section all of the various forms of breast cancer are described, beginning with ductal carcinoma in situ (DCIS), a lesion that has not broken through the duct. (The term *in situ*—pronounced *in SYE-tew*—means "in place.") DCIS has been brought increasingly into medical prominence over the past two decades because of screening mammography. These abnormalities are often far too small to feel as lumps. What would seem to be the lobular counterpart to DCIS, lobular carcinoma in situ, or LCIS, turns out not to be cancer at all but a possible harbinger of cancer—cells marked by irregular growth patterns. Although these cells are not cancerous, they have the potential to transform into malignant ones.

In addition to the in situ conditions, invasive cancers—both ductal and lobular—are explored in this section. Next comes a section on rare tumors, and after that are sections on understanding the pathology report and on how breast cancer is staged.

DUCTAL CARCINOMA IN SITU

DCIS lesions are so stealthy they can exist for decades without your having the slightest clue that something may be amiss. They are also controversial because some are capable of evolving into full-blown invasive cancers while others are not. At the moment, doctors cannot distinguish between the two, so all cases of DCIS are treated as if they have the potential to invade. (See the sidebar "DCIS Indecision" for more about this.) It is important to note that the term *invasive* means breaking through the duct and invading surrounding healthy tissue. The word *invasive* is not synonymous with *metastasis*, which means spreading to another site in the body.

The vast majority of DCIS lesions are brought into view through mammography because of their small size. Others can be felt as a lump because they may reach about 1.5 centimeters or more, but remain inside the duct. Since the advent of mammography the number of DCIS diagnoses has skyrocketed.

The American Cancer Society estimates that roughly fifty thousand cases of DCIS are diagnosed annually. Before the widespread use of mammography, doctors diagnosed fewer than five thousand a year. DCIS lesions are composed of malignant cells. Some are called *DCIS-MI* (DCIS with microinvasion) because of the sprinkling of malignant cells in the margin of healthy tissue surrounding the affected duct.

DCIS Indecision

Dr. Judah Folkman, a Harvard theoretician who first postulated that cancers spread by creating a blood supply for themselves (a process called angiogenesis), has addressed one of the more enduring mysteries about DCIS. Speaking at a meeting of the American Association for Cancer Research, he noted that in a series of autopsies on elderly women who had died of causes other than breast cancer, a large proportion had DCIS lesions. In some cases, the lesions had been present for many years, some possibly as long as forty years. Dr. Folkman was intrigued because these lesions never erupted into invasive cancers. Instead, they remained inactive for decades. What this suggests, he said, is that a significant number of women develop DCIS that never becomes invasive. Why this is true remains puzzling to researchers such as Folkman. More important still, he said, is developing a way to distinguish between lesions that can become invasive and those that will remain harmless throughout much of a woman's life.[2]

Even though DCIS has been studied extensively in recent years, these lesions remain profoundly mystifying because there is still so much about them that doctors and cancer researchers do not know. Among their questions is whether DCIS is a single entity or part of a spectrum of malignancies that can affect a duct.

Clearly, some DCIS tumors come equipped with the genetic ability to break through healthy tissue, while others have no way of ever acquiring those genes. Definitive research in this area ultimately could affect who receives aggressive treatment and who does not. Change has already begun to surface, because even the vocabulary once used to categorize DCIS abnormalities is fast becoming obsolete. For years, pathologists divided DCIS into "comedo" and "noncomedo" types. Doctors thought these two terms, which referred to the way DCIS appeared under a microscope, gave them some power of prediction over a lesion's fate, letting them know which ones might advance to invasive disease.

Comedo refers to the bunching of so many malignant cells in a duct that those in the center can no longer survive. Doctors once thought comedo cell types were more likely to lead to invasive ductal cancer. *Noncomedo* refers to cancer cells that do not completely fill the duct. In fact, DCIS cells are usually of the papillary and micropapillary configuration that do completely fill the duct. So researchers are certain of one major point—that the potential invasiveness of DCIS cannot be easily diagnosed. Those of the noncomedo type have led to invasive disease as well as recurrences. (Remember that the term *invasive disease* refers to breast cancer that breaks through the wall of a duct.)

Cancer specialists such as Dr. Beryl McCormick, a radiation oncologist at Memorial Sloan-Kettering Cancer Center who has treated hundreds of patients with DCIS, says the terms *comedo* and *noncomedo* are used less frequently nowadays because of newer scientific information that is advancing the general understanding of DCIS.

DCIS is found in both pre- and postmenopausal women, Dr. McCormick says, and the lesions are often accompanied by tiny calcifications within breast tissue. The calcifications—micro calcifications as they are often called—are literally bits of calcium that show up as fine white flecks on a mammogram.

Dr. Frank Vicini, a radiation oncologist and professor of medicine at William Beaumont Hospital in Glen Oak, Michigan, says that contrary to popular belief, DCIS is not a precancer. Some well-respected books about breast cancer aimed at lay readers often refer to these lesions as precancers. This gives the impression that DCIS is not to be taken as seriously as other forms of breast cancer.

One of the key issues involving these lesions, Dr. Vicini emphasizes, is the lack of scientific ability to distinguish between the kind of DCIS that will remain quietly within a duct for decades and the type that will become invasive. Many more years of study are needed before those facts become known. "A DCIS is also called intraductal carcinoma of the breast," Dr. Vicini says. "It is not a precancer. It is cancer. The controversy is whether or not it is preinvasive. This means whether or not it will become an invasive breast cancer, which has the capacity to spread if left untreated. DCIS does not by itself have the ability to spread [to distant organs] even though it is cancer. That is the distinction made between the typical invasive ductal carcinoma and DCIS, a noninvasive carcinoma."

But even though DCIS does not spread to distant sites, these lesions have been known to recur in women who have undergone lumpectomies. Researchers are studying how much healthy tissue should be removed along with the affected duct in a lumpectomy. As will be explained in greater detail in the chapter on surgery, some women treated for DCIS undergo mastectomies because of the diffuse nature of the DCIS and the microcalcifications that are found throughout the affected breast. In other words, sometimes DCIS is found in multiple sites within the breast, necessitating a mastectomy.

Doctors are predicting that within the next several years enough information will have been gathered on DCIS to determine which lesions will require aggressive treatment and which ones patients and their doctors may decide can be minimally treated. With current standard treatment—either lumpectomy and radiation; or lumpectomy, radiation, and tamoxifen (a hormonal drug therapy)—the cure rate approaches 100 percent.

Women treated for DCIS say that despite the minuscule size of the lesion, their memories remain vivid of having weathered cancer.

Sister Mary D., a nun and retired teacher, says the discovery of her breast cancer came on her birthday.

I made a practice of getting a mammogram on my birthday or as close to it as possible. That way I wouldn't forget. So this was some birthday present. The doctor told me that even though I was sixty-six, I would be able to get through this just like a woman ten or twenty years younger. I think I was most surprised the cancer they found was so small. But I got through it with flying colors.

Barbara G., a high school teacher diagnosed with DCIS in her early forties, comments that with a tumor so small it is difficult to comprehend that something as serious as cancer has taken hold.

You don't feel anything. You don't even feel sick. There's no lump, either. But they're telling you it's cancer. This is not most people's idea of what cancer is like, at least not at first, not until you get to the treatment part of it.

DCIS Doesn't Count

Here is a startling fact about DCIS: It is treated medically like any other breast cancer, but it is not counted in official breast cancer statistics. Many patients treated for DCIS find that fact shocking. What is the reason for it? Epidemiologists say this form of cancer is not tallied annually in government databases because it is noninvasive, despite evidence that an estimated fifty thousand people a year are found to have this form of breast cancer. Other noninvasive forms of cancer, such as common skin cancers, also are not tallied in government cancer-incidence statistics.

Patients who have been treated for DCIS often beg to differ with epidemiologists about this distinction because the treatment for DCIS is serious. Activists often have spoken out on the issue, saying that sorting the data so finely is unfair to the legions of patients who have the cancer. Separating the numbers, they say, implies that DCIS is not a serious cancer even though patients face surgery and a full regimen of additional treatments. Activists also complain that separating the statistics suggests that there are fewer breast cancer cases than there are in reality.

Caren C. also was diagnosed as having DCIS and was shocked when she was told she would have to undergo cancer therapy. The physician's opening remarks, she says, seemed to suggest that DCIS was not dangerous. As the physician continued her explanation, Caren found she was facing a more sobering reality.

> She didn't use the word *tumor*. She said it was preinvasive. In my mind that translated into: not cancer. You hear somebody use "pre-" and that starts your mind clicking. I'm immediately translating that into "precancerous." But she kept talking, and the more she talked the more I started getting this completely different picture. I'm saying, "Hold on. Let's back up. Let's go over this again." Then she told me I would need surgery and radiation. When she said surgery I knew there was no getting out of this the easy way.

LOBULAR CARCINOMA IN SITU

The word *carcinoma* is a frightening one to most people because it usually means cancer. In the case of lobular carcinoma in situ (LCIS) it does not. LCIS is not cancer. It is not the lobular counterpart to DCIS. It usually is found in a more diffuse pattern than DCIS; that is, it is often located in the lobules (milk-producing glands) of more than one part of the breast.

Differences between DCIS and LCIS abound. DCIS can directly lead to invasive cancer; LCIS's abnormal cell development is a marker lesion, a sign of elevated risk. Pathologists see these abnormal cells under the microscope.

There are several other differences between DCIS and LCIS. First, DCIS affects both pre- and postmenopausal women. LCIS usually is detected primarily in women who are premenopausal. Second, LCIS is usually found incidentally, most often during a biopsy for other types of breast abnormalities. It is not always imaged well on mammograms; however, the increasing use of mammography has helped bring more cases to the attention of doctors. DCIS, on the other hand, can be readily detected through mammography. Third, if LCIS is found in the right breast, then chances are likely it will also be found in the left. And while some experts now refer to LCIS as lobular neoplasia, a definition that more strongly suggests its cancerous potential, the statistics have not changed in terms of the percentage of women who ultimately develop the disease.

The good news is that a majority of women diagnosed with LCIS never go on to develop invasive breast cancer. Upon discovering a case of LCIS, doctors usually recommend close monitoring of the patient through periodic checkups. In some cases, preventive therapy with a hormone-based drug is prescribed.

Dr. Lisa Newman, of the University of Michigan, says that quieting patients' alarm is the first task when LCIS is discovered. Equally important is getting them to understand that it is a marker lesion, not preinvasive cancer.

INVASIVE DUCTAL CARCINOMA

Whether your doctor calls it invasive or infiltrating, a cancer that has broken through the duct and entered the surrounding tissue is the kind likely to be associated with the most dreaded of symptoms: a lump. Invasive ductal carcinomas account for 80 percent to 85 percent of all breast cancers (see Figure 3).

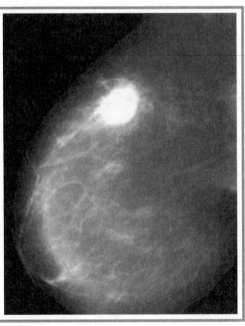

Figure 3. *Mammogram of a large invasive ductal carcinoma in a 73 year-old woman. The cancer has invaded surrounding breast tissue and is seen developing close to the breast's surface.*
(Credit: Photo courtesy of Southern Illinois University / Photo Researchers, Inc.)

An interesting fact about lumps is that as a cancer proceeds through its doubling times, increasing in size, the body produces fibrous scar tissue around it. Even though the tumor is growing, it is smaller than the lump that is felt. The encircling mass of scar tissue helps doctors better spot the location on a mammogram. What can be palpated by touch generally is reported by both doctors and patients to be a "hard" and "unmoveable" mass that feels "anchored in its place." In Chapter 1 Lynne J. described her lump as feeling "gravelly," a term many women have used.

Gayle-Marie A. says even though she initially ignored the lump and did not seek medical attention for many months, she could not completely escape its hard, unyielding presence.

> Cancer never crossed my mind, even with all of the things I've heard about lumps and mammograms and early detection and all of that. I might have noticed it when I was nursing the baby, but I really can't say for sure. If I noticed it then, I'd have to say it really wouldn't have struck me as unusual. I only really noticed it after I had gotten him on a bottle. That's when I thought it was some kind of holdover from nursing. I would notice it when I'd get dressed or undressed; I'd notice it when I was taking a shower. I can't say that it felt like it was getting bigger. It was just there. Cancer just never crossed my mind. And no, I didn't mention it to my gynecologist. But I would say to myself, "Why doesn't it just shrink like everything else and go away?"

Invasive ductal carcinomas affect both pre- and postmenopausal women. Again, just because a tumor is called invasive doesn't mean it has spread to distant sites in the body. Invasive breast cancer can refer to the tumor having infiltrated surrounding tissue and to the cancer's migration into nearby lymph nodes.

Having a tumor that has already migrated to the lymph nodes (a condition known as regional spread) does not mean your disease cannot be brought under control. Lynne J. recounts her bout with breast cancer right after she reached menopause.

> My oncologist told me that I had a mixed bag of risk factors. I had been looking at everything as black and white, good or bad, live or die. He didn't make light of the fact that I had four lymph nodes positive—a fact I'd been despairing about—but

he put that in perspective. He said, "You have positive lymph nodes, which isn't so good. You have more than one or two. However, four is still a relatively low number. You have a relatively small tumor." (Two centimeters—it sounded huge to me.) "You have positive hormone receptivity, which is a good thing to have since it gives you more treatment options. However, it's borderline positive, not strongly positive. The aggressiveness of your tumor is pretty low." He then told me his recommendation for treatment based on the combination of those factors. Mastectomy seemed worse than the cancer.

Sometimes a ductal tumor develops so deeply within breast tissue it cannot be easily palpated. The first alert to its presence may come as the result of a routine mammogram. There also may be other symptoms. For instance, a tumor might cause the retraction of the nipple or it may cause a nipple discharge. In Lynne's case, the tumor caused the nipple to "point off center," as she explained it. There is also a possibility the cancer can cause the breast to appear dimpled. Invasive ductal cancers will be discussed further in the chapter on surgery.

INVASIVE LOBULAR CARCINOMA

One of the most difficult and unsettling breast cancer diagnoses is that of invasive—also called infiltrating—lobular carcinoma. It does not make its presence known by way of a solid lump but rather spreads through the lobules as masses of malignant cells. Unfortunately, there is a strong possibility of this type of cancer existing in both breasts at once. Such is not always the case, but when the cancer is found on one side, chances of it being on the other side are fairly high. When cancer is found in both breasts it is said to have occurred bilaterally.

Doctors cannot overemphasize the difficulties involved with this form of breast cancer. Infiltrating lobular carcinoma cannot always be detected early, and its diffuse nature makes it difficult to image on a mammogram. It also is not a form of breast cancer that women think of—or for that matter have even heard of—unless they have strong reasons for a higher than usual degree of suspicion.

Perhaps a close relative had the cancer and you know about it that way, or maybe you had it in the past.

On the whole, this form of breast cancer has not garnered much of the spotlight in the popular media. The media tend to focus only on the generic disease popularly called "breast cancer," as if it were a single condition linked to a simple set of controllable risk factors. Invasive lobular carcinoma accounts for an estimated 10 percent to 15 percent of all invasive breast cancers that occur annually in the United States.

In addition to the differences already mentioned between invasive lobular carcinoma and invasive ductal carcinoma, you may want to note yet another. Along with invasive lobular carcinoma's tendency to spread through the lobules is its other tendency to cause abnormal thickenings in these structures. Teams of scientists in the United States and abroad are studying this form of breast cancer, and high on the list is developing more effective methods of detecting it.

Dianne B., who has been coping with metastatic breast cancer, says the discovery of invasive bilateral lobular cancer is difficult news to handle. When she was told she had this form of breast cancer, she describes her reaction as one of feeling dazed for what seemed like weeks.

> It feels like walking under water. I had had a lot of problems since I was a teenager. Lumpy breasts, painful breasts, a whole lot of things. I also had very small breasts, so I got implants to—how should I put it—to improve my profile. That's when I was twenty-eight. I got them out when I was thirty-three because I was having a lot of problems with them. They found the cancer when I was thirty-seven. I think it wouldn't have been so hard to take if it was just one tumor in one breast. But this kind of cancer is very ornery in how it affects you. It creeps everywhere, through both breasts and under your arms. It was in my lymph nodes, too.

There was no evidence that Dianne's implants led to her cancer, something her doctors have told her. But it is a possibility that often makes her wonder.

When pathologists examine tissue specimens from patients with invasive lobular carcinoma, they are essentially asking the same kinds of scientific questions they ask with invasive ductal carcinoma. Are the cells aggressive? Are lymph nodes affected? What is the hormone status?

When patients are diagnosed with estrogen-positive invasive lobular cancers they, like their counterparts with estrogen-positive invasive ductal carcinoma, have more treatment options. Specifically, they have the option of taking hormone-based drugs.

Rare Forms of Breast Cancer

The trouble with some rare forms of breast cancer is that they can mimic noncancerous conditions. Inflammatory breast cancer, which is difficult to diagnose in many women who develop it, sometimes is mistaken for a breast infection. Paget's disease, another rare form of breast cancer that affects the nipple and areola, causes itchiness and scaling that is akin to dermatitis, a fairly common skin disorder. Having any of the rare forms of breast cancer, some survivors say, can be an especially isolating experience. It is not easy finding others who are similarly affected and who share your very special concerns.

INFLAMMATORY BREAST CANCER

The sad and frightening story of inflammatory breast cancer is that it is often detected only after it has advanced. While this form of breast cancer affects just 1 percent to 4 percent of women with breast cancer in the United States, doctors find it particularly worrisome.

Because the disease initially can be mistaken for something other than cancer, time is lost from the point of discovery to that of diagnosis. One far less dangerous condition for which it can be mistaken is mastitis, an infection of the breast. An obvious symptom of inflammatory breast cancer is a reddening or a deeper discoloration on the chest, depending on your complexion. A similar reddening is a primary symptom of mastitis. Doctors now know that the reddening associated with inflammatory breast cancer is not a result of inflammation but is caused by the spread of cancer cells through the lymphatic system just below the surface of the skin.

Inflammatory breast cancer causes the skin to take on what is sometimes called a *peau d'orange* (orange peel) appearance. A dramatic swelling of the breast is another important symptom. In some cases there may be itchiness along with the other symptoms, giving this form of breast cancer a series of hallmarks that are very much unlike those associated with other forms of the disease. As is the case with invasive lobular carcinoma, inflammatory breast cancer is another cancer for which mammography is not very useful. As a result, the road to diagnosis can be fraught with frustration.

In many instances, the metastatic disease in the bones, liver, or elsewhere in the body is diagnosed first. In young women, doctors may not initially think in terms of cancer when they encounter these symptoms. Their suspicions, at least at first, may be something far less life threatening. When a woman in her thirties complains of pain in a joint, as was Pat G.'s case, the doctor may first want to rule out all other causes of the discomfort—many in keeping with the activities of young women—such as strain caused by jogging or other forms of vigorous exercise.

For some women, doctors have to perform very rapid investigations to track down the source of the symptoms. Such was the case for Pat G., a mother of a child in elementary school. After an initial misdiagnosis, Pat's life was defined by a series of aggressive treatment regimens. One of her most ardent hopes is that primary care doctors will learn more about inflammatory breast cancer in order to suspect it. She also thinks it's vital that patients with this form of breast cancer seek each other out and correspond with one another.

> This is the most difficult kind of breast cancer to diagnose and treat. And because it's so rare, you don't meet many other women like yourself. It is important to compare notes and help each other get through this. It has been a roller coaster for me. But I'm a fighter. I guess that's why somebody up there gave me the worst form of breast cancer. I think they gave it to me so I can fight it. A lot of people probably would have given up by now—but not me.

For some patients with inflammatory breast cancer, finding an effective treatment can prove to be nearly as frustrating as the initial difficulties proved in getting the right diagnosis. The first physician Pat saw thought she had a minor orthopedic problem. The second one quickly recognized her symptoms as inflammatory breast cancer and realized the strong possibility that the disease had already spread to her bones. As far as treatment is concerned for anyone with this form of breast cancer, mastectomy is not an initial option because of the pervasive nature of cancer cells throughout the chest wall. Usually the first line of treatment is chemotherapy. Survival rates are improving for inflammatory breast cancer as doctors try a variety of medications and drug combinations.

PAGET'S DISEASE

This very rare form of breast cancer makes itself known by symptoms on the outside of the breast, usually affecting the nipple and areola. In some women it can cause itching and scaling, and can be mistaken for eczema.

CYSTOSARCOMA PHYLLOIDES

Seen most often in women under age fifty, this form of breast cancer makes itself known by way of a lump that can grow to significant size. It is not a carcinoma; it falls into the category of cancers called sarcomas. Until biopsy, it may be mistaken for a fibroadenoma, a benign condition. Some doctors say this tumor only technically meets the definition of breast cancer.

BREAST CANCER IN MEN

Male breast cancer is very rare, accounting for less than 1 percent of all breast cancers and less than 1 percent of all malignancies that affect men. Breast cancer in a man poses a special set of emotional and psychological issues, making many feel especially isolated. Having cancer certainly is a tremendous burden. Having a form of cancer for which no other member of your gender can be found in support groups, or in much of the literature about the disease, might make it even more difficult to handle.

Tumors of the breast manifest in men just as they do in women, usually signaling their presence with the development of a lump. Unfortunately, breast cancer is often discovered at a much later stage in men than it is in women. As mentioned in Chapter 1, this time lag is due to several factors. Men do not regularly examine their breasts as women are encouraged to do monthly. Nor do men undergo mammography during their annual physicals.

Understanding the Pathology Report

If the only notation on your pathology report were the type of breast cancer affecting you, then the document would be fairly easy to understand. But having undergone a biopsy for breast cancer, you're well aware that your doctors wanted a long list of questions answered. A pathologist—a medical doctor trained in the study of diseases at the tissue, cellular, and genetic levels—subjects samples of tissue to highly sophisticated tests and can tell fairly quickly whether malignant cells are present.

Your specimens are processed in a variety of ways, and information is gathered both pre- and postsurgery, which means there will be more than one report. Of course, if you would like to seek a second opinion about your diagnosis, that step is best taken immediately

---

Mystery Cancers

A rare and startling cancer phenomenon is one called an unknown primary tumor, or UPT. It occurs when runaway cancer cells establish new tumors in other organs. Many forms of cancer have been known to form a UPT. For example, breast cancer may be first discovered developing in a distant site, but there is no evidence of cancer in the breast. Doctors know they are dealing with a breast cancer when they find its cellular hallmarks elsewhere in the body. The bloodstream is the conduit to new sites.

Dr. Vincent Vinceguerra, chief of oncology at North Shore University Hospital on Long Island, says theories abound as to why the UPT phenomenon occurs. A UPT may be a stealthy tumor that reaches enough heft to metastasize, and perhaps then is destroyed by the immune system. Or the original may be so small it evades detection. Mastectomy remains the "gold standard" treatment for a UPT.

after your initial mammograms and the biopsy. How to go about seeking a second opinion will be discussed later in this chapter.

When your samples were sent to the laboratory some of the cells were stained and transferred to slides so they could be better studied under a microscope. Doctors are interested in answering numerous questions about your cells' appearance and how they compare to normal, noncancerous cells. One such question they hope to answer is the degree of "differentiation." Cells that are "differentiated" and appear most like normal ones suggest a slower-growing cancer. Those that are "undifferentiated" and appear more abnormal tend to suggest a more aggressive cancer.

Your specimens were also subjected to tests that zeroed in on the cancer-cell surface to hunt for the presence of estrogen and progesterone receptors. Hormone receptors are proteins that stipple the surface of cancer cells and essentially serve as the lock into which the hormone "key" fits. Once lock and key are united, the hormone can enter the cancer cell and rev up its growth. Fortunately, drugs exist to block the hormone from latching on to a receptor site. Patients with hormone-receptor-positive cancers—men and women—tend to have a better prognosis.

What Pathologists Seek from Your Tissue Specimens

1. *Hormone-receptor status*—When receptor proteins are present on the surface of the cancer cells, that means the cancer is estrogen-receptor positive (ER+). The same goes for progesterone (PR+). There are more treatment options for receptor-positive cancers. Tumors can also be hormone-receptor negative.

2. *Proliferation rate*—You may see this written as "S-phase fraction" or "MIB-1." This test determines the rate at which the cancer cells are growing. The slower the rate, the better the prognosis.

3. *Cell grade*—This test determines how cells appear under the microscope. The closer to normal, the better the prognosis. Tumors are graded based on this test on a scale of 1 to 3. Grade 1 has the best prognosis.

Another test to which your tissue was subjected revealed DNA activity in the core of the cancer cells by determining the size of the nucleus in those cells and the percentage of cells in the process of dividing. And a highly sophisticated "biomarker" test is conducted to search for the presence of the HER-2 oncogene, which, if present, suggests an aggressive cancer. About one-third of all breast cancers are HER-2 positive. The oncogene can spur abnormal cell growth.

As you familiarize yourself with the contents of the report, there are several key points you probably will want to grasp: How aggressive or nonaggressive is your cancer; what is its hormone status; and, most important, what kind of breast cancer do you have?

Anne S., an obstetrics nurse who developed breast cancer at fifty-one, was given a copy of her pathology report by her physician so that the two of them could peruse it together as the doctor explained the findings.

> This wasn't done because I'm a nurse and she thought I would understand it better than her other patients. She does this for everybody. Mine was DCIS [ductal carcinoma in situ], so there was no spread; the lymph nodes were clean. If it weren't for the fact we were talking cancer, I'd say everything looked great. The best thing was my doc taking the time with me. She went over the technical aspects step by step and I found this to be very helpful. I took it home and read it carefully again. Do I think this is a good idea for everybody with breast cancer? Yes and no. It wasn't too difficult for me because my case was straightforward. There was no reason to be frightened about its spreading. She kept emphasizing that. But I can imagine if it had been more advanced I probably wouldn't have been prepared to hear the technical findings at that time.

Lourdes R. was told she had a two-centimeter mass, based on findings from her pathology report. Beyond that, Lourdes' daughter Magdalena, again translating for her mother, says the oncologist wanted Lourdes to understand that breast cancer is not a death sentence.

> My mom had a doctor who spoke Spanish and he kept saying, "Don't worry so much, Mrs. R., because you have early cancer and that's very good." He said that many times. He said the lab gave her good news and he kept trying to make

my mom understand she wasn't going to die. The things the lab found meant my mom had a small cancer and she was not going to die. That's how she understood what the lab found, because he told her.

The take-home message about test results from your biopsy specimens is simple: The pathology report is a pivotal document and profoundly influences the kind of cancer care you receive. As mentioned earlier, teaching hospitals, which house some of the nation's top cancer and breast centers, are among the best institutions for your treatment. In large institutions, pathologists have the enviable position of being able to confer with several colleagues, some of whom may have published extensively in major medical journals on diagnostic aspects pertinent to your case.

A Lesson on Tumor "Staging"

When Bev Parker of Y-Me remarked earlier in the chapter that having an advanced degree seemed necessary to understand the contents of her pathology report, she was referring to the technical nature of the report's language.

> ### Additional Important Tests
>
> 1. *Margins*—After surgery, the pathologist examines the rim of tissue removed with the cancer to determine if there is a clear rim of healthy tissue or evidence of cancer surrounding the tumor and, if so, how much is in the margin.
>
> 2. *Lymph node status*—This is one of the most important tests. The samples can be obtained surgically or through sentinel node biopsy.
>
> 3. *Staging*—This occurs after the tumor is removed. Specific rules govern how breast cancer is staged. These rules are based on tumor size, the number of lymph nodes involved, if any, and whether there is metastasis (spread to distant organs).

Nowhere in your report does the sense that you're dealing with a foreign code come more into play than in the description of your cancer's stage. It is a combination of numbers and letters that have very specific meanings. Although your "stage" may not be known until after your cancer is removed and examined in the laboratory, staging is important for several vital reasons: It is a way to describe and categorize a tumor, a way to gather all of the evidence known about a particular cancer so that the most appropriate treatment regimen can be prescribed. All breast cancers are classified according to their stage.

Staging begins with numerical designations, starting with 0 and ranging through Roman numerals I through IV. The higher the number assigned to your tumor, the more serious your case.

THE TNM SYSTEM

It would be much simpler to understand staging if the Roman numeral designations were the end of the process. But as it turns out, there is more. The TNM system of classification is used to further define tumor size and any possible spread into the lymph nodes and beyond. The system also is known as the AJCC system, named after the American Joint Committee on Cancer, which developed the method of classifying breast cancers.

Basically, T stands for tumor, N for lymph nodes, and M for metastasis. In addition to these letters and the Roman numerals mentioned earlier, there is another set of numbers, ranging from 0 to 4. Don't let your eyes glaze—it gets easier, and I've included a chart below that breaks it down.

As part of staging, your doctors will approximate the size of your tumor. They will take into account the number of lymph nodes—if any—that are affected. They also will take into account the results of bone scans and tests involving other organ systems. In so doing, doctors can determine whether there have been any obvious metastases to other parts of your body. All of these factors are taken into account to stage your cancer.

For instance, a tumor designated T1 would measure two centimeters or smaller; T2 refers to a cancer that is up to two centimeters but not more than five centimeters; T3 refers to a cancer that is larger than five centimeters. T4 refers to a cancer of any size that has metastasized into the chest wall or into the skin.

N is designated as N0, N1, N2, or N3. N1 means the cancer has spread to anywhere from one to three lymph nodes. N2 means that more than three but fewer than ten nodes are affected. N3 refers to cancer having spread to ten or more nodes.

With the letter *M*, which stands for *metastasis*, M0 means no spread to distant organs. M1, the only other M category, means that cancer has spread to a distant site, such as to the liver, lungs, or bones.

There are numerous possibilities when it comes to staging. If you have DCIS, for example, much of the complicated nature of staging does not pertain to you because your cancer is small and contained within a specific site. Your cancer would be categorized as Stage 0 because your tumor would be staged as follows:

- ❖ Tis, for in situ

- ❖ N0, for zero lymph node involvement

- ❖ M0, for zero metastases

Invasive cancers are a different matter altogether because they can develop in a range of characteristics. See the chart below.

It may take several perusals of the various stages to grasp their meaning, but it is important to get an idea of what the categories convey about the disease because of the kinds of treatment recommended as a result of the designation. The treatment for DCIS would be far different from that of Stage III B breast cancer. For further information on the TNM system of classification you can peruse the website of the National Cancer Institute at http://cancernet .nci.nih.gov/clinpdq/soa.html.

The Importance of Pathology

Just as the skill and experience of a surgeon has an impact on the results of a delicate operation, the experience of the pathologist has an impact on the precision of the pathology findings. Ultimately, that level of skill has a bearing on the kind of surgery and medications you receive.

Pathologists in large academic centers who have diagnosed numerous cases, ranging from those that might be considered textbook cases to those of challenging levels of difficulty, know all too well that subtleties are to be expected from tumor specimens. At major cancer centers, pathologists regularly take part in staff meetings where each brings his or her most difficult slides. All of the doctors at the meeting study the specimens and comment about various cellular features. In some instances, one of the pathologists in attendance may have published widely on various cellular characteristics of a cancer being presented as part of the discussion, which may prove to be an added plus for the patient.

Dr. Lee Tan, a pathologist at Memorial Sloan-Kettering Cancer Center in New York City who specializes in the pathology of breast cancer, cites the importance of having a pathologist study your tissues who has studied the special microscopic features of breast cancer as well as other forms of cancer. Even though she specializes in breast pathology, Dr. Tan also is intimately familiar with the nature of other types of tumors. That knowledge sometimes has a bearing on what she is able to conclude about some patients' breast cancer. She says:

How Breast Cancer Is Staged

General Stage	T group	N group	M group
Stage 0	Tis	N0	M0
Stage I	T1	N0	M0
Stage II A	T0	N1	M0
	T1	N1	M0
	T2	N0	M0
Stage II B	T2	N1	M0
	T3	N0	M0
Stage III A	T0	N2	M0
	T1	N2	M0
	T2	N2	M0
	T3	N1	M0
	T3	N2	M0
Stage III B	T4	Any N	M0
Stage III C	Any T	N3	M0
Stage IV	Any T	Any N	M1

When patients come here from the outside, the medical oncologist always has us review the pathology. And it's a good thing we do. There was one case that was said to be an invasive breast carcinoma. It had the characteristics of invasive breast carcinoma. But I also knew that it resembled something else. There is a highly aggressive form of lung cancer, and we recognize it by certain [cellular] features. There is also a very rare form of breast cancer with the same kind of features. It is very important to recognize the similarities because of what this means in terms of treatment. Now if I hadn't seen these features in lung specimens I probably wouldn't have recognized them in breast [tissue].

There are other instances in which tissue specimens can give the impression of more aggressive disease, according to Dr. Tan, when in reality a patient has a much milder form of breast cancer. "We have also recognized a pattern that sometimes DCIS [ductal carcinoma in situ] can be involved with a benign lesion in the breast, and in those cases it mimics invasive ductal carcinoma. We recognize that so easily here because we see so many cases."

Dr. Stuart Schnitt, the director of surgical pathology at Beth Israel–New England Deaconess Medical Center in Boston, also emphasizes the importance of having slides examined at a major center. Subtleties at the cellular level can mean the difference in the kind of care a patient receives. To the untrained eye, a common precancerous condition called borderline atypical ductal hyperplasia can easily appear as if it were a form of breast cancer that is confined to a milk duct. He says, "Sometimes we see borderline atypical ductal hyperplasia, which can be difficult to distinguish from low-grade DCIS. It's a nuance of difference, but you have to recognize it because there are important clinical implications if the pathologist makes a mistake. Atypical ductal hyperplasia means there is a risk for breast cancer. DCIS *is* cancer."

There exists enough conformity in medical judgment to limit the likelihood of wide discrepancies when any two pathologists diagnose the same specimen, according to Dr. Schnitt, but he acknowledges that discrepancies do occur, citing what is known in medicine as "observers' reproducibility."

Second Opinions on Pathology Specimens

Either you or your oncologist can obtain a second opinion on your tissue specimens if you want one. This is not a difficult task to undertake. If you are going into this mission with the idea that a second pathologist will overturn the findings of the first and declare you cancer-free, then you may not want to get your hopes too high about what a second or even a third opinion might offer. However, errors can occur. A pathologist who is not as keenly aware of microscopic subtleties as Drs. Tan or Schnitt may not notice the slight nuance of difference between atypical ductal hyperplasia and DCIS. You may be told that you have an elevated risk for cancer when in reality you already have the disease. With such a fine line of difference, it would be wise to seek a second opinion. There are numerous reasons to consider another pathologist's expertise.

Maybe you're a patient at a small, nonteaching hospital and you (or your doctor) have concerns about the level of skill of your hospital's pathologists. Perhaps your physician is concerned about the conclusions drawn on some of your tests. Sometimes a pathology report can raise more questions than it answers. Maybe your oncologist wanted substantially more information than the pathology report revealed. Perhaps you are the one flush with questions. There were tests you had hoped to see but that were not run by the pathology department.

You might even wonder whether your oncologist has made the right treatment recommendations based on the findings in your pathology report. If you're facing the possibility of a mastectomy because of information contained in the report, and you want to know if you can undergo less extensive surgery, then certainly do not hesitate to seek a second opinion.

Highly trained pathologists are acutely aware of the numerous subtleties in breast cancer pathology. Renowned New York breast pathologist Dr. Paul Peter Rosen, of Cornell Weill Medical College in New York City, describes the breast and the many types of malignant manifestations that can occur there by saying, "It is an organ with the most complexities in tumor types."

The author of several well-regarded textbooks on breast cancer and breast pathology, including the book *Rosen's Pathology*, Dr. Rosen consults with breast cancer patients about their biopsy specimens. He has found that most of the patients he sees are well aware "of the enormous impact" a pathology report can have on the type of cancer therapy a doctor recommends. So most patients, he says, give considerable thought to what they want out of a consultation with him before seeking one. "There are a number of motives for doing this," he says. "They are not just looking for a diagnosis. Most of these patients want to know if the treatment [recommended by their doctors] is correct. And they want to discuss their cancer with someone who does not have a vested interest in the case."

Dr. Rosen renders second opinions for either physicians or patients. If you were to seek a second opinion from Dr. Rosen—or other pathologists like him—your doctors would not have to be involved in the discussions. Dr. Rosen estimates that more than 25 percent of the two thousand cases he reviews annually are from patients who bring in their own pathology specimens. The remainder of the cases for which he offers a diagnosis come from other physicians seeking his expertise.

Because his practice is so specialized, Dr. Rosen does not diagnose other forms of cancer. He began his practice in 1998 after more than thirty years as a staff pathologist at Memorial Sloan-Kettering Cancer Center in New York City. His type of medical practice, however, is not unique.

Conferring with a Consultant

At St. Mary's Hospital in San Francisco, the Breast Cancer Consultation Service also works directly with patients. Dr. Michael Lagios (pronounced LYE-ose) founded the service in 1981. Dr. Lagios' website helps patients understand some of the finer points about second opinions. His service accepts pathology data from patients anywhere in the world.

Dr. Lagios has been in the vanguard of diagnosing DCIS and has written extensively on this form of cancer in major medical journals. He does not limit his practice to DCIS. All forms of breast cancer are diagnosed at his consultation service.

In the southeastern United States, a similar consultation program is operated at Vanderbilt University in Nashville, Tennessee.

Overseen by Dr. David L. Page, a professor of pathology and preventive medicine at Vanderbilt School of Medicine, the Breast Consultation Service accepts biopsy data and supporting materials from patients anywhere in the world. The service also consults with pathologists and oncologists on particularly difficult cases.

Like Dr. Rosen, Dr. Page is an author of textbooks on breast pathology. His book *Diagnostic Histopathology of the Breast* is a text widely used in North America and abroad. Biographies of Dr. Page and his staff, as well as descriptions of how the program functions, can be viewed on the website at www.breastconsults.com.

In addition to consulting with these physicians, there are several other ways to obtain a second opinion. If, for example, your cancer was not diagnosed at a major medical center, you can have your physician forward your slides and specimens to the pathology department of an institution of notable rank. You will first have to determine if the institution even bothers with cases other than those of their own physicians. Some centers do not have the time or personnel to devote to outside cases. If the center does accept your case for a second opinion, there will be a charge that may or may not be covered by your insurance.

There is yet another avenue to pursue if you want a second opinion on your pathology specimens. You can take advantage (also at additional cost) of services offered by the Armed Forces Institute of Pathology in Washington, D.C. Because the AFIP works only with physicians, your doctor will have to see that specimens are forwarded to the program. By the same token, once the AFIP has completed its review of your case, the pathology report will be sent to your physician, not to you.

An Activist Comments on Second Opinions

Pathologists generally agree that breast cancer patients have become extremely knowledgeable over the years about the disease they are facing. Women with breast cancer also have become increasingly motivated, many of these doctors say, to seek second and third opinions on pathology data, something they attribute to media reports and the growing influence of breast cancer advocacy groups.

Diane deLara, project coordinator for the advocacy organization Breast Cancer Action, based in San Francisco, says the importance of second opinions can never be overlooked. The issue of second opinions, she says, is a topic often broached in the group's newsletter. BCA reaches an international audience through its newsletter and website.

Breast cancer patients also are encouraged to call BCA when they have questions. Women newly diagnosed with the disease are frequently among the callers seeking advice on how best to handle their diagnosis. It isn't just the pathology report that women are encouraged to seek second opinions about, but any aspect of their cancer care. DeLara says, "We think second opinions are important, especially when someone is uncomfortable or disagrees with what a doctor says. Just this morning a woman called to say she felt she needed another opinion, but she didn't know if that was the right thing to do. We told her of course it was. If that's what she believed to be the right thing, then by all means, go ahead and do it."

❧ ❧ ❧

Even though pathology departments are often tucked away in areas of treatment centers where patients are less likely to encounter them, the impact that pathologists have on cancer care is profound. If before now you were unaware of the wide scope of the services performed by pathologists, you may want to take a few minutes to think about their role—and what the pathology findings mean with respect to your case.

Chapter 5

A Primer on Risks, Part I: Age, Genes, and Ethnicity

Dr. Silvana Martino, a breast cancer specialist and associate professor of medicine at the University of Southern California, has conducted hundreds of studies on breast cancer and written prolifically on the subject in prestigious medical journals. She has presented results of her studies at major scientific gatherings, such as the annual meeting of the American Association of Clinical Oncology and the San Antonio Breast Cancer Symposium. But when asked about breast cancer risk factors, Dr. Martino, who is also an adjunct faculty member at the John Wayne Cancer Center in Santa Monica, California, takes a deep breath and offers her most learned opinion: "Just being female and growing older are the biggest risk factors. Everything else is secondary."

For years, medical scientists have said that approximately three-quarters of all breast cancer cases diagnosed each year in the United States cannot be explained by the known risk factors. That means most women simply cannot be told what may have led to their cancer. Still, doctors have some good hunches, despite a lack of convincing evidence that would allow them to tell each individual the precise reason why her cancer occurred.

More than 75 percent of all cases of the disease occur in women over the age of fifty. By itself, age does not cause the disease. The risk comes from DNA-damaging exposures that happen throughout life. Beginning your menstrual cycle early or entering menopause late are both breast cancer risk factors, as are having your first child later in life or never having children at all. These and similar risk factors are associated with tumor development because they directly affect the number of years you are exposed to the cycles of your own hormones.

For a comparatively small percentage of patients with a family history of breast cancer, the cause may be obvious and related to one of the so-called breast cancer genes, BRCA1 or BRCA2. Mutations in these genes can initiate a cascade of molecular events that lead to tumor development. The genes can be inherited from either your mother or father. And just as genetic flaws can lead to breast cancer in women, the same holds true for men.

This chapter examines how genetic damage—inherited or accumulated over time—can lead to breast cancer, why some people call themselves members of cancer families, and how they cope. The discussion then turns to ethnicity and breast cancer, taking another look at BRCA1 and 2. It also addresses why African American women are sometimes diagnosed younger and have a poorer prognosis than their white counterparts.

Understanding Risk

Along with the two major breast cancer risk factors mentioned by Dr. Martino—female gender and advancing age—several other factors can be added to the list. These are the so-called known risk factors for breast cancer. Most, such as early menarche (the start of menstrual periods), late menopause, having your first child after age thirty, and drinking more than one alcoholic beverage daily, are moderate risks. High-risk factors include having a personal or family history of the disease or carrying one of the gene mutations.

Here is a list of the known risk factors:

1. A personal history of breast cancer

2. A family history of breast cancer or ovarian cancer

3. A biopsy that reveals atypical hyperplasia or LCIS (see Chapter 4)

4. A mutation in BRCA1 or BRCA2

5. Starting your periods before age twelve

6. Starting menopause after age fifty-five

7. Having your first child after age thirty

8. Never giving birth

9. Drinking more than one alcoholic beverage per day

10. Currently taking hormone replacement therapy

11. Postmenopausal obesity

What Is a Gene? (Part I)

A gene is the smallest single unit of DNA (deoxyribonucleic acid) capable of transmitting a trait. It is thus the tiniest unit of heredity, an infinitesimal molecule. Genes are responsible for your height, your hair and eye color, the shape of your nose, and to some extent even your athletic capability or your musical talent. Genetic traits can be conveyed by a single gene or through several genes acting in concert with one another. High blood pressure, a potentially devastating vascular disorder, occurs when multiple genes produce the trait. Cancer occurs when mutations occur in the genes governing cell growth.

Breast Cancer and Genetics

Breast cancer occurs when genes in cells that make up breast tissue accumulate mutations. This takes a very long time, possibly decades. If you imagine a gene as a sequence of words literally spelling out what is supposed to happen in a cell, then you can also imagine mutations as serious "spelling errors" in those sentences. Errors mean the cell lacks proper instructions for growth. When a vast number of cells carry mutations, then normal growth and development are impossible. Each time a cell divides and creates two new progeny—daughter cells—the spelling errors are carried into each of the newly created cells. With each cell division, the errors can be recreated in hundreds, then thousands, and, ultimately, millions of other cells.

Dr. Patricia Ganz, director of cancer prevention and control research at UCLA's Jonsson Comprehensive Cancer Center, says mutations alter the function of healthy cells, a transformation that changes their growth patterns, eventually leading to the mass of rogue cells called cancer. Cancer cells are not invaders like bacteria or viruses. They are normal cells that have become irrevocably changed. The mutations may be inherited—passed along in your family—or they may be acquired through assaults that alter the normal function of your genetic material. These assaults can come from a wide range of sources, including the body's own hormones. Hormones can damage the function of genes after many decades of exposure.

Mutations, Dr. Ganz explains, are responsible for virtually all forms of cancer. And understanding that fact, she adds, illustrates how subtly cancers evolve. "Breast cancer is a genetic disease," she says, "and that is because it occurs after you have mutations in the genes of many cells. This does not happen overnight. It takes many years to acquire these mutations. This is as true for breast cancer as it is for any other form of cancer. Take skin cancer. A child may be overexposed to the sun, and that exposure causes a mutation in one cell, causing it to grow a little faster than its neighbors. When that cell divides, the mutation is transmitted to the daughter cells. There may be another serious overexposure

> **What Is a Gene? (Part II)**
>
> At its most basic level a gene is made up of the chemicals adenine, tyrosine, cytosine, and guanine, which biologists abbreviate as *A, T, C,* and *G*. These letters are the alphabet of genetics. Nature strings them together in various ways, in countless lengths and permutations, to spell out sequences of genetic code—sentences that direct the body to do something specific. There is a code commanding the body to make more enzymes to digest lunch and dinner, and another one to make fresh proteins to repopulate the immune system or suppress the genesis of a tumor. When a wrong letter appears in a genetic "sentence," or when a letter is missing, the sequence is said to have a mutation. Mutations are the source of hundreds of diseases, including breast cancer.

as a teenager and again in the twenties, each producing mutations that are passed on in successive cell divisions. By the time the person is sixty, or even before that time, these accumulated mutations may result in skin cancer."

Different types of assaults, Dr. Ganz continues, can cause damage leading to mutations that underlie other forms of cancer. In lung cancer, for instance, it is often the combustion products from cigarette smoking that attack healthy genes in the lungs. "Lung cancer is related to length and dose," Dr. Ganz says, referring to the number of years a person smokes and the average number of cigarettes smoked during that time. So the longer someone has the habit, the greater the potential to have smoked hundreds of cigarettes, and to have seriously damaged genes in the lungs. In the case of thyroid cancer, Dr. Ganz continues, it is often radiation exposure that has damaged the genes in thyroid cells.

In breast cancer, the assaults to cells are often subtle, which is a reason why doctors cannot always say with any certainty that A, B, or C caused a patient's tumor. Instead, they look at what risk factors the patient might have. For women with a family history of the disease, doctors may suspect one of the known breast cancer genes. As Dr. Ganz sees it, inheriting a genetic predisposition to breast cancer often means developing the disease decades before women whose mutations occur by chance. "People with a genetic risk start out with a mutation from birth. That is why their breast cancer occurs in their thirties, forties, or early fifties. But for the rest of us, the mutations may not occur until the second or third decades of life, which is why for the majority of women, breast cancer occurs much later."

The Link Between Estrogen and Breast Cancer

Doctors have known for more than a century that when women's ovaries were removed early in life, they faced a life free of breast cancer. Figuring out why this was so took the better part of the twentieth century. But doctors now have a strong base of knowledge linking the hormone estrogen to the disease.

Estrogen stimulates normal cell division and growth in a variety of target tissues: the breasts, ovaries, uterus, heart, and bones. The hormone's specialized effect upon breast tissue is the reason why breasts develop during puberty. Estrogen is a miraculous chemical because it possesses the ability to influence the rate of cell division. Yet any estrogen-influenced mutation can be repeated over and over—thousands upon thousands of times—as estrogen drives the growth and replication of cells, but this process can take decades. That is why Dr. Ganz underscores that women at average risk of breast cancer often develop the disease much later in life. It takes a very long time for enough copies of a mutation to be spread among countless cells to, in turn, produce the problematic circumstance we know as cancer.

Still, that isn't the sum of the estrogen story. As a growth stimulator, it also possesses the ability to drive the growth and development of tumor cells—those with estrogen receptors—once a cancer develops.

BRCA1 and BRCA2

The National Cancer Institute estimates that inherited gene mutations that are known to cause breast cancer account for only 5 percent to 10 percent of the 211,000 cases that occur in the United States annually. That means a large majority of cases are what scientists refer to as "sporadic." These cancers occur for reasons that cannot be easily explained, if explained at all. Most sporadic cases are diagnosed in women past the age of fifty. On the other hand, Dr. Martino, from USC, says there is at least one signal that a case of breast cancer may be related to a gene mutation: "We've known for many years that in families with [hereditary] disease, women tend to get breast cancer when they are younger."

Not only are women who inherit a predisposition to breast cancer typically younger when they get the disease; they also tend to have more aggressive tumors that lack—or have lost—hormone receptors on the cells' surface, a feature that often makes breast cancer in younger women more difficult to treat.

Genes dubbed BRCA1 and BRCA2, when mutated, are associated with breast and ovarian cancers that run in families. A major hallmark of these genes is cancer's occurrence at a young age, often under forty. The letters *BRCA* are an abbreviation for b̲reast c̲ancer. The number 1 refers to the first gene that was identified; the number 2 refers to the second.

Scientists suspect that there are many more genes associated with hereditary breast cancer. The first scientific evidence that breast cancer could be inherited came in 1990 from studies conducted by Dr. Mary-Claire King while she was on the faculty of the University of California at Berkeley. She postulated that a single gene could lead to breast cancer. Four years later researchers at the University of Utah found the precise chromosomal location of BRCA1.

BRCA1 is a fairly large gene, residing on chromosome 17. By *large* I mean there is a complex combination of ATCG sequences spelling out the gene's function (see the sidebar "What Is a Gene? Part II"). BRCA2, located on chromosome 13, is an even larger gene. It also consists of a complex series of sequences. Dr. Kenneth Offit, chief of clinical genetics at Memorial Sloan-Kettering Cancer Center in New York City, and a team of researchers discovered BRCA2 in 1996. There are at least two specific mutations on BRCA1 and one well-described (and possibly at least one other) mutation on BRCA2.

When healthy, both genes function as tumor suppressors. That is, they serve as "brakes" to stop unfettered cell division, the kind of unchecked division associated with cancer. Anyone with a "misspelling"—a mutation—in either BRCA1 or BRCA2 is at greater risk for breast and ovarian cancers because the mutations allow tumors to develop and flourish.

An analysis of more than a thousand women of Ashkenazi Jewish descent found that mutations in either BRCA1 or 2 confer an 82 percent chance of developing breast cancer over one's lifetime. The study, which is considered confirmatory, also found that when BRCA1 is mutated, an individual has a 54 percent lifetime risk of contracting ovarian cancer. The lifetime risk for ovarian cancer for those possessing a mutated BRCA2 is 23 percent.[1]

The research, conducted by a consortium of researchers known as the New York Breast Cancer Study Group, additionally discovered that women who were most physically active during adolescence could delay cancer's onset. Exercise reduces the level of estrogen available to cells. As discussed above, the hormone has a profound influence on cells, and the longer a person is exposed to estrogen throughout her life, the greater the likelihood of damage to the genes governing cellular growth. The study, which was reported in an October 2003 issue of the weekly journal *Science*, was led by Dr. King and is considered to be the most extensive analysis of the two genes in a high-risk population.

Mutated BRCA1 and 2 genes are not exclusive to Ashkenazi Jews, an ethnic group whose ancestral roots are in Eastern Europe. The genetic miscodes have also been found in studies of other ethnic groups, particularly women of Icelandic, Dutch, Norwegian, and Korean descent.

Cancer in the Family: Survivors Speak

Even before the discovery of the two breast cancer genes, those who had seen breast and ovarian cancers occur time and again in their families knew without such stunning scientific discoveries that breast cancer could be passed on as readily as traits for height and eye color from one generation to the next.

From a fairly young age, Betsey W. felt that breast cancer was stalking her. Although she tried to stay a step ahead of her pursuer, she knew it would eventually catch up.

> I always knew someday I would get breast cancer. I was forty-seven years old when I was diagnosed with bilateral breast cancer [cancer in both breasts]. Not really much of a surprise, but an awful shock!
>
> My mother was forty-two years of age when she was diagnosed with breast cancer in one breast. Radical mastectomy was the obvious treatment for her during that era,

because her lymph nodes were involved. She declined chemo and did well with no treatment for twenty years, when she had a recurrence in the second breast. She died in 1999 of a ruptured brain aneurysm.

My father was diagnosed with prostate cancer in 1993 at the age of seventy-one. It is possible that there is some kind of BRCA genetic mutation or some other genetic mutation that may be implicated in prostate, breast, and ovarian cancer. My mother's brother had prostate cancer; my mother's aunt Cora had breast cancer.

Judy B., another woman in whose family breast cancer has occurred in multiple generations, believes the genetic deck was stacked heavily against her and that breast cancer was inevitable.

Our family history showed that no female on my father's side, through my generation, ever escaped breast cancer. We knew about this risk and knew that it was being inherited long before doctors announced the discovery of breast cancer genes.

With such a family history, it became a personal mission for Judy to learn as much as possible about breast cancer as well as other forms of cancer. Colon and lung cancers were other common malignancies in her family, going back several generations.

Here's a rundown of what we know. On the paternal side, my grandmother died of breast cancer. She and her husband, my grandfather, had four sons and two daughters. Neither daughter lived to adulthood. The four sons all married and had children. Three of the four sons lived to their eighties, but all died with cancer, two lung and one colon. The fourth son died in his forties of lung cancer.

The children of those four sons included four girls and four boys. All four girls were diagnosed with breast cancer in their thirties. Two died during or shortly after treatment. Two remain alive today. One of the boys developed brain cancer and died during treatment in his thirties. Another of the boys developed tongue cancer and died in his fifties.

The next generation includes eight children who are presently in their thirties, six boys and two girls. One of the girls, my daughter, has been diagnosed with breast cancer.

Judy is deeply concerned about the history of cancer in her family and worries about her four grandchildren. Judy and her family run a website (www.cancersurvivors.org) to educate others about cancer and familial risk. She cautions others affected by breast cancer not to believe that genes for increased risk flow only from the maternal side of the family. She has no doubt that she inherited her exceptionally elevated risk for the disease from her father. That risk was compounded by the fact that her mother was diagnosed twice with breast cancer.

Many who develop breast cancer after other close family members have had the disease say they recognize similar patterns of development. Although this is purely anecdotal, they say they've noticed that the ages of cancer onset are often similar, or that a lump is found in a similar location. However, some people appearing to have an elevated familial risk are confused when the type of breast cancer affecting them differs from that of a close relative. Julie B. discussed that matter with her doctor.

> My mother was diagnosed with breast cancer when she was thirty-six. I was thirty-three when I was diagnosed. Her breast cancer was of a different type from mine; hers was Paget's disease, which is rarer. I initially thought this might rule out any hereditary connection. But my surgeon is of the opinion that breast cancer is breast cancer, that it just manifested itself differently in me than in my mother.
>
> I am not certain about the validity of this. It may just be one doctor's opinion. Frankly, I do suspect a genetic link. My mother's father died of melanoma that spread to the brain, and there is also a history of cancer on my father's side.

Breast cancer specialists point out that Paget's disease affects the areola and is typified by scaling. However, the visible scaling in some cases may be from an invasive ductal cancer that developed close to the nipple. Technically, this form of breast cancer would not be Paget's disease, but the more common form of breast cancer, invasive ductal carcinoma.

Donna O. and her sisters underwent genetic screening and discovered that two of the three women carried a BRCA2 mutation. It was a test result that spoke volumes about their family's medical history.

> We always said among ourselves that we belong to a cancer family—kind of a bad joke and reality check rolled into one. My two sisters and I got tested around the same time. My younger sister and I have the gene, and we've both had breast cancer. My sister who turned out not to have BRCA2 had skin cancer three times—not the serious kind. But she lives in Florida so maybe that explains that.
>
> My younger sister was diagnosed with breast cancer first, three years ago, and I was diagnosed after that. Our mom died of breast cancer in '97. Her mom had breast cancer but died of a stroke. A paternal aunt had ovarian cancer and died; and her daughter, a first cousin of ours, has breast cancer now. My daughter is twenty-four and hasn't been tested for the gene. There's a fifty-fifty chance she might not have it. So I am praying and keeping my fingers crossed.
>
> Some of the men have had cancer, too—not breast cancer. But that's the short list, which sort of gives you an idea why we've called ourselves a cancer family.

Cathy R., the aerobics enthusiast whose love of exercise and broccoli we discussed in Chapter 3, also uses "cancer family" to describe her own situation and that of her close relatives. Having a family history of the disease, she says, gives you a different perspective on life.

> I treat each day as precious, as a gift. And I try to do the best for my health, because I know that something is ticking away in there that wants to do otherwise. I'm still worried. Will I have a recurrence? Will I not have a recurrence? I don't know. I also want to say that because so many people I love very dearly have been stricken with breast cancer or ovarian cancer, we are more forgiving of each other's faults and shortcomings. If somebody says something that's a little bit mean,

that's okay. We don't stop speaking to each other or stop sending birthday cards or whatever. We realize that life's a gift. None of us has been tested for the breast cancer genes. I don't think getting tested was on anybody's radar because we already knew.

Zora K. Brown, a breast cancer activist, survivor of the disease, and founder of the Breast Cancer Resource Committee in Washington, D.C., says she too has a long family history of the cancer, and because of it she has participated in major scientific studies. She hopes to help advance the understanding of breast cancer's hereditary nature.

Her family, however, was among only a handful of African Americans participating in the major BRCA1 and 2 research projects. Because so few black participants were recruited into the studies, she says scientists really do not have a strong sense of how pervasive the major susceptibility genes are in African Americans. Zora says she would like to see medical researchers focus more attention on breast cancer in African American women.

Men and BRCA2

Scientists have confirmed that men as well as women can pass along genes that predispose their offspring to breast cancer. Researchers additionally have confirmed that men who develop hereditary breast cancer are likely to carry the BRCA2 mutation. New York state representative Cameron Alden, a breast cancer survivor, said he implored his physicians to consider his family history of breast cancer. Doctors initially were reluctant even to test him for breast cancer despite a palpable lump. He told his physicians of two close female relatives who had developed breast cancer, evidence to him that breast cancer genes can be passed as readily to sons as to daughters.

I know we carry the BRCA1 gene because our family was in the original Mary-Claire King study. The National Cancer Institute also had done a study on my family. My mother, grandmother, and great-grandmother had breast cancer. On my father's side of the family there was also a high incidence of breast cancer. I remember as a young girl my mother cautioning us about breast cancer in our family. My mom used to tell us, "Science will have to catch up with us."

I was age thirty-one when I was diagnosed. One of my sisters was diagnosed at age twenty-seven, and another was diagnosed under the age of forty—she was thirty-six, I believe. And just last week one of my nieces underwent a bilateral mastectomy for breast cancer, and another niece was diagnosed at age twenty-nine.

I don't think there has been the will to really look at the African American community in terms of genetic susceptibility. I run a support-group program, and the data we have collected are compelling enough to suggest a strong genetic component for many breast cancer cases.

Additional Mutations

Not all genetic mutations are passed from one generation to the next. Sometimes they are acquired during an individual's lifetime. Scientists have pinpointed major classes of genes that play critical roles in breast cancer development. One group is composed of tumor suppressor genes that are endowed by nature to protect a person from developing cancer when these genes are healthy. When these genes are mutated, they can lead to the disease. Another class is known as oncogenes, which are altered genes capable of triggering unregulated cell growth.

To get a better sense of what is meant when it is said that not all mutations are passed from one generation to the next, it may be a good idea to become acquainted with genes in which mutations can be acquired. This is where things may seem a little confusing, but try to bear with me. As you learned earlier BRCA1 and 2 are tumor suppressor genes that when mutated can cause breast cancer. These mutations are inherited. By contrast, other kinds of tumor suppressor genes pick up mutations at various times throughout your life.

One such gene in this category is p53, once dubbed by *Time* magazine as Molecule of the Year. When p53 is mutated (or in some instances when it is missing), cancer—any kind of cancer—can occur. Researchers have implicated mutated or missing p53 genes in 50 percent of all types of cancer, from breast cancer to prostate malignancies to tumors that infiltrate the colon.

When it is healthy, p53 suppresses tumor growth, just as BRCA1 and 2 are known to do when they are healthy. What helped p53 earn the title Molecule of the Year was its *other* ability, to protect DNA and to maintain the orderly nature of cell division—and to do so in a variety of tissues, not just breast tissue. When it is mutated or missing, however, cell growth can occur without any of the usual robust checks and balances.

Another critical gene involved in breast cancer is HER-2, which, more precisely, is known as an oncogene. Unlike BRCA1 or 2 there is no familial pattern involved with HER-2; therefore, anyone can carry it. Earlier in the book I referred to HER-2 (sometimes written as HER-2/neu) as a biomarker because this gene and its protein are found on the surface of tumor cells. To go a step further, as an oncogene HER-2 can trigger abnormal cell growth.

HER-2 is present in about one-third of all cases of breast cancer. Pathologists test for its presence during a patient's biopsy studies because its overexpression usually means a more aggressive cancer with a greater likelihood to spread. HER-2 is endowed with growth-propelling properties, which can drive the production of cancer cells. Later in the book we will discuss how the drug Herceptin, which directly targets the HER-2 oncogene, is being tested in combination with other medications to stave off metastatic disease in some women.

Additional mutations involving other tumor suppressor genes are also being studied for their roles in breast cancer, as are other oncogenes. And even as such analyses are occurring, scientists are still maintaining an aggressive search for genes that can be passed along in families to cause the disease.

Scandinavian scientists, working with geneticists at the National Human Genome Research Institute in Bethesda, Maryland, found evidence of another hereditary breast cancer gene, the kind of gene in which susceptibility is passed from one generation to the next. The study focused on women who live in Nordic countries and hail from families in which three or more female family members have had breast cancer. Dr. Olli Kallioniemi, a senior scientist at the National Human Genome Research Institute, wrote in the *Proceedings of the National Academy of Sciences* that the "BRCA3 candidate" gene may help explain cases of obviously hereditary breast cancer for which there is no clear link to either BRCA1 or BRCA2. Scientists are not yet convinced that this candidate for BRCA3 will eventually prove to be a cause of breast cancer, but their early evidence seems compelling.

This suspected mutation, like BRCA2, resides on chromosome 13. Even though BRCA2 and the candidate for BRCA3 are located on chromosome 13, they are not related. Dr. Kallioniemi, working with thirty-five colleagues in fourteen laboratories in the United States and Europe, reports that their candidate for a breast cancer susceptibility gene is a significant distance away from BRCA2—essentially the genetic equivalent of several miles. The distance strongly suggests the two genes are not related and function independently of each other.

Scientists suspect the mutation may account for one-third of all hereditary breast cancers that cannot be explained by either BRCA1 or 2, at least in Nordic populations. This does not mean the mutated gene causes breast cancer only in Northern European women. Rather, it means that this population, in which the mutation is prevalent, has helped scientists pinpoint a potential hereditary mutation. Future studies, of course, will enable researchers to determine the mutation's prevalence in other groups and whether it should be officially titled BRCA3.

Geneticists worldwide are on the hunt for additional breast cancer genes that can be passed along in families. It is very likely that many more may be found. When word was released from the National Human Genome Research Institute that at least a candidate for another breast cancer gene had been found, Dr. Francis Collins, the institute's director, put the discovery in perspective. "I greet these research findings with a combination of excitement and caution," he said. "We've suspected for some time that hereditary breast cancer is triggered by many susceptibility genes. Once we have most of them identified and understood, we'll be able to tailor diagnosis and treatments much more effectively than we are able to do now. However, lots [more] research remains to be done."[2]

Should You Seek Genetic Counseling?

Genetic counseling allows you to discuss your family medical history with a trained genetic counselor. You may wish to do so simply for your own edification, or prior to undergoing genetic screening. If you have been diagnosed with breast cancer, you may be seeking genetic counseling to better understand breast cancer's risk factors, and to help put into perspective what your cancer means in terms of your children's or grandchildren's future. The Susan G. Komen Breast Cancer Foundation, a patient-advocacy group, recommends genetic counseling if you are at particularly high risk for breast cancer based on the following criteria:

a) [If you have] a personal history of breast or ovarian cancer

b) [If you have or] had two or more close relatives with cancer

c) [If you have or] had a relative with breast cancer at an early age (i.e., before menopause)

d) [If you have or] had a relative with bilateral (both sides) breast or ovarian cancers

e) [If you have or] had a relative with more than one type of breast or ovarian cancer

f) [If more than one generation of your family has or had] a pattern of breast or ovarian cancer

The Susan G. Komen Foundation further outlines what genetic counseling includes:

a) Obtaining detailed family, medical, and lifestyle histories

b) Documenting cancer-related diagnoses

c) Constructing and analyzing pedigrees (family history)

d) Providing risk assessment and counseling

e) Discussing risks and benefits of gene testing

For more information on breast cancer and genetic counseling, contact the Susan G. Komen Breast Cancer Foundation, (800) I'M

AWARE (800-462-9273); the American Cancer Society, (800) ACS-2345 (800-227-2345); or the National Cancer Institute's Information Service, (800) 4-CANCER (800-422-6237).

Genetic Screening: Pros and Cons

Undergoing genetic screening for breast cancer is a highly personal and difficult decision, because many of the potential benefits of such testing can be outweighed by the drawbacks. If you are pondering a decision about genetic testing, you might want to think about to whom you will convey the information you receive, and what kind of emotional impact such knowledge could have on you and loved ones.

You may also want to give some thought to the possibility of the potential misuse or abuse of genetic information. Although legislation has been enacted to provide some protection for people who have undergone genetic testing, activists feel that the available laws are not nearly strong enough to effectively protect those who test positive.

Blood tests are commercially available to determine whether you carry a mutated BRCA1 or BRCA2. If you are positive for one of the mutations, you then know that each of your children—male and female—has a 50 percent chance of also being a carrier. If you're still of childbearing age, this information can help with future family planning. And if you are the parent of grown children, the information may serve as a reason for your children to consider testing.

Besides being linked to breast and ovarian cancers, BRCA2 mutations have been linked to two devastating pediatric conditions, Fanconi's anemia and a rare brain tumor known as medullablastoma. These conditions occur when both parents carry copies of the gene. BRCA mutations also have been associated with colon and prostate cancers.

Unfortunately, the development of genetic screenings has outpaced the approval of legislation aimed at protecting people who get screened. In 1996, measures included in the Health Insurance Portability and Accountability Act (HIPAA) offered the first legal protections against health insurance discrimination based on information from genetic testing. The law prevents genetic test results from being regarded as a "preexisting" medical condition. The legal protection also prevents genetic test information from being used as a reason to hike insurance premiums. Activists who support the causes of people with cancer say being aware of this law is important because its guidelines can be easily skirted. If you suspect its rules have been violated, you should contact your state insurance commissioner.

In addition, you should also be aware that the Department of Health and Human Services has established standards ensuring the privacy of health information. These guidelines regulate methods of disclosure and access to medical information by health insurance companies.

In 2003, the U.S. Senate passed its version of the Genetic Nondiscrimination in Health Insurance and Employment Act, which prevents genetic test information from being used as a basis for firing, not hiring, or failing to promote people who have tested positive in a genetic screening. Many major advocacy organizations have not strongly supported the act because they feel its enforcement provisions lack strength. A House version of the Genetic Nondiscrimination in Health and Insurance Employment Act, sponsored by Rep. Louise M. Slaughter, a New York Democrat, contains language on workplace protections that advocacy organizations find more appealing. Among groups endorsing the House version are the National Breast Cancer Coalition, the National Organization for Rare Disorders, and the American Academy of Family Physicians.

Survivors Discuss Genetic Screening

Understandably, many with a family history of breast cancer have voiced a wide range of concerns about genetic screening. While some people diagnosed with breast cancer—or who are at high risk for the disease—have gotten the tests, others have shied away from them, citing fears that their privacy would not be adequately protected.

Julie B., who was diagnosed with breast cancer when she was thirty-three, believes in the importance of the tests, especially for research purposes. However, she is uncertain about how gathering such information advances the search for a cancer cure.

> I have mixed feelings on the issue. From everything I've read—and believe me since being diagnosed, it's almost an obsession—a woman may be diagnosed as having the gene, but it's still unknown what exactly sets it off. It's still unknown what the catalysts are. A woman who has the gene may very well go through life without developing the disease.
>
> On the one hand, knowing that one possesses the gene may result in a constant vigilance. For example, knowing my mother's history served me well, as I performed constant self-checks, and in fact discovered the lump myself, and fortunately early enough that it had not spread. On the other hand, there is a price to be paid emotionally for knowing that you "might" possess this ticking time bomb, not to mention the issues of insurance, employment, etc.

Judy B., whose family sponsors the website for people with all forms of cancer, underwent genetic testing along with other relatives because she felt it was important to get a sense of exactly what kind of genetic flaw had affected her family for several generations.

> We had the genetic testing done during a BRCA1 and 2 study, and we felt that our involvement might help the overall pool of knowledge brought to bear on breast and other cancers. Additionally, my daughter and I had already been diagnosed when we were tested, so the issue was almost moot for us in terms of medical care.
>
> I personally believe that technology in this area has grown so fast that there is not sufficient protection for medical privacy (assuming that medical privacy exists at all). While I do not personally know of a single case where someone's employment or insurance has been compromised because of the release of genetic information, I can see the potential for great damage.

Ethnicity and Breast Cancer

No population of women anywhere in the world is immune to breast cancer. No diet, ethnic delicacy, amount of strenuous exercise, magic chant, or voodoo spell can eliminate it—at least not yet. What differs from one country to the next is the rate at which the disease occurs. The rate is lower in the underdeveloped world compared with industrialized nations, and even among industrialized countries rates differ.

A microcosm of breast cancer's global demographics can be seen in the population of the United States. Some groups are less susceptible than others. Throughout the United States, breast cancer is the most commonly diagnosed cancer in women, regardless of ethnicity. On the whole, Caucasian women have a higher incidence of the disease than any other group in the United States, but the death rate for this population continues to decline. According to data from the Surveillance, Epidemiology, and End Results (SEER) program, the five-year survival rate for white women is 88 percent, compared with 73 percent for African Americans. The SEER program has monitored cancer occurrence and survival in 10 percent of all U.S. patients diagnosed with all forms of cancer since 1973.

Ethnicity and Breast Cancer in the United States

White women have the highest incidence of breast cancer in the United States, followed by Hawaiian and African American women. According to data from the Surveillance, Epidemiology, and End Results (SEER) program, Hispanic, American Indian, and Asian women have significantly lower rates.

The CDC's division of Cancer Control and Prevention estimated the incidence among various groups as seen below. (Note these figures do not separate Hawaiian women from a larger ethnic grouping that includes Asians, who have very low rates.) Each value is per one hundred thousand women:

All races: 127.2

White: 129.9

Black: 106.7

Hispanic: 86.6

Asian/Pacific Islander: 78.1

Let's take a look at how issues related to breast cancer affect certain ethnic groups within the U.S. population.

LATINAS AND BREAST CANCER

People of Latin American heritage now comprise the largest minority group in the United States, and while they have a greater propensity for some conditions, such as diabetes, Latinas have a comparatively low incidence of breast cancer. For women of Latin American heritage, both the incidence of breast cancer and death rates from the disease are consistently lower than they are for either black or non-Hispanic white populations.

But lower incidence does not mean zero risk, and major advocacy organizations want women to be aware of that fact and to educate themselves about the disease and its treatment when they are diagnosed. The National Alliance for Hispanic Health is one such group that stresses the importance of learning about breast cancer. The organization posts information about the condition on its website (www.hispanichealth.org) to inform women about the disease and its therapy.

Aurelia G., who was diagnosed with breast cancer at age sixty, has become a vocal advocate in her family for breast cancer screening. She found the lump herself and within a week of its discovery was scheduled for a mastectomy. "My life changed overnight," she says. Aurelia's experience also inspired her to learn as much as possible about the disease. She was learning about breast cancer, however, as she was being rapidly inducted into the complex system of cancer care.

> Everything happened so fast. The first week I had one medical appointment after another. My head was spinning. I had to get a mammogram. I had to see my doctor. I had to get my lab work. I didn't have a lot of time for questions. I didn't have time to say, hey, I am a person, not a number.

Having to learn about breast cancer on the fly while meeting appointments and coping with the thought of a life-threatening condition is not in the best interest of the patient, Aurelia says. She recommends taking a week or two to gather your thoughts.

> My oncologist told me around the time I was getting chemo that things really didn't have to move so fast. He said I could

have had a breather. Well, great. He's telling me this when I'm almost done. He's telling me that I came across like a no-nonsense lady, like somebody ready to be done with cancer as fast as possible. He got the impression I wanted to get everything on the ball and rolling. I don't know how he came up with those ideas. I was just scared.

Aurelia, who was born in Puerto Rico but has lived in the United States for most of her life, says she has often wondered how women fare who do not speak English, particularly in the kind of whirlwind diagnosis and treatment experience she had. She wonders if everything is being properly explained and whether patients have time to slow down and have the entire process spelled out slowly in Spanish. Her concerns are timely. The Institute of Medicine (IOM) in Washington, D.C., found in a study on health disparities that language barriers have an impact on the care patients receive. The insitute, a division of the National Academies, was chartered in 1970 to advise both Congress and the nation on matters of health and health-care delivery.

As a result of the IOM finding, many health-care advocates suggest that people who do not speak English have someone fluent in it accompany them to appointments whenever possible—even when the hospital offers translators. That way, patients are ensured of clear channels of communication, which is especially important when the diagnosis is a potentially life-threatening one such as cancer.

JEWISH AMERICANS AND THE BRCA GENES

Among Ashkenazi Jews, scientists estimate that possibly 2 percent of the population—men and women—carry a mutation in one of the BRCA genes. More than 90 percent of the Jewish population in the United States is Ashkenazi, descendants of mostly Eastern European immigrants. Scientists attribute the prevalence of the BRCA mutations to an ancient "founder" effect, which means the genetic changes date back centuries to several original families who carried the DNA flaws. These genetic miscues were easily passed through numerous succeeding generations, experts have theorized, because of the close-knit nature of Jewish culture.

As advocates have strongly underscored and evidence from around the globe continues to demonstrate, BRCA1 and 2 mutations may be far more prevalent in other populations around the world. Only with time, after dozens of additional populations have been tested for the genes' presence, will medical science have a more complete grasp on how many other ethnic groups carry the mutations.

Studies conducted by researchers around the world demonstrate that early and consistent screening is the key to promptly detecting breast cancer caused by the two known inherited mutations. When carriers are routinely screened, cancer can be caught at a treatable stage. For carriers of either mutation, risk has been estimated to be as high as 85 percent from age twenty-five onward.

Barbara (who didn't want her last initial used) is a BRCA1 carrier. She says the prevalence of the BRCA mutations was identified among Ashkenazi Jews because so many volunteered to be in the scientific studies. The volunteers were determined to help scientists solve one of the biggest genetic questions of the twentieth century.

Yet Barbara has deep concerns about a number of issues involving genetic risk. As the mother of a teenage daughter, she laments that so few options are available to help her daughter avoid cancer, if it turns out that the youngster is a carrier as well. "I absolutely do not believe that prophylactic mastectomy [voluntary surgical removal of the breasts for the purpose of preventing breast cancer] is an option most young women would even want to consider," she says.

Her concerns are also riveted on another key issue: the privacy of medical information. She wants to know how carefully it can be guarded. If one family member is found to be a carrier, she asks, how well protected is the medical information of other relatives who then must undergo routine cancer screening as a result?

Even if her daughter does not choose to be tested for the gene, Barbara says, her medical records would be a red flag because "here you would have a young girl coming in on a regular basis for mammograms. It's crazy. Her records would be a dead giveaway, even without BRCA stamped all over them." And she has other questions. Barbara wonders whether routine cancer screenings of women at high risk are identifying enough breast cancers in the early stages. Barbara had a bilateral mastectomy after she was diagnosed at age forty-one.

Dr. Ellen Warner, of the Sunnybrook Regional Cancer Center in Toronto, Canada, wrote in the *Journal of the American Medical Association* that women with the mutations are advised to begin routine screening for breast cancer at twenty-five. Screenings for the general population usually begin around forty.

In her study, Dr. Warner reported that even with breast examinations being performed by a doctor every six months and mammography once a year, cancers were still not being detected at an early stage in some women with the BRCA genes. In her analysis of 236 women aged twenty-five to sixty-five, all of them carriers of one of the two genetic mutations, Dr. Warner found that among those who were screened by MRI (see Chapter 1), cancers were caught earlier.[3]

ASIAN WOMEN AND THE MIGRATION STORY

In migration studies of women who have moved from Japan to the United States, medical scientists have found that the incidence of breast cancer increases sixfold. (Although a 500 percent increase is shocking, it still does not bring Japanese immigrants anywhere near the higher rates of breast cancer seen in other segments of the U.S. population.) Researchers have speculated that the switch from traditional Japanese dietary habits to the average American diet may help explain the dramatic difference. To date, however, there is no proof that dietary changes alone fully account for the striking increase in the number of cases.

What is noteworthy, though, is that the sharp jump between lower rates of breast cancer in Japan and higher rates when Japanese women move to the United States is something researchers have seen time and again for more than two decades, which suggests that it is real and not a statistical fluke. Does that mean women in Japan have special defenses against breast cancer? Some scientists say there is a possibility that Japanese women carry genes that predispose them to lower risk. This trait, coupled with a traditional

Japanese diet, may help explain the lower rates of breast cancer in Japan. Whatever provides the protection is vulnerable to loss upon migration, and therein lies the deepest part of the mystery.

Given the fact that lower rates of breast cancer are prevalent in Japan, are similar rates of low incidence seen elsewhere in Asia? While the answer, generally, is yes—and those low rates continue to be seen when women from other Asian countries immigrate to the United States—new studies suggest Korean researchers are finding evidence of BRCA mutations.

Doctors in Korea are seeing a notable number of younger patients—women under age forty—with invasive breast cancer. The youth of these women is an indication that mutated genes may underlie the upsurge. Again, the number of cases comes nowhere near the proportion of women in the United States of all ethnicities who develop the disease, but the increasing number of cases being detected in Korea is helping medical researchers better understand the pervasiveness of gene mutations that can lead to breast cancer.

Doctors at the University of Ulsan Asian Medical Center in Seoul, found mutations in BRCA1 and BRCA2 in 12.7 percent of 173 patients being treated for breast cancer.[4] The study was published in 2004 in the *Journal of Korean Medical Science*. The analysis also found in a control group that 2.8 percent of cancer-free women possessed one of the two genetic flaws. In high-risk patients, BRCA1 and 2 mutations were found to be most prevalent in those with a family history of breast and ovarian cancers, male breast cancer, bilateral breast cancer, and multiple organ cancer, including breast cancer. The findings are surprising because in the United States Koreans have the lowest breast cancer incidence of all ethnic groups.

AN AFRICAN AMERICAN DILEMMA

One of the biggest conundrums in the demographics of breast cancer is the high mortality among African American women. Black women with breast cancer are more likely to die of the disease than any other group in the United States. Government figures show a death rate for African American women of 31.4 women per 100,000, compared with 25.7 per 100,000 for Caucasian women. As the death rate has continued to decline for whites it has gone up for blacks. Overall, African Americans have a lower incidence of the disease than Caucasians. But a small segment of the black population—women under forty—has a higher incidence than whites.

A majority of cases among white women occur past the age of fifty. Among African Americans, the disproportionate number of younger women with the disease has triggered the alarm of activists who want to know why. Breast cancer is a difficult diagnosis regardless of the age at which it is diagnosed. However, it can be far more difficult for the patient to cope with and for the physician to treat when the woman is young. Older women are more likely to have hormone-receptor-positive cancers, for which there are a number of very effective treatments. Hormone-receptor-negative cancers—the type often seen in younger women—tend to be more aggressive and often more difficult to treat. Overall, regardless of race, about eleven thousand women age forty and younger develop breast cancer annually in the United States, accounting for about 5 percent of invasive disease cases.

Among premenopausal African American women, studies have found that the disease can be particularly virulent. Thus, it comes as no surprise that issues involving black women and breast cancer have produced a very complex picture.

Researchers reporting in the June 2003 issue of the journal *Cancer* found that African American women under the age of fifty had lower survival rates than their white counterparts, even when the type and stage of their cancers were identical. Yet the same study found no discernable differences in treatment or survival among blacks and whites sixty-five and older who were on Medicare. The findings suggested that treatments were essentially equal under Medicare.

The analysis, led by Dr. Kenneth Chu, program director of the Center to Reduce Cancer Health Disparities, a division of the National Cancer Institute, used the vast SEER database to identify cases and to determine what kinds of treatments patients received.[5] Dr. Chu and his colleagues compared tumors between black and white women according to hormone-receptor status and cancer stage. That way, women with Stage II, estrogen-receptor-positive (ER+) cancers were compared with other Stage II, ER+ patients, and Stage III, ER– patients were compared with other Stage III, ER– patients, etc. The study concluded that it is not just the biology of the disease that is important, but that access to health care also makes a difference, especially for younger women. The research underscored that a lack of health insurance among younger black women was linked to poor outcomes. The study was commended for its insight and hailed as the kind of research that added context to a long-standing problem.

Other studies have suggested that African Americans are more likely to seek treatment only after a tumor has advanced. Still others have shown that black women generally do not avail themselves of screening programs, which suggests that tumors are not being detected at an early, treatable stage.

What Do Advocates Say?

Advocates for African American patients say the higher death rate and trend toward younger black women developing the disease is one of the biggest issues facing the cancer research community today. Reona Berry, a breast cancer survivor and cofounder of the African American Breast Cancer Alliance in Minneapolis, notes that many of the women seeking membership in and information from the organization are pre–middle age. She says, "We've noticed ever since we started out that a lot of the women are thirty-five, forty, certainly under forty-five. We thought, Why isn't that information getting out; why don't people know this? There are more and more younger African American women being diagnosed all over the country. It has been proven that black women have a more aggressive type of breast cancer. The biology of the disease is more difficult." The alliance, which began its work in 1990, runs support groups in Minnesota and reaches a larger population through its website and biannual newsletter.

Dr. Lovell Jones, a professor of gynecologic oncology and molecular biology at M.D. Anderson Cancer Center in Houston, believes that focusing only on problems of health-care access misses larger, more complex matters. The notion that African American women are not seeking treatment early in the course of their disease does not explain all cases, he says, and also essentially blames an entire ethnic group for poor outcomes:

> The problem facing black women is one that largely affects other women of color. There is an attitude of blaming the victim. I think the inadequate-access argument has been overplayed. We really don't know much about the genetics of the disease in black women. The tide is beginning to change a little. I've been speaking about the need to study the genetics of breast cancer in African Americans as being more of a concern than access to care, but it has been like beating one's head against a stone wall. When you look at the things the government spends money on it really begs the question where health care fits in. Health care is not a priority in this nation—for anyone. The research budget for the National Institutes of Health is twenty-four billion dollars. But eighty-seven billion dollars was spent on Iraq for just one year. So where is the priority?

Dr. Jones, who is also director of the Center for Research on Minority Health at M.D. Anderson, believes that scientists need to frame new research questions to better understand why African Americans are more likely to die of breast cancer. He says:

> We need to change how we do research. We can no longer afford to just define the problem. We can no longer do the same kinds of studies that were done in the twentieth century. As medicine has moved more toward managed care, time and money have become bigger issues in health care, and there is still a tendency toward "patient profiling." If you're African American or Hispanic some doctors automatically assume you may not be able to pay for certain therapies. So the kind of care you're prescribed can be based on what you look like, and that of course can have an impact on your survival. The Institute of Medicine documented this. So researchers must look at those kinds of issues as they frame the questions that their studies will explore.

Zora Brown, founder of the Breast Cancer Resource Committee in Washington, D.C., says the disproportionate number of young African American women developing breast cancer suggests that a genetic link may underlie the higher incidence. The only way to be certain, she says, is to conduct the research to find out. "One of the things I get very disturbed about is that the only studies we have say that [African Americans'] cancers are much more virulent. What we don't have are enough data to understand why. I think researchers definitely need to understand why the cancers are more aggressive. They can't just say it's obesity or the environment or poverty, or there was a lack of compliance [with the regimen of care]. The women in our group are very compliant; insurance is not an issue. We need to know why so many young black women are developing breast cancer."

In 2004, a collaborative effort by researchers at the Fred Hutchinson Cancer Research Center in Seattle, Emory University in Atlanta, and the CDC found abnormal p53 genes in tumors of a group of black patients with the disease. The research also discovered—as previous studies have found—that black women had particularly aggressive tumors. Meanwhile, Dr. Olufunmilayo Olopade, a physician-scientist at the University of Chicago, has been studying breast cancer in African American families to determine which genes may be related to aggressive disease at younger ages. Dr. Olopade has been researching the possibility that BRCA1 and BRCA2 may play a prominent role in the breast cancers of African American women because of the virulence of the cancers and the youth of the women who are being diagnosed. As Zora Brown mentioned earlier in this chapter, few African American families were studied in the original BRCA1 and 2 research projects.

Cassandra Y., an African American breast cancer survivor who developed the disease at thirty-six, was stunned when her doctor told her she had breast cancer.

> I didn't want to believe it. I didn't think I fit the image of somebody with breast cancer. When I thought of breast cancer I thought of someone very rich, very glamorous, and white, like Suzanne Somers.

Cassandra's doctor helped her understand that there is no "image" of someone with breast cancer. All women, the doctor said, are vulnerable.

> My doctor, who is one of the sweetest people in the world, told me I had to throw that image out of my head. She said she was at risk. Every woman I had ever seen and will see is at risk. She told me to stop worrying about what somebody with breast cancer should look like, and to start paying attention to how I was going to fight it.

Another Look at Hormones and Risk

When Dr. Patricia Ganz noted earlier in this chapter that those who carry a genetic risk for breast cancer start out with a predisposing mutation at birth, she alluded to the fact that most other people acquire mutations later in life. Random mutations triggered by hormone exposure are a substantial part of the story in breast cancer risk factors. You are exposed to your natural hormones throughout life, yet, as vital as they are, doctors theorize that in some instances they can help promote the development of cancer. Note that this does not mean that your hormones are bad and that you should have done something early on to suppress them.

Throughout life hormones influence a wide range of biological functions. Estrogen, the blanket name given to several chemically similar compounds, is the primary female sex hormone. It is produced largely by the ovaries. It has dramatic effects throughout the body. In the skeletal system estrogen maintains bone density and strength. In the vascular system estrogen keeps blood vessels pliable and influences the function of high-density lipoproteins, the so-called good form of cholesterol. After menopause, hormones produced by the adrenal glands (which lie just above the kidneys) can be converted into estrogen.

A major function of estrogen is to trigger the thickening of the uterine lining during the first phase of the menstrual cycle. It is then that it also activates cellular growth in the breasts, increasing the density of the tissue. Progesterone, another key female hormone, prompts changes in the uterine lining during the second phase of the menstrual cycle. These changes facilitate implantation of a fertilized egg.

Lesbians and Breast Cancer Risk

For years medical researchers have recognized that women who are lesbians have a higher risk of breast cancer than do women who are heterosexual. The increased risk has nothing to do with sexual orientation but rather with several underlying reasons, one of which is key: Lesbians are less likely to seek regular medical care. The Mautner Project: The National Lesbian Health Organization notes that lesbians are less likely to seek routine health care because of their discomfort with disclosing information about their sexual orientation. As a consequence, women who partner with women also are less likely to undergo routine gynecologic exams, which generally include a clinical breast examination and encouragement for routine mammography. Other reasons cited by the organization are that lesbians are less likely to give birth by the age of thirty, if at all. Delaying childbirth and not having children are breast cancer risk factors (see the section "Estrogen, Aging, and Breast Cancer Risk"). The Mautner Project underscores another important point: Lesbians are more directly affected by women's lower earning potential, and they lack the benefit of a spouse's health-insurance coverage. Among the group's recommendations are getting routine mammograms after age thirty-five, establishing an open relationship with a health-care provider, and visiting that provider on a regular basis.

Estrogen, Aging, and Breast Cancer Risk

The role of estrogen as a breast cancer risk factor revolves around one simple issue: time. The longer a person is exposed to the hormone, the greater her risk for breast cancer. This increased risk is evident among women who began their menstrual cycle before they reached the age of twelve or whose menopause began after the age of fifty-five. Dr. Ganz emphasizes that, as important as estrogen is in the monthly cycle, it can have a deleterious effect on the breast tissue over time. "Every month," she says, "a woman's breasts are responding to the estrogen level present in the first half of the cycle and progesterone in the second half. The cells are responding as if there will be a pregnancy. The estrogen in the blood goes to the nucleus of cells in the breasts and the uterus and tells them to up-regulate growth and cell division. So there's a repetitive stimulation of the tissue. When rapidly growing and dividing in this way over periods of many years, a chance mutation can occur."

In fact, the longer the exposure the greater the likelihood that many random mutations can occur. Beginning menstruation early or starting menopause late are not the only ways in which a woman can be overexposed to estrogen. Waiting until after age thirty to start having children or never giving birth at all are two other ways. (During pregnancy the monthly menstrual cycle halts, and estrogen's activity in the body is much more concentrated.) Historians and anthropologists have supported the credibility of the medical literature by adding their accounts about breast cancer prevalence in certain populations. For instance, breast cancer occurs in higher than average frequency among Roman Catholic nuns because their vows of celibacy mean they do not bear children. Nuns' predisposition to breast cancer has helped scientists further bolster theories on how prolonged estrogen exposure might lead to the disease. Medical evidence involving nuns and breast cancer has been documented for more than three hundred years.

In this chapter we have explored the nature of breast cancer risk as it relates to genes and hormones. In the next chapter we'll address the concept of risk again, looking this time at a few risk factors that are currently drawing exceptionally bright spotlights. The aim of both chapters is to underscore the fact that risk is an elevation of chance. It is not to be confused with a direct cause-and-effect relationship.

Chapter 6

A Primer on Risks, Part II: Obesity, Hormone Replacement Therapy, and Other Exposures

If you are unaware of what is being called the growing prevalence of obesity in the United States (it's even a "global pandemic" according to some who are prone to hyperbole), then surely you have been vacationing on another planet. Daily reports are of a crisis so big, so outsized, so out of proportion, that the only things matching the enormity of the problem are the growing backsides of average Americans.

Generally, the debate over obesity is a welcome one in the ongoing discussions about how body weight can affect health. The links between excess weight and heart disease, diabetes, and stroke are well known. A developing body of knowledge has been finding links between excess body weight and cancer. An unfortunate outgrowth of all this attention, however, is that some journalists and many Internet "bloggers" have elevated the results of some preliminary studies to the weight of final scientific word, missing, it seems, some of the nuances contained in the studies themselves. The trend is particularly disturbing when it comes to breast cancer.

Many lay writers with access to the public's eyes and ears have seized on an attention-capturing sound bite: Obesity causes breast cancer. Indeed, anyone with access to cable TV probably has seen news reports where the subject is breast cancer but the cameras are trained on paunchy stomachs and bulging, big butts as the voice-over announces the killer consequences of fat.

The truth about obesity and breast cancer is this: It is a moderate (not a major) risk factor for women who develop the disease after menopause. It is also a "modifiable" one, which means you can lose weight to avoid its becoming a risk factor for a recurrence. Body fat by itself does not trigger the disease, so obesity does not "cause" breast cancer. The link between excess body fat and breast cancer resides in the fact that body fat is one site where postmenopausal estrogen is produced (muscles are another site). As mentioned in the last chapter, estrogen over time can stimulate certain breast tumors to develop and grow. The effect, therefore, is cumulative. It is not a situation where someone could in a year or two overeat her way into a breast cancer diagnosis.

Having excess padding, as it turns out, is an unusual card in the deck of breast cancer risk factors. Not all overweight postmenopausal women develop the disease, and in younger women being overweight appears to provide *protection* against breast cancer, something that stands out as a mystery in the ongoing discussions about cancer and body fat. No doctor anywhere in the world would encourage a premenopausal woman to gain weight to acquire breast cancer protection. But rest assured, reasons for the phenomenon are being vigorously researched.

This chapter examines the obesity debate as it relates to breast cancer. Activists, as you'll soon read, take issue with the charge that obesity causes breast cancer. Reports of obesity's link to breast cancer, they say, are aimed at a general audience that is cancer-free. For people in the general population the underlying message is how to reduce the risk to prevent the disease. For those who've been diagnosed, they add, the message can be interpreted quite differently: You caused your cancer. You pigged out so much that you ate your way into a life-threatening disease. Activists worry about the fallout from such reports, especially about how the news may affect the resolve of patients trying to overcome cancer. However, Dr. Mary Jane

Massie, the mental health expert, says that even though women who are overweight have anxieties about their size, most are able to put those worries aside as they face down the disease that has changed their lives.

Following the discussion about body fat, the issue of hormone replacement therapy is explored. Prescribed for decades to treat not only hot flashes and menopausal mood swings, HRT was touted as a veritable cure-all for some of humankind's most dreaded afflictions: heart disease, strokes, and Alzheimer's disease. A massive study by the Women's Health Initiative debunked those beliefs and at the same time raised a red flag about breast cancer risk. The chapter ends with a look at other moderate risk factors, including alcohol consumption.

The Role of Obesity in Breast Cancer

One of the more complicated issues in medical science is the role of obesity in breast cancer. The National Cancer Institute defines obesity as fat constituting "an abnormal proportion" of overall body mass. It is defined more precisely as having a body mass index— BMI—of thirty or above. The Nurse's Health Study, an ongoing research project that explores health issues involving women, found that postmenopausal women who gained at least forty-four pounds after age eighteen had twice the risk of developing the disease as did women who gained fewer than five.

A study published in an August 2003 edition of the *Journal of the National Cancer Institute* showed that postmenopausal women who had a BMI of thirty or more had blood-estrogen concentrations ranging from 60 percent to 219 percent higher than thin women. The breast cancer rate, the researchers found, increased at an average of about 18 percent per five-point increase in BMI. On average, this study found that obese women had a 19 percent risk of developing breast cancer.[1]

But when these same researchers adjusted their data for the specific types of estrogen in circulation (as mentioned earlier, there is more than one type of estrogen), the 19 percent risk had to be lowered to a 2 percent risk. What this means is that additional studies must be conducted to further ferret out the links between excess weight and breast cancer.

In another area that is being investigated, Dr. Larry Norton, physician-in-chief at Memorial Sloan-Kettering Cancer Center in New York City, says overweight postmenopausal women tend to have larger tumors at the time of diagnosis than do those who are thin. Again, the theory is that estrogen produced in fat tissue can serve as a stimulus for growth, and larger tumors tend to have a poorer prognosis.

Still, Dr. Silvana Martino, an associate professor of medicine at the University of Southern California in Los Angeles, says that among risk factors, obesity does not rank nearly as high as would a genetic predisposition caused by one of the known breast cancer mutations. As Dr. Martino sees it, the issue of being overweight and its relationship to breast cancer still leaves some important questions unanswered.

> Obesity is an issue for women who are postmenopausal but not for women who are premenopausal. And I don't know that anyone can give you a good answer why that is so. Remember, fat becomes a major source of estrogen when women get older [because of an enzyme called aromatase that converts certain hormones—prohormones—into estrogen]. While this conversion occurs in premenopausal women, it is really quite minor compared to what the ovaries are able to make. In postmenopausal women, this conversion provides the only source of estrogen, and this can be viewed as a problem because the more fat a woman has, the more estrogen she is able to produce. The way to reduce risk is to get the woman to lose weight, to reduce the body's fat content, which should lead to less estrogen production.

Among the newer classes of breast cancer drugs are those called aromatase inhibitors, which will be discussed in greater detail in Chapter 10. These medications, designed for postmenopausal women, are capable of shutting down all estrogen produced by way of the enzymatic conversion in fat and other tissues in the body.

Aromatase inhibitors are prescribed to women who are normal weight, overweight, and obese.

Dr. Martino, one of the country's leading breast cancer researchers, has been looking into the benefits of yet another type of drug aimed at treating women with postmenopausal breast cancer. Her work will be discussed at greater length in Chapter 10.

What Do Activists Say?

Activists, meanwhile, want answers to a long list of questions regarding weight, body fat, BMI, and breast cancer. Why is breast cancer seen across a spectrum of BMIs, they ask. And what are the risk factors for slimmer women who exercise regularly but who still develop the disease? As people who work closely with the newly diagnosed through support groups, activists are concerned about the psychological issues associated with breast cancer and the effect that provocative but still inconclusive reports have on patients undergoing treatment.

Geri Barish, executive director of Hewlett House, on Long Island, has been one of the most vocal advocates for more than a decade. Geri waged her own battle against the disease, and as an activist helped call national attention to the higher than usual rate of breast cancer in her region of New York. Geri believes that a number of issues involving weight and breast cancer need to be addressed—none of them flashy enough to lead the evening news but nevertheless of enormous concern to those with the disease. On her wish list would be more studies that seek ways of helping women who gain weight while undergoing cancer therapy.

Weight gain during breast cancer treatment is common, she says, and it's a reason for anxiety among some patients. Some women eat to ease symptoms of nausea. In other instances the effects of certain medications, such as steroids, influence weight increase. Geri says one woman she knew craved ice cream and ate it constantly during chemotherapy. Another ate only carrots throughout her treatment; she was following what she believed to be a cancer-prevention diet.

Geri is also concerned about how breast cancer is reported on by the media. Casting the nation's problem with breast cancer as part of the obesity epidemic, she says, is a disturbing throwback. She would like to see news agencies report studies with more context and caveats, and with less emphasis on sensationalism.

> It's as if we've returned to the dark ages of history. You ate the wrong thing, you drank the wrong thing. You're the problem. That's why the [activist] organizations began in the first place. We wanted genuine answers. There are women in our support groups of all shapes and sizes. They certainly are not all overweight. There are people who really watch their weight, who exercise regularly and do all of the right things, and they still wind up with breast cancer.
>
> So this angers me when I hear this [that obesity causes breast cancer]. If you went into a room with a thousand people and all one thousand of them had breast cancer, you wouldn't find two people sitting at any of the tables who were the same size, same shape, or same waist measurement. I've spoken to many scientists about breast cancer, and they say there's not any one single thing causing this disease. It's multifactorial. That's why they feel looking into the genetics of breast cancer will help them come up with strong answers.
>
> We would hate to hear someone say, "I caused this. I gave myself breast cancer." This is such a complex disease that I don't think any one factor can explain it. Also, the concept of who is obese keeps changing. It used to be that size twelve was a pretty reasonable size. Now there are gyms everywhere and young women are working very hard to be size one and size zero. I think fashion is helping to drive some of the concepts of who's fat and who's not.

Zora K. Brown, founder of the Breast Cancer Resource Committee in Washington, D.C., agrees that the types of tumors seen in cases of invasive breast cancer are extremely complex and probably cannot be explained away by a single risk factor. She says:

> We haven't been given good answers about how obesity relates to breast cancer. I hate even the word *obesity;* what does it mean? It really says, "Let's blame this person's breast

cancer on her for being overweight." Yes, we see larger women in support groups, but we see a larger population [throughout the United States] in general. I think it's an insulting word, and using it really doesn't compel people to change their behavior. I sat on an advisory panel that examined the link between obesity and breast cancer [during which scientists presented their data on obesity to panelists]. After they finished, they said they wanted members of the advisory panel to develop programs that would allow the scientists to come and lecture the women [in support groups] about obesity and breast cancer. Lecture. That's the word they used. Lecture.

Zora says the scientists' aim was to tell women diagnosed with breast cancer how obesity relates to the disease. As executive director of an organization that sponsors support group meetings, she says that she would not allow them to burden women trying to fight the disease with imprecise data while offering no way to help them as patients. "I said no way. No way were they coming to lecture us about obesity and breast cancer. On the one hand they explained that obesity had a protective effect—that it helped prevent breast cancer. On the other they said postmenopausal women were at higher risk. They couldn't explain why. That's what was important, explaining *why* there was such a difference. I think if we are ever going to get people to change their behaviors, we have to talk about the health of the individual, about survivorship, and not about what they may or may not have done to cause their disease."

Which Is the Real Risk Factor: Body Weight or Seeing a Doctor Too Late?

While scientists are still trying to work out the finer details that would explain obesity's role in breast cancer, particularly how it might protect younger women but provide the fuel to harm older ones, medical experts have collected other compelling data on weight and cancer. For more than a decade doctors have documented evidence showing that overweight and obese women are less likely than their slimmer counterparts to undergo breast cancer screening and that they are equally less likely than thinner women to seek a physician's care for any kind of medical complaint.

In one of the earliest studies on the issue of screening and being overweight, researchers at Beth Israel-New England Deaconess Medical Center in Boston found that not only were overweight women less likely to be screened for breast or cervical cancers, but they were also more likely to die of the two disorders.[2]

The study, which appeared in the *Annals of Internal Medicine*, analyzed data from 8,394 women between the ages of eighteen and seventy-five. When the data were adjusted for factors such as socioeconomic status, ethnicity, and education, researchers still found lower rates of screening among those who were overweight.

In the group of women ages fifty to seventy-five, 62 percent in the obese group and 64 percent in the overweight group had received a mammogram in the two years preceding the study. These percentages compared with 68 percent of thinner women in the same age group who had received a mammogram during the same period of time.

Even though the study was not designed to explain why overweight and obese women are less likely to be screened, the study's lead investigator suggested that attitudes toward these women by health-care professionals could be one explanation. Additional possibilities are a general feeling of low self-esteem and possessing a poor notion of body image. These psychological barriers may dissuade women from undergoing medical tests that involve getting undressed.

Psychological Issues and Obesity

Women who are overweight, with and without breast cancer, usually are burdened with anxieties because they live in a culture that not only admires thinness as a virtue and constantly promotes the health benefits of a low body mass index, but elevates it as a symbol of beauty. Dr. Mary Jane Massie, of Memorial Sloan-Kettering Cancer Center, says despite the psychological and emotional issues associated with being overweight, most women facing breast cancer do not let their problems with obesity get in the way of cancer treatment.

> People who struggle with real obesity do not feel good about themselves because of their obesity. But do people who have serious weight problems blame their cancer on their weight? No. I think that women today know that a very small percentage of breast cancers are hereditary, and that scientists are not really able to explain the rest.

> You can't go back and lose the ten pounds that you should have lost ten years ago. What you have to reduce now is stress. Breast cancer sometimes is an opportunity for arranging a more manageable life. Some women say in the aftermath of the diagnosis and treatment, "I realized how precious my life is." Some women will say cancer is a wake-up call. The past is thrown out with yesterday's newspaper and half-eaten sandwich. They'll say, "Today is what I have to deal with, and if I can make positive changes in my life, isn't that good?"

> I certainly have met and worked with many women who have been very careful about what they've eaten, careful about exercise, and careful about their weight, and who still have gotten breast cancer. Those women are sometimes very, very disappointed. They say, "I've been very careful; I've done all of the right things."

> I think for a lot of women who have breast cancer the real issue is "Now, what's ahead for me?"

What Do Patients Say?

When Carla D., fifty-eight, was diagnosed with breast cancer a decade ago, she weighed 210 pounds.

> If you're going to print what I have to say, I don't want you to give people the impression I look like a blob. I'm five-foot-ten—not petite by any stretch—but I've lost about thirty pounds since being diagnosed with breast cancer, and I've kept it off. Do I think obesity put me at higher risk for breast

cancer? I never considered myself obese to begin with. Over-weight, yes; but not obese. Others in my family—my Dad, my cousin—had cancer and were rail thin. No one else has had breast cancer.

So, to answer the question, Do I think obesity put me at higher risk? Okay, this is how I want to answer that question, and don't get me wrong, I'm very pleased to tell my story. But to be honest, we're talking about weight, and there's a lot more to me than just size, like, how I got through cancer treat-ments and how I'm a ten-year survivor. That's what I'm most proud of, and my family. Ask anybody who's had breast can-cer and who has made it to this point, and they'll probably say the same thing: surviving is what's most important to them. I don't know how I got breast cancer. I don't think any-body knows. The doctors certainly aren't concerned about that. I just know I got past it.

Maryanne B., who had trouble convincing a physician to order a mammogram for a lump she found in her breast, believes some physicians do not treat overweight patients with the same amount of respect accorded those who are thin. Scientific studies have cor-roborated that notion. Maryanne says when doctors focus on their patients' weight, it becomes difficult for the patient to concentrate on her medical issue.

He said to me, "You're extremely large on top, kiddo." Or he would say something that would kind of sound like a joke but really wasn't. The last time I went there he said, "Oh, the Bobbsey twins are back." It was really frustrating, not to men-tion insulting. I was always leaving that place feeling insulted. I even asked, and I asked politely, that he not make references to me like that, but he ignored me. You would think when your patient is coming in trying to find out if she has breast cancer, the doctor would not be so fixated. But what could I do? I couldn't just throw up my hands and say to hell with it. I couldn't stop trying to figure out what was wrong, just be-cause I didn't like the doctor. I had to get a diagnosis and I had to go to his office because he was our primary care physi-cian. He's the guy the insurance company was paying.

Helen S., who admits only to weighing over two hundred pounds, believes her weight probably contributed to her breast cancer because her doctors have connected other nagging health conditions to her weight.

> The diabetes diagnosis came first, seven years ago, and I was diagnosed with high blood pressure a couple of years after that. Then came the breast cancer, so there was a progression of things, none of them good. My doctor is always saying lose weight, reduce, reduce, reduce—get serious. I *am* serious. I'm telling you, I've done Weight Watchers and Jenny Craig, NutriSystem, mall walking—you name it. I'm on Atkins now. No one told me being overweight makes breast cancer more likely. None of my doctors ever said that. But why am I not surprised? Nothing surprises me about being heavy.

Why Has Weight Become a Breast Cancer Issue?

In addition to studies that have linked postmenopausal estrogen exposure to breast cancer, others have suggested that insulin, a pancreatic hormone, may help drive the growth of cancer cells in those who carry extra weight. It is another theory researchers are investigating. When more fat tissue is present, higher levels of insulin are in circulation. With weight loss, insulin levels are lowered. While weight can be changed as a breast cancer risk factor, other moderate risk factors cannot, such as when you began menstruating and when you entered menopause.

Yet some experts say more definitive answers regarding breast cancer and its relationship to obesity may be a long time coming, because scientists have yet to answer many important questions about obesity itself. Some people have an extremely difficult time losing weight, especially as they age. And the subject of obesity is so intricately intertwined with social values, social perceptions, and concepts of morality that some activists say they first would like to see some of those layers peeled away as scientists embark upon new rounds of study.

In a report appearing in the July 2004 *Tufts University Health and Nutrition Letter* that addressed concerns involving obesity, nutrition therapist Heather Bell, MPH, R.D., of the Tufts-New England Medical Center, said obesity is as much a physiological problem as it is a social one. "We're told over and over, explicitly and implicitly, that obesity is a character flaw," she said.[3]

The article explored themes that have surfaced repeatedly in the obesity debate: Why can't people simply eat less and exercise more? According to Bell, that perception is "overly simplistic," and one that has become particularly "moralistic." Even nutritionists, she suggested, have not yet fully figured out why some people tend to gain large amounts of weight and maintain it, while others who consume similar diets and expend similar amounts of energy through exercise do not. "With some people," she wrote, "once they have gained a lot of weight there could be something in their physiology that vigorously defends the higher weight in the face of significant behavioral changes."

Hormone Replacement Therapy (HRT)

In July 2002, the principal investigators in the Women's Health Initiative, a large nationwide study group, announced that hormone replacement therapy was not as beneficial as doctors had once thought. The combined pill of equine (horse) estrogen and synthetic progesterone that women took to ward off hot flashes, night sweats, and other symptoms of menopause apparently raised the risk of breast cancer and other dangerous health disorders.

The announcement did not come as an eye-popping surprise. Many smaller, statistical studies conducted throughout the 1990s in the United States and Britain had found evidence of elevated breast cancer risk among women who took HRT. These smaller studies were being reported even as many doctors continued to tell women that HRT protected them from heart disease, Alzheimer's, and osteoporosis. Doctors weren't doing this because they were shills for the pharmaceutical industry. They did it because there were still other statistical studies—and anecdotal data—that strongly suggested that HRT had a long list of benefits.

As results ultimately would reveal, the pills actually contributed to heart attacks and strokes. Muddling the matter even further, HRT did nothing to protect the brain from Alzheimer's disease. The hormones provided a modicum of protection against osteoporosis and colorectal cancer, but the risk associated with taking the pills to prevent those conditions was greater than the small amount of protection that was offered.

The actual day-to-day regimen for participants in the Women's Health Initiative, a government-sponsored research project, involved taking either the daily hormone tablet or a harmless placebo. More than sixteen thousand women at forty centers in the United States participated. When researchers found that women taking HRT had higher rates of breast cancer, heart attack, and stroke, they stopped the study prematurely to let women outside of the study know that the risks outweighed the benefits. The study, reported in the *Journal of the American Medical Association*, found a 26 percent increase in breast cancer, a 29 percent increase in heart attacks, and a 26 percent increase in strokes. Heart attacks and strokes increased because HRT elevated levels of blood clotting.[4]

Drs. Suzanne Fletcher and Graham Colditz, writing in an editorial in the journal, invoked words from the Latin Hippocratic oath in an effort to change the prescribing habits of doctors around the country. "We recommend that clinicians stop prescribing this combination for long-term use," they wrote. "*Prinum non nocere* [first do no harm] applies especially to preventive medicine."

Later in 2002, a British study of more than one million women produced similar results. Dr. Valerie Beral, lead investigator of that project, reported that the use of HRT had produced twenty thousand cases of breast cancer in Great Britain that otherwise would not have been expected. Finally, Swedish researchers in 2004 found that women who took HRT after being treated for breast cancer experienced higher rates of cancer recurrence than women who refrained from taking the pills.

A Patient and a Physician Ponder HRT

Jeanne G., sixty-three, whose breast cancer was diagnosed shortly before she and her husband were to retire to Florida, had her first and only child at age thirty-eight and experienced menopause in her late forties. She was on and off hormone replacement therapy for several years. Jeanne has wondered whether HRT contributed to her cancer, but she says there is no way to be certain.

> Who knows? I mean, who really knows? My most basic instinct was to fight the cancer and to put that entire episode in the past tense. I was a very motivated patient—motivated like you wouldn't believe. Now I'm a motivated survivor. That means I definitely don't want to travel the cancer road again. I watch what I eat. I get a lot of exercise. I'm doing everything conceivable to stay healthy. Maybe HRT was a mistake, I don't know. Really, I can't dwell on that.

Dr. Mary Jane Massie, of Memorial Sloan-Kettering Cancer Center, says some women who took HRT and later developed breast cancer are not sorry they were on hormones. "Many of those women who had been taking hormones are happy they did it. Breast cancer occurs in women who have never taken hormones. There is a slight increase in breast cancer in those who took HRT. I think women who read the results of the studies are aware of that. And the women I've seen are saying, 'My hormones may have done it, but I'm glad I did [take hormone replacement therapy].' I don't think this is a devastating thing to women. I think the press made a big deal out of it."

Lifestyle Issues and Breast Cancer Risk

Over the years reams of studies have pointed to a veritable laundry list of potential risks for breast cancer. Many studies of lifestyle issues have failed to produce compelling enough evidence to warrant considering them a serious threat. One lifestyle issue, the consumption of fatty foods, has received considerable scientific attention, but medical researchers have yet to find what the connection between dietary fat and increased breast cancer risk might be.

Here are a few lifestyle risk factors for which studies have shown at least how a biological mechanism might enhance the risk of breast cancer:

- ❖ Consumption of alcoholic beverages

- ❖ Smoking

- ❖ Consumption of broiled and pan-fried meats cooked at high temperatures

- ❖ Lack of exercise

Does Alcohol Consumption Raise the Risk of Breast Cancer?

There is one thing about which scientists are certain: Alcohol consumption may play a beneficial role for those who consume it to prevent heart disease. Taking a daily sip, nip, or shot of your favorite spirits can be a surefire way to keep the old ticker intact. However, alcohol and its relationship to breast cancer, studies reveal, is a completely different matter. Drinking alcohol, study after study has shown, can increase the risk of the disease. Here's the sixty-four-thousand-dollar question: How much is too much?

Researchers at Harvard School of Public Health reported as long ago as 1998 that women who regularly drink alcoholic beverages are at elevated risk of breast cancer when compared with teetotalers. Although several smaller studies have come out since the late 1990s, the Harvard study remains the largest of its kind, having analyzed alcohol-consumption data from 322,647 women in the United States, Canada, Sweden, and the Netherlands. Among those women, more than 4,300 developed breast cancer. Researchers concluded that women who drink two to five alcoholic beverages a day have up to a 41 percent higher risk of developing invasive breast cancer than women who abstain.[5]

In the study, researchers reported that virtually any regular amount of alcohol consumption drives up the risk of breast cancer. Scientists demonstrated that for every ten grams of alcohol a woman consumes per day, her breast cancer risk goes up by 9 percent. In terms of glasses of wine or bottles of beer, the amount in grams works out this way: Thirty to sixty grams of alcohol equals 2.8 to 5.6 glasses of wine or 2.3 to 4.5 bottles of beer. In terms of hard liquor, such as whiskey, that amount of alcohol is consumed in a mere two shots.

Although scientists are not certain, they theorize that several possible biological mechanisms may come into play to make alcohol a breast cancer risk factor. One is that alcohol may influence the activity of hormones in the body, particularly estrogen. As mentioned earlier, lifetime estrogen exposure is a primary risk factor for the disease. What has yet to be determined is whether blood alcohol drives up estrogen levels, or whether alcohol prevents estrogen's breakdown. Because of questions that remain unanswered about how alcohol directly influences estrogen, and through which precise biological pathways, scientists at least for now are not calling it a major risk factor.

Foods and Breast Cancer Risk

Scientists at the National Cancer Institute (NCI) have looked at high-heat grilling of meats and have found a potential risk for breast cancer. Results of the NCI work, along with similar analyses from several other researchers, were presented during a meeting of the American Association for Cancer Research. Dr. Rashmi Sinha, an NCI epidemiologist, said it is not the meat that increases breast cancer risk, but rather compounds produced in high-temperature preparation. Her study looked at high-heat frying, flame-broiling, and grilling of a variety of meats.

A suspect compound produced when meats are cooked at high temperature is 2-amino-1-methyl-6-phenylimidazol pyrimidine, known as PhIP for short. The World Health Organization considers PhIP a possible human carcinogen, and animal studies further bolster that notion because animals fed meats containing PhIPs develop tumors.

Dr. Sinha analyzed dietary surveys from women participating in the Iowa Women's Health Study. The group of study subjects included 273 women with breast cancer and 657 controls (women without the disease). All study participants were asked questions about meat preparation and were shown pictures of meats cooked in various ways. The idea behind the pictures was to get a sense of how the women preferred their meats cooked. Results showed that women who ate flame-broiled, pan-fried, or grilled meats were more likely to have breast cancer.[6]

Additional data suggesting that PhIP plays a role in breast cancer have been reported by scientists from Johns Hopkins University in Baltimore. Dr. Kala Visvanathan, reporting at the same cancer research meeting, said some people carry a gene that accelerates the breakdown of PhIP-like substances consumed in meats. Women who carry this gene, she said, have a lower risk of breast cancer. Dr. Visvanathan's study of 88 women with breast cancer and 92 controls without the disease showed that women without the gene who consumed flame-broiled meats had double the risk of breast cancer.[7]

❧ ❧ ❧

Our discussion in this and the preceding chapter focused on several risk factors that are linked to breast cancer. Of course there are others that this book has not explored and that deserve a mention. Potential environmental exposures, as mentioned in Chapter 3, have long drawn public concern. And who among us has not given even passing thought to the possibility that pollutants play a role in breast cancer?

The Sprecher Institute of Comparative Cancer Research at Cornell University has been investigating possible environmental links to breast cancer since 1995. The reason? The known risk factors, as discussed earlier in this and the previous chapter, do not explain all cases of the disease. Among the institute's suggestions is a cautious use of common household products that are used for a variety of purposes from disinfecting kitchen countertops to erasing grease spots from driveways. These products should never be inhaled nor should there ever be direct skin contact. Institute experts cite pesticides used to kill bugs, weeds, and molds at the top of their list of harmful products.

For more than a decade studies have suggested that organochlorines, the kind of compounds that make up pesticides, may act weakly as estrogen in the body and possibly trigger the type of DNA mutations that set the stage for breast cancer. Many of these analyses remain indefinitive, but scientists have not given up their research. And as those studies continue, scientists elsewhere are taking a radically different approach in the search for environmental links to the cancer.

In the fall of 2004 the National Institutes of Health embarked on a ten-year project to provide answers in a study aimed at analyzing environmental and genetic associations to the disease. Called the Sister Study, the project is unusual, seeking out fifty thousand healthy volunteers whose sisters had breast cancer. Researchers are particularly interested in finding exposures that may be similar between siblings, because sisters of women who have had breast cancer are known to be at elevated risk for developing breast cancer.

Going into the study, researchers hypothesized that while siblings share genes, they also share similar eating habits and, equally important, shared a common environment during their youth. Many continue to share a common environment in adulthood and probably also have many of the same interactions with the environment.

Through the analysis of urine, house dust, and toenail clippings (certain pollutants concentrate in toenails), scientists may well find new secrets about an old and very frightening disease. The research has been greeted with applause from environmentalists and breast cancer activists, two groups that have long argued that a search for environmental associations to breast cancer has taken a back seat to other forms of study.

Chapter 7

Surgery

Surgery is the primary treatment for most forms of breast cancer. The type of surgery a patient undergoes depends on the size and location of the tumor and how extensively the cancer has invaded the breast and lymph nodes. Surgery for breast cancer has become progressively refined over the years and is far less debilitating than it used to be. It nevertheless is invasive surgery, even in the case of the minimally invasive procedure known as lumpectomy (when only the tumor and small amounts of surrounding tissue are removed).

Preparing for surgery is a task that almost all breast cancer patients must face, and, as mentioned in Chapter 2, it involves choosing the surgeon who will remove the cancer. You and your surgeon will discuss the type of operation that will most effectively treat your disease. In some cases a surgeon may not even recommend surgery right away, suggesting chemotherapy first as a way to shrink the tumor, rendering it more amenable for surgery later. If your operation is a mastectomy (removal of the whole breast), you will probably also discuss whether to undergo a reconstructive operation. Reconstruction can begin immediately after cancer surgery, or you can delay it until sometime in the future. Questions probably abound. You may have concerns about the hospital stay, how postoperative pain is managed, and how soon you will be able to return home.

This chapter opens with a discussion on the various surgeries performed for breast cancer, beginning with the lumpectomy, also known as breast-conservation surgery. Also addressed is the debate about margins—how much healthy tissue should a surgeon remove along with the cancer. The discussion advances to an explanation of the mastectomy and why it is performed, and an analysis of the timing of surgery, which may play some significance in surgical outcomes for premenopausal women. The chapter ends with a primer on the hospital stay: admission, the consent form, the nursing staff, meeting the anesthesiologist, what to expect during surgery, and, finally, preparing for the next step in your care.

Which Operation Is Best for You?

Only two operations are performed for breast cancer: breast-conserving surgery and mastectomy. Breast-conserving surgery (or lumpectomy) is usually followed by daily radiation treatments (for five to seven weeks), in a combination that has proven highly effective in clinical trials. When preservation surgery is followed by radiation treatments, the combination is known as breast-conserving therapy.

Variations on what doctors call breast-conserving operations may give the impression that there are numerous surgical procedures available for the treatment of breast cancer. You've probably also heard of partial mastectomy; wide excision and segmental techniques; excisional biopsy; lumpectomy; and breast-preservation surgery. All, in actuality, are what are popularly known as breast-conserving operations or lumpectomy. Because *breast-conserving surgery* is a term that is widely used by physicians, for the purposes of familiarity we'll use that term.

The surgery you undergo is chosen to treat the underlying disease. It is recommended based on information that your surgeon learns from your tests. You are not left out of this process, or at least you should not be. In discussions with your surgeon about your operation, you certainly should have some say in what type of operation you prefer. If you're seeking less extensive surgery, be aware that your preferences will have to be in line with your medical realities.

If you are to undergo a breast-conserving operation, your surgeon undoubtedly will explain that breast preservation does not necessarily mean you will emerge from surgery with a breast that looks as it always has appeared, although surgeons strive for the best aesthetic result possible. Conservation surgery, nevertheless, has become an option for a wide range of patients, including men.

A mastectomy, removal of the entire breast, can be performed as either a modified radical mastectomy or as a total (also called simple) mastectomy. The modified radical involves removing the breast and the fatty tissue in the chest wall associated with it. Affected lymph nodes in the armpit are also removed in this operation. The modified radical is the surgery of choice for large tumors, for small tumors accompanied by extensive calcifications in the breast, and for instances of bilateral breast cancer.

The simple or total mastectomy involves removing the breast alone. This type of mastectomy, a limited version of the modified radical, generally is performed for treatment of DCIS and other tumors believed to have little chance to spread beyond the breast. Doctors also recommend this form of mastectomy to patients who undergo what is called prophylactic mastectomy, a voluntary surgery undertaken to prevent breast cancer that may occur as a result of family history or other predisposing factors.

Among the side effects associated with lumpectomy and mastectomy are infection and fluid accumulation in the surgical wound. These issues can be cleared up quickly should they arise. With mastectomy, a more difficult side effect is numbness in the arm on the side of the body where the mastectomy was performed. The condition is known as lymphedema; it will be discussed in greater detail in the "Potential Problems with the Modified Radical" section later in this chapter.

Breast-Conserving Surgery

The history of breast conservation—lumpectomy—spans no more than a generation. The surgery garnered the spotlight in its earliest years because of patients' activism, which helped bring it into standard practice. Breast-conserving surgery now is an option for most women. In the 1970s, however, the procedure wasn't widely embraced by doctors; few surgeons would buck the medical establishment to perform a more conservative operation.

In the next few sections we will look at both the history of breast-conserving surgery and today's debate over margins (normal tissue surrounding the tumor that is also removed during the breast-conserving operation). The question among some experts is how much surrounding tissue—how much of a margin—should be taken.

The idea behind the lumpectomy is to conserve as much of the breast as possible. But the operation your surgeon performs, even if he or she calls it "breast preserving," may not be the same as the surgery your friend or relative received for breast cancer. Tumors differ in size and location, and those factors affect how the surgery will be performed and what the aesthetic outcome will be.

Keep in mind that in addition to the tumor, the surgeon is also removing a rim of healthy tissue. So the larger the tumor, the greater the surrounding margin of tissue your doctor will probably want to remove. If a tumor is very large the cosmetic outcome may not be attractive. Your surgeon should have some idea of the potential cosmetic result in advance, based on the positioning and size of your cancer.

As much as surgeons strive to offer breast-conserving surgery to patients with breast cancer, it is not a possibility for everyone. When cancer is in more than one position in the breast or when there are multiple areas of calcification, the breast-conservation operation usually is not an option. Pregnancy is another reason why the more limited operation cannot be considered. With radiation therapy, the routine follow-up to breast-conserving surgery, the fetus would be endangered.

Additionally, if your tumor is five centimeters (two inches) or more and is not easily diminished by tumor-shrinking chemotherapy, then a lumpectomy would be ruled out. Women who have disorders such as lupus erythematosus, discoid lupus, scleroderma, and other disorders of connective tissue are also ruled out as candidates for breast-conserving surgery. The follow-up radiation treatment can adversely affect connective-tissue disorders.

As part of the lumpectomy your surgeon may also remove affected axillary lymph nodes (those in the armpit), if cancer has spread there. A lumpectomy is routinely followed by a course of radiation therapy and, for some women, hormone treatments or chemotherapy. Radiation therapy, chemotherapy, and hormone treatments will be discussed in greater detail later in the book.

In addition to the medical considerations involving your surgery, be aware that many health insurance companies do not list a procedure called a lumpectomy as a reimbursable form of surgery. In fact, your doctor may not even use the term *lumpectomy*. Your insurer or surgeon may refer to your operation as a partial mastectomy or quadrantectomy. Either way, the reference is still to breast-conserving surgery or, in the more common terminology, a lumpectomy.

PATIENTS TALK ABOUT THEIR LUMPECTOMIES

Women who choose breast-conserving surgeries cite numerous reasons for doing so. Most are concerned about keeping their body intact while having the tumor and surrounding tissue removed. They also cite their preference for a more limited form of surgery.

A lumpectomy can have a range of cosmetic effects from one patient to another. In women with large breasts, there may not be too much of a change in appearance if the tumor is very small. Bear in mind that the body does not regrow tissue in the area of the surgical site to re-create the original contour. If you have a very small breast, you may notice an even more dramatic difference in appearance after surgery because you had less tissue to begin with.

Doctors interviewed for this book say there is a strong trend toward breast-conserving surgery, and it is offered when it is the most feasible approach to treat breast cancer.

Candace S., forty-two, is pleased with the outcome of her surgery, despite now having breasts of different sizes. She does not want reconstruction.

> I really don't care about the difference. It would be silly to
> think that you could have surgery for something as serious as

cancer and come out looking as if nothing ever happened. I am happy to have my health again. With the lumpectomy I didn't have to have plastic surgery and I didn't want it. I've been cancer-free for more than five years, and that's what really counts with me.

There were women in my support group who had tumors the same size as mine, and they preferred mastectomy. I thought it odd when we first talked about it. I thought, Why would somebody ask for a mastectomy? But they're happy with their choice.

Maryanne B., who fought mightily just to have her lump diagnosed, believes her struggle to convince doctors that as a young woman she indeed could have breast cancer served only to strengthen her. She considers her lumpectomy a victory won through self-advocacy.

If I hadn't gotten the diagnosis when I did, things could have turned out a lot worse. But I got the lumpectomy and I'm fine now. In fact, I'm great. I tell people I am a cancer survivor. Going through surgery is a lot easier than trying to get a diagnosis from a doctor who doesn't believe you have breast cancer.

Helen S., fifty-six, a homemaker, underwent a breast-conserving surgery for DCIS. She recalls reacting with surprise when her physician explained that in the not so distant past a radical mastectomy was the accepted form of treatment for tiny tumors such as hers.

When I saw the mammogram, I was shocked. No—stunned! It was just a speck, an itsy-bitsy speck. It didn't even look like a lump, but that's what he kept calling it. I said a lumpectomy is definitely overkill. It seemed like there should be a pill to get rid of something that small. That's when he said a few years ago he was doing mastectomies for specks like that.

Helen says her surgery was not debilitating and that she is certain a lumpectomy was the best choice for her.

The lumpectomy was a breeze. I was in the hospital a lot longer than most people who have a lumpectomy because I have diabetes and high blood pressure, and my blood pressure was very high. I was in for three days. They kept checking my blood sugar and blood pressure.

A SURGERY BORN OF ACTIVISM

As an accepted and routine form of surgery, breast conservation did not have its beginnings along medicine's traditional paths. It is a minimalist's operation born in an era when most surgeons preferred the radical mastectomy developed in 1894 by Dr. William S. Halsted of Johns Hopkins University. Until the 1970s, a radical mastectomy was the primary operation a majority of women in the United States could expect when treated for breast cancer.

Known simply as the Halsted, the radical mastectomy was a surgical procedure synonymous with disfigurement. It also was a key target of breast cancer activists who first rose vocally during that time, hoping to rid medicine of several frightening practices: aggressive, disfiguring surgery, as well as the practice of conducting a biopsy (which was performed under anesthesia) followed immediately by a mastectomy when cancer was found. When women emerged from the anesthesia they had already undergone the Halsted. The emotional trauma was immeasurable. Patients' laments from a generation ago are the polar opposite of comments many breast cancer patients now make when referring to their surgeries.

Retired nurse Hettie T., seventy-six, who worked in hospitals throughout the Southeast for nearly forty years, knew firsthand about the debilitating effects of radical breast cancer surgery because of the patients she cared for. She knows even more intimately about the effects of breast-conserving surgery because of her own lumpectomy.

> Sometimes I think if I could just go back in time and let those patients know a better day was ahead, I would do that. To tell them that what they went through was really helping their daughters, their granddaughters, and their great-granddaughters. Doctors don't treat patients with certain medicines or certain kinds of surgery because they're barbarians or because they're stupid. They're giving their patients what ev-

erybody in that particular time thinks is best. I know this because I was a nurse and I saw a lot of changes.

As for me, there were no problems. I don't see too much of a difference in the before and after, so I guess that means my surgeon did a good job. I got radiation afterwards to get the cancer he couldn't see. My surgeon is a real nice young man. He told me after the operation, "Hettie, we took such good care of you, your husband will never know the difference."

Among the activists who paved the way toward less aggressive surgery for breast cancer was the late Rose Kushner, a Maryland writer who became a feisty advocate for women with breast cancer after her own diagnosis in 1974.

Rose's struggle is detailed in her book *Why Me*, but much of her story was also captured in headlines of the day and on television news. Her name is synonymous with activism. She is best known for her passion and was considered a firebrand. Rose refused to allow a surgeon to perform a radical mastectomy immediately following her biopsy—as was standard practice at the time. Like other activists of her day, Rose was adamant that doctors find a more humane way of treating breast cancer.

Yet Rose didn't even want a lumpectomy, an operation doctors would have considered outrageous. She simply wanted a modified radical mastectomy—the loss of her breast but without the additional loss of the supporting muscles. Even though the modified radical was coming into vogue in 1974, it was not yet widely embraced by the medical establishment.

Dr. Barron Lerner, an associate professor of medicine and bioethics at Columbia University's College of Physicians and Surgeons in New York, wrote in his book *The Breast Cancer Wars* that Rose's tumor was only one centimeter in diameter (less than half an inch). All of the lymph nodes in her armpit were free of disease. Dr. Lerner nevertheless documented the days leading to lumpectomies as highly contentious ones, with women such as Rose squarely in the vanguard. "Kushner was able to convince her family surgeon to perform only a biopsy," he wrote. "Kushner later recounted the surgeon's anger at having biopsied a breast cancer without performing an immediate mastectomy. Rattling the bars of her bed in the hospital recovery room, he snapped, 'I never should have let you get away with it.' Kushner's problems with physicians were only beginning. When she [tried to seek] out a surgeon who would be willing to perform a modified radical mastectomy, she got eighteen straight rejections."[1]

A landmark study from the late 1970s, overseen by the National Surgical Adjuvant Breast and Bowel Project and headed by the renowned Dr. Bernard Fisher of the University of Pittsburgh, showed that breast conservation, when followed by radiation therapy, is just as effective as mastectomy. Rose Kushner, a growing number of other activists, and the physicians who joined with them were right on target about the effectiveness of less aggressive surgery for breast cancer.

In a series of additional studies that continued into the 1990s, Dr. Fisher and his colleagues would repeatedly find that lumpectomies are very effective in the treatment of breast cancer. For more than twenty years, Dr. Fisher's analyses trained a spotlight on the lumpectomy and its effectiveness.

THE MARGIN DEBATE

The issue of how much healthy tissue to remove in a lumpectomy is a vital one, and the thinking among many doctors can be broken down simply to this: The wider the margin, the more likely it is that errant cancer cells will be captured during the lumpectomy.

Over the years, however, patients and doctors alike have argued that taking too wide a margin impairs the cosmetic outcome of the surgery. Despite those arguments, there remains a key issue of concern: The cancer can recur if cells from the tumor are left behind in the breast. In this section and the next one we examine several issues in the debate about margins, including arguments regarding how much healthy tissue should be removed with tiny, nonpalpable tumors.

Ever since surgeons began routinely performing breast-conserving surgeries there was a fact that was abundantly clear: Some women experienced recurrences of their cancers; some did not. Those who experienced recurrences were patients whose surgeons removed the smallest rims of healthy tissue with their tumors.

In her book *Advanced Breast Cancer: A Guide to Living with Metastatic Disease*, breast cancer activist and author Musa Mayer contends that such local recurrences are believed by many doctors to be the result of insufficient surgery. Recurrent cancers in the same breast, Mayer reports, undoubtedly relate to a lumpectomy in which surgeons removed too small a margin of healthy tissue.

> A local recurrence can happen when tumor cells remain in the original site and, over time, grow to become a measurable tumor. While requiring further treatment, a local recurrence doesn't by itself mean the disease has become systemic and life threatening. A percentage of women who elect to have breast-conserving surgery (lumpectomy or similar limited surgery which removes the tumor and enough surrounding tissue to provide clear margins) will have some part of the tumor cells grow back from cancer cells that were left behind, despite radiation therapy to the remaining breast tissue.
>
> Residual cancer cells, over time, can grow a new tumor without spreading through the circulatory or lymphatic system. One extensive study, published in the *Journal of Clinical Oncology*, found that 10 to 20 percent of patients will have locally recurrent disease one to nine years after lumpectomy and radiation. Doctors generally treat local recurrence as a failure of the initial treatment, and do not consider it a true spread of the cancer.[2]

MARGINS AND DCIS

Some of the strongest arguments about margins and breast cancer have risen over DCIS (ductal carcinoma in situ; see Chapter 4). With such localized tumors, some so small they cannot be palpated, why should much healthy tissue be removed at all? Many prominent breast cancer experts view the matter differently. Dr. Freya Schnabel, a surgical oncologist and director of the breast cancer service at New York-Presbyterian Hospital/Columbia University Medical Center in

New York City, says that, with all due respect to those of opposing points of view, securing a wide margin around DCIS is important. "To those people who say you don't have to do much at all, I say the whole point rests in the business of predictability. It's impossible to say whose DCIS will behave nicely and whose won't. But with DCIS we are dealing with a heterogeneous group of lesions, and I personally think DCIS must be treated with respect. Because when you don't treat it with respect, you have to treat it more than once, and when that happens you're taking something that is curable and allowing it to turn into something else entirely."

Dr. Schnabel credits the work of a growing number of cancer researchers with helping to demystify some of the issues involving DCIS and how best to treat these cancers surgically. She especially credits Dr. Mel Silverstein of the University of Southern California with advancing scientific knowledge about the issue of margins and DCIS. His studies, reported in the *New England Journal of Medicine* and other prestigious medical publications, are influencing the thinking of many surgeons about the matter of surgical margins in a lumpectomy. Dr. Schnabel believes surgical oncologists owe a great deal to Dr. Silverstein and his pioneering studies. She says:

> The treatment of DCIS has really evolved in recent years, thanks largely to Mel Silverstein. He started to struggle toward an understanding of who could qualify for breast conservation. What he's also come to now is recognizing that the core concept of a lumpectomy is a complete and thorough removal of the disease from the breast. And the more thorough you are, the better the results are going to be. When you get this good, wide margin, the radiation really doesn't add much to the results. But there's more to this. Sometimes you can do a lumpectomy and you can't get as wide a margin as you would like because of cosmetic reasons; then you can compensate with radiation.

Dr. Frederic Waldman, a cancer researcher at the University of California, San Francisco, contends the wider the margin, the more insurance a patient has that the cancer will not come back. Dr. Waldman argued in an issue of the *Journal of the National Cancer*

Institute that surgeons should secure a margin of at least ten millimeters (about half an inch) around a DCIS to insure that indolent cancer cells (those that are slow to develop) are captured in the lumpectomy. DCIS, he said, has the potential to recur, so why not eliminate as much of that potential as possible?[3]

Dr. Bernard Fisher and his son Edwin, also a breast cancer researcher, countered Dr. Waldman in an editorial appearing in the same issue of the *Journal of the National Cancer Institute.* The Fishers argued that taking a ten-millimeter rim of healthy tissue provided no proof that one specific measurement of tumor-free breast tissue is better than another. In fact, if surgeons adhered to such a policy, it would impair the cosmetic result for many patients, the Fishers said.

Additional evidence favoring a wide margin comes from studies conducted by Dr. Frank Vicini, a radiation oncologist at William Beaumont Hospital in Royal Oak, Michigan. He found that DCIS is more likely to recur in younger women whose lumpectomy involved removing only a small margin of tissue with the tumor. By comparison, recurrences were less likely in older women who had undergone a similar operation.

In his study of 146 women, reported in the *Journal of Clinical Oncology,* Dr. Vicini found that women under the age of forty-five were more likely to have a DCIS recurrence than women older than forty-five. His analysis confirmed a series of prior studies, which also showed a higher rate of DCIS recurrence in younger women.[4]

Dr. Vicini contends that the surgical excision plays a key role. The higher rates of cancer recurrence were in younger patients who had the least amount of tissue removed in their lumpectomies.

> With respect to the issue of margins, virtually all studies that have looked at factors that predict for recurrence of DCIS indicate clearly that patients do better if you perform adequate surgery, meaning obtaining a clear negative margin. The only controversy is how much of a margin. It is very easy to say just give a big margin around the cancer. Unfortunately, the bigger the surgery, the worse the cosmetic result. In effect, surgeons have to "balance" the extent of the surgery. On the

other hand they want to guarantee the cancer won't recur by performing a larger surgery while at the same time not destroying the appearance of the breast. This is what is being argued at the present time.

Results of his study showed recurrences in 26.1 percent of the younger women compared with recurrences in only 8.6 percent of older women. Age apparently is a salient factor in the rebound of DCIS, according to Dr. Vicini, because younger women have denser breast tissue and thus deeper sites for indolent cancer cells to hide.

Dr. Waldman, in a molecular study, found that recurrent cancer bears a striking genetic relationship to the original DCIS. He said this suggests the recurrent cancers were offshoots of the original tumor and not evidence of new cancers taking hold.

Mastectomy

Mastectomy means removal of the breast. It is a form of surgery commonly performed in the United States for breast cancer. The history of this surgery is a long one in the United States and other Western countries, dating back to the nineteenth century. However, the surgeries performed today are not like those of the past. Today, there is an emphasis on conserving the patient's upper-body strength and mobility. The prospect of immediate reconstruction following today's mastectomy also helps to extinguish some of the anxiety caused by a cancer diagnosis and the loss associated with it.

If your surgeon has suggested a mastectomy, you will want to know which of the procedures is being recommended. There are two: the modified radical mastectomy, and the total or simple mastectomy.

There are numerous reasons why doctors recommend the modified radical procedure. Usually it is the surgery of choice for large tumors, lesions accompanied by calcifications, and other forms of extensive disease. The total mastectomy generally is recommended less often and usually is reserved for cases in which cancer is not expected to extend beyond the breast.

MODIFIED RADICAL MASTECTOMY

The modified radical mastectomy, though it still involves the loss of one's breast, is a far less disfiguring surgery than what used to be performed. Like the lumpectomy, it also came about as a result of patients making demands on the medical profession. Credit does not go completely to the activists, however. Medicine was moving increasingly toward less radical operations in general. "Less invasive" were the buzz words for surgeries ranging from those for heart disease to those performed for appendicitis and knee injuries.

Doctors began their move toward the modified radical in the late 1970s as studies continually demonstrated survival rates equal to the more aggressive operation, but with an advantage of better cosmetic results. Though the patient loses a breast, lymph nodes, fatty tissue associated with the breast, and the lining of the chest muscle, there remains more skin and what doctors call a "mound," which can be used to construct a new breast, if desired. Some women are satisfied to leave the surgical site as it is.

A modified radical entails removing the entire breast, some of the axillary (armpit-area) lymph nodes, and the lining over the chest muscles. Subclavicular lymph nodes, just below the neck, are left intact.

The operation is performed by way of an elliptical (oval) incision, usually about six to nine inches long, across the chest. However, in some cases the procedure can be performed with a considerably smaller incision (about three inches). This minimalist approach is called skin sparing, as more skin is left available for reconstruction.

WHO UNDERGOES A MODIFIED RADICAL?

Generally, a modified radical mastectomy is performed in the following medical situations: for large tumors with or without lymph node involvement; for bilateral breast cancer; for multiple tumors; and for single small tumors, including DCIS, accompanied by multiple calcifications or other abnormal pathology. The surgery also can be performed shortly after a lumpectomy when pathologists find evidence of disease in tissue margins removed with the tumor.

Sometimes a lumpectomy reveals cancer in the margins that suggests more extensive disease than the initial biopsy studies revealed. In such cases doctors strongly recommend mastectomy. Additionally, in cases of recurrent breast cancer, surgeons would not perform a second lumpectomy on the same breast. That's because a course of radiation therapy is part of standard lumpectomy care, and, for a variety of reasons, including potential damage to the heart, doctors do not offer patients therapeutic radiation twice.

Even some women with small, noninvasive tumors elect to have a mastectomy, embracing the idea that more extensive surgery provides greater assurance the cancer will not recur. Reconstruction can begin immediately after the mastectomy, even while the patient is still on the operating table.

POTENTIAL PROBLEMS WITH THE MODIFIED RADICAL

Patients report a range of problems following their operations, from discomfort immediately following surgery to chronic problems of numbness, swelling, and fatigue that can last anywhere from weeks to years. Among the most common complaints are swelling and numbness in the arm from which lymph nodes were removed. Numbness also can occur in the surgical region of the chest.

Swelling in the arm occurs because lymphatic fluid is no longer able to drain properly. Refined surgical techniques are aiding in the prevention of this side effect, which is known as lymphedema. The condition can cause a patient's arm to swell slightly or to enlarge several times its normal size, necessitating drainage by a physician. Lymphedema is a continuing problem for many women who underwent mastectomies many years ago, before surgical techniques reached today's level of refinement, although the condition is not exactly passé. Women who have had mastectomies in recent years are quietly living with less dramatic swelling caused by lymphedema.

Another consequence of lymphedema is poor mobility of the arm and hand affected by fluid collection. Diane Sackett Nannery, the late Long Island breast cancer activist, coauthored a book about the condition titled *Coping with Lymphedema*. She said in an interview for this book that it is difficult for doctors to predict which patients will develop the condition. More perplexing, she explained, is predicting when the disorder will manifest. For some patients it occurs immediately after surgery, but for others it may occur months or even years later.

Numbness in the arm comes as a result of nerves under the arm being cut during lymph node dissection. This loss of sensation may last for a while or it may be permanent. A loss of feeling also can occur in the region of the mastectomy scar because large nerves serving the breast were cut during the operation.

Problems affecting the arm are most bothersome, especially when they occur on the side of one's dominant hand. Some women who have undergone a modified radical and lymph node dissection say feeling returned to their arms, while others say the numbness never recedes. Liisa M., a journalist and mother of three, said she was miserable after her mastectomy because of the degree of numbness in her arm. However, eventually—and surprisingly—the numbness faded and mobility returned.

SENTINEL NODE BIOPSY

In a landmark study, medical researchers have found that removing just one to three key lymph nodes at the time of breast cancer surgery is just as effective as removing more than a dozen, as is common with the conventional lymph node dissection that accompanies modified radical mastectomy. The less aggressive procedure is known as a sentinel node biopsy. Like the conventional operation, it is designed to determine whether cancer has spread beyond the breast. The less aggressive technique, doctors say, can prevent permanent arm discomfort, which can be one of the side effects of the conventional dissection.

Results of the sentinel procedure were reported at the San Antonio Breast Cancer Symposium, a major annual meeting of physicians and scientists who specialize in breast cancer. Doctors found that the less aggressive biopsy has a high degree of accuracy and is believed to be at least 97 percent effective.[5]

Although the sentinel node biopsy has been an option for many years, some doctors have not performed it because there was no scientific proof that it equaled the conventional procedure, which has been considered the "gold standard." There were also questions about some surgeons' skill in performing the newer method.

A sentinel node biopsy is based on a simple principal: If cancer has spread to the nodes, it will most likely go to those involved in draining the tissues nearest the tumor. The biopsy involves injecting a weak radioactive dye or a nonradioactive blue-colored dye in the region around the tumor. Basically, when there is no evidence of cancer in the sentinel nodes, cancer has not spread and no further lymph node removal is warranted. When cancer is found in a sentinel node or nodes, then a more extensive lymph node dissection will be performed.

TOTAL (OR SIMPLE) MASTECTOMY

The simple or total mastectomy involves removing the breast alone, and in some rare instances a few lymph nodes. This type of mastectomy, a limited version of the modified radical, generally is performed for treatment of DCIS and other tumors believed to have little chance of spreading beyond the breast. It is neither performed nor recommended very often because it is too limited for larger tumors and more extensive disease. Doctors do recommend this form of surgery to patients who wish to undergo prophylactic (preventive) mastectomy to prevent breast cancer that may occur as a result of family history or other predisposing factors.

This operation removes only the breast itself. It leaves behind all breast tissue along the chest wall and under the arms. Breast tissue, as will be explained in greater detail in the section "Talking to Your Surgeon," later in this chapter, is extensive throughout the upper body. For women with large tumors and a more complicated disease, a simple mastectomy would not provide enough insurance against a recurrence.

PATIENTS DISCUSS THEIR MASTECTOMIES

Women who have undergone modified radical mastectomies cite a wide range of experiences and emotions about the operation.

Gloria B., sixty-five and retired from her administrative position of more than forty years at a major university, underwent a modified radical nearly a decade ago. She is pleased that she agreed with her doctor about the benefits of the surgery. At the time of her diagnosis, she felt the mastectomy recommendation was a very radical suggestion.

> My doctor advised me that the mastectomy was the best way to go. One reason was my age. I was fifty-six. The other reason was because he wanted to be sure that he got all of the cancer. And I guess he did, because it's almost ten years later and I've never had a recurrence.
>
> It is a little frightening. They took the whole breast, the lymph nodes—everything. Quite a while after the mastectomy my left arm swelled. I had the mastectomy on the left side. That arm is still a little larger than my right arm.

Yvonne M., fifty-three, had a modified radical after first undergoing a lumpectomy. Juggling single motherhood and a job as an instructor at a major California university, Yvonne says she did not have time for a second surgery. A mastectomy, she says, sounded a lot more frightening than a lumpectomy.

> It was right after my lumpectomy, just a few days. They told me they found cancer cells in the margins. It seemed that every time I went for the next step it was always worse than I thought. So they decided it was best to do a mastectomy. I was scared to death. I had a lot of denial going on. At the time, I felt like they were going in for the kill and I would never be the same again.
>
> Now, however, I feel like I've gotten a new lease on life. I feel better. I feel like I look ten times better. Cancer makes you see things differently

Liisa M., fifty-one, also underwent a modified radical after first having a lumpectomy. She found out about her need for a second surgery on the day of her first postoperative checkup.

> I had gone in expecting him to examine the lumpectomy site and to get, at the very worst, a recommendation that I have another mammogram in six months. The lumpectomy had

been about six days before. But they found calcifications in the margins that were related to the half-inch tumor. The really bad news was that the tumor had broken out of the duct. My doctor said a mastectomy would be necessary and that he would look at my lymph nodes as soon as possible.

My recollections of the mastectomy are that it was quite routine—if you can call such a life-changing thing routine. I had tubes in me to drain lymph fluid and a suction pump. There was very little pain. Maybe that was because a very nice nurse in recovery named Blanca gave me morphine. I was in the hospital overnight, had a bowel movement, and was discharged the next day.

Coping with some of the medical realities of a modified radical, Liisa says, were both startling and trying.

I guess most shocking was the numbness in my arm. My doctor had explained there would be no way to save the nerves, but I wasn't prepared for the extent of the numbness. He explained that sometimes feeling comes back and sometimes it doesn't. About three months into chemo, my arm would start to itch, usually at night. The next day I would find that some feeling had returned. It was gradual—little by little. Now I have enough feeling that I don't notice the numbness.

Lula F., the retired nurse who at first did not tell her daughter about the lump, says her surgeon, whom she had known for years as a colleague at California Hospital in Los Angeles, took several factors into account before offering her a choice of surgeries. She was sixty-one at the time of her diagnosis, had a tumor that measured about an inch, and had lymph nodes affected by the cancer.

When he told me I had cancer, he said he had some good news and some bad news. First, the good news was that breast cancer is very curable. Then he said the bad news was that I could have surgery. He said I could have a lumpectomy or a mastectomy. And then he asked me if I needed time to think about it. I said no. I didn't want to waste time thinking about it. I'd rather have the mastectomy, and I wanted it as soon as possible. After the surgery he said he had gotten it all. He said, "We went as deep as we had to go." They also removed the lymph nodes from under the arm. I still have some swelling in my arm.

In retrospect, Lula believes she made the best choice, given the circumstances and her deeply held belief that she was more interested in saving her life than preserving her bust line.

I was sixty-one when I was diagnosed, and I didn't have a problem with having a mastectomy. I was not that vain. Maybe if I had been in my forties I would have considered a lumpectomy.

Having worked for years as a nurse in high-risk obstetrics, she'd cared for a number of patients who developed breast cancer during pregnancy and was very familiar with the concerns of breast cancer patients. Life seemed infinitely more difficult, however, when she became the patient.

I was in the hospital for only a few days. I had the surgery on a Thursday and they sent me home on Saturday. I was very upset about that. I asked my doctor, "Why are you sending me home so early? I just had my breast removed." They didn't even give me any pain medication. He said to take Tylenol, and if I needed anything stronger to give him a call. I knew him on a nurse-doctor basis, and on that level I had a lot of respect for him. But when I had to be a patient I had different thoughts about him. I thought he was not being kind sending me home in just a few days.

Among the most difficult adjustments after a mastectomy is summoning the courage to look at the surgical site—that is, to begin the path of accepting how you look without a breast. Lula believes that step was her most challenging.

It's difficult to remember how long it took to look at it. I can't remember. When I went to have the dressing changed, I asked him, "Is it normal, not to want to look at it?" He said, "Of course it is. You feel disfigured." It must have taken at least three weeks to summon up the courage. I went to the mirror and said, "Okay, you're going to have to face this." So I looked at it. The drainage tube was still in. I was really depressed. It was a very difficult experience.

Janice R., forty-four, who also had a modified radical, found solace in Internet chat groups. She says it was a boost to "talk" to others who had undergone "the most devastating thing in their lives."

> I was in the hospital only a couple of days, so I was back home in no time, and that's when reality really began to set in. I'm home, everything is as it always has been. The cat is still on the windowsill; dishes are still piled up in the sink. My sons are fighting over the remote. Everything is the same— except me. I'm different now. My mom came over to help out and chat after my husband went to work and the kids were at school. But when she would leave, that feeling would come back, that everything is normal, but I'm not. With the dressing on and the tubes in I felt like I had been wounded by life itself. I have never felt so sad, or so down.
>
> The medical center offered support groups, but that was such a long drive and I just didn't want to go that far. That's when I said to myself, "There must be somebody like you sitting around in her old chenille bathrobe and slippers feeling sorry for herself, wondering why this has happened to her." So I got on the computer, and that's where I found a lot of new friends who were just like me.

Talking to Your Surgeon

As a vital part of patient education and presurgical planning, whether you'll be undergoing a lumpectomy or a mastectomy, you should be included in frank discussions with your surgeon about your operation a week or two before it is scheduled. As surgical oncologist Dr. Rajiv Datta explains, having an open, one-on-one talk about your surgery is important for both you and the surgeon. Doing so allows you and your surgeon time to become better acquainted and allows you to ask any questions you may have about your cancer, no matter how trivial you think they may be.

Dr. Datta, who specializes in the treatment of breast cancer at the breast center of South Nassau Communities Hospital, on Long

Island, believes the patient should be allowed to see the mammogram so she will have a sense of the tumor's whereabouts in the
breast. Then, in the case of a lumpectomy, patients can discuss how
the surgeon plans to remove it, how long it will take for the surgical
site to heal, and how much of a scar will be present afterward.

If your surgeon is recommending a mastectomy, then talking to
her or him will help you understand the operation more fully so that
you will know what you are facing. It's your health; ask any question
that comes to mind. Ask about nerves that might be cut during the
operation. Ask about numbness and swelling in the arm and chest.
Ask about drainage tubes and how long they may have to remain in
place.

Dr. Datta says it is important that patients see illustrations or
scale models of the areas that will undergo surgery. He also believes it
is vital for patients to understand that breast tissue isn't located only
in the breast. Breast tissue extends throughout a substantial portion
of the upper body—front, back, and side. As Dr. Datta explains it,
"Anatomically, we say breast tissue and fatty tissue extend from the
clavicle [the collarbone] and medially to the breastbone as well as
along the lateral [side] part of the body and to the lattisimus dorsi,
which is in the back. We cannot leave any of the fatty tissue behind
because there is a possibility of the cancer remaining in fatty cells
and recurring."

It is also important that patients be fully grounded in their understanding of a lumpectomy when that is the operation they are
about to undergo. Tumor location differs from one woman to the
next. Tumor size is another variable, as is breast size. All of these factors play into how a lumpectomy will be performed. They also affect
the aesthetic outcome of surgery.

Prior to surgery, the mammogram and other diagnostics have
provided a map, giving surgeons the tumor's precise location. The
question remaining, Dr. Datta says, is whether all women who want
a lumpectomy can successfully undergo a breast-conserving procedure.

> Pre-op we have a pretty good idea of what we're going to do,
> and the majority of women we see say they want breast

conservation. But let's say that I see a woman with a very large lump and she insists on breast conservation. We can offer neoadjuvant chemotherapy [chemotherapy delivered before surgery] to her to reduce the size of the cancer. This allows us to save the breast, and we have done this many times, especially for young women. When the tumor is smaller, then breast-conservation surgery can be offered.

Always, our first aim is to see if we can provide breast-conservation treatment. Today, we detect many, many nonpalpable masses with mammography. That means many of the women we see can be offered breast-conservation surgery, and that includes some women who come in with palpable masses.

Patients' Bill of Rights

Patients' rights have been recognized for more than three decades. They are among the measures adopted by the American Hospital Association. More recently, sweeping congressional legislation—the McCain-Edwards-Kennedy Patients' Bill of Rights—was passed to guarantee a host of rights, including access to specialists and a fair review process when disputes arise. The American Cancer Society endorses AHA's patients' rights. Here is a synopsis of them:

❖ The right to considerate and respectful care

❖ The right to current and understandable information about your diagnosis and prognosis

❖ The right to know who is involved in your care: physicians and nurses, as well as students and other trainees

❖ The right to privacy

Health-care institutions must advise patients of their rights.

With respect to cosmetic results, Dr. Datta adds, it is important that women understand what is meant by breast-conserving surgery. When a woman with a large breast and another with a small breast have identical amounts of tissue removed in a lumpectomy, the cosmetic outcomes can be dramatically different. The woman with a larger breast is losing less of her overall breast tissue. With the exception of the surgical scar, women with large breasts may not notice much of a difference after a lumpectomy; women with smaller breasts may notice a significant difference.

Amid explanations of what to expect, your surgeon will take a detailed medical history, asking about other medical conditions, medications you may be taking, and any family history of breast cancer or other malignancies.

The list is longer, but this gives you an idea of the patient's role in maximizing the effectiveness of treatment when being treated in a health-care institution.

Your Hospital Stay

As surgical procedures have become less drastic over the years, the amount of time required for hospitalization has been reduced. One reason for shorter hospital stays is that with less debilitating surgery, patients are on their feet sooner, requiring less day-to-day medical and nursing care. Another reason, of course, is the trend among health maintenance organizations and other insurers to curtail costs by limiting the amount of time patients spend in the hospital.

There are no hard and fast rules regarding how long patients should be hospitalized for mastectomies or breast-conserving surgeries. Practices

Patients' Responsibilities

Besides having rights, the American Hospital Association and the American Cancer Society say that patients have a role as well:

❖ You have the responsibility to inform clinicians about past illnesses, medications, hospitalizations, etc.

❖ You must take the initiative to ask for additional information or clarification when you do not understand your health status, treatment, or doctors' orders.

❖ You should inform clinicians when you cannot follow the prescribed regimen of care.

differ from one center to the next. Some "routine" lumpectomies can be performed on an ambulatory-care basis—that is, in an outpatient or "short-stay" surgical center. If you have additional medical conditions, such as heart disease, diabetes, or kidney failure, for example, your hospital stay may be somewhat longer. Assuming there are no additional medical conditions or other complications, you can expect your stay in the hospital to be approximately as follows:

❖ Modified radical mastectomy: one to two days

❖ Modified radical mastectomy with reconstruction: three days or more

❖ Total mastectomy: one day

❖ Breast-conserving surgery: on an outpatient basis, with no overnight stay

ADMISSION

Whether you are admitted to a hospital or will have your procedure performed in an ambulatory-care setting, the initial step toward surgery is meeting with personnel in the medical center's administrative department. There, you will answer questions about insurance and next of kin; provide information about where you live and work; and receive a plastic ID bracelet. The bracelet has a patient-identification number that corresponds to the number that also is on your surgical chart. Most medical centers have converted the numbering to bar codes, like those used on items in supermarkets. No matter how it's done, hospitals need to identify patients in order to keep track of who is in-house and to make certain that each patient receives the correct medications and the right surgery. For patients who undergo same-day lumpectomies, the admissions officer will also inquire about arrangements you've made to return home.

INFORMED CONSENT

Prior to any surgical procedure, you must give your written consent for the operation. Before you can do that, your doctors must explain the operation to you, as well as its risks, benefits, and any alternatives. While it may seem that signing such a form is a mere formality, you can look at it another way. The consent form is a way to insure that you undergo a procedure that is in the best interest of your health, and by signing it you will receive exactly what you are admitted for.

You may find it interesting to note that you don't have to accept a consent form as it is written. Patients have rights, and as a patient you can ask to change the consent form to better reflect your concerns and wishes. You can do this by writing directly on the form or by having a sheet attached to it. For example, if you do not want to be treated by students (medical students, nursing students, etc.), you have the right to say so and to make that known to the center or hospital where you are being treated. You can also refuse transfusions with blood and blood products (although there rarely is a need for transfusions in surgeries involving breast cancer).

Of course, your wishes have to be within the realm of common sense. If, for example, you indicate that you do not want any procedures other than those involving breast cancer, you may be setting yourself up for problems down the road. Helen S., who spoke of her lumpectomy earlier in this chapter, received more treatment for diabetes and hypertension than for breast cancer while she was in the hospital. Her blood pressure was a dangerously high 180/110, something she was unaware of until the workup leading to her lumpectomy. Doctors at the Atlanta hospital where she was undergoing treatment generally treated lumpectomies on an ambulatory basis. Her other medical problems, however, necessitated a hospital stay that included evaluations by cardiovascular specialists. As Helen's example illustrates, if you plan to modify the surgical consent form, do so with your own best interests at heart.

NURSING

Dr. Glennie Metz, R.N., Ph.D., professor of nursing at Stony Brook University Hospital in New York, says that although impending surgery may seem daunting, nurses can help ease your admission into the hospital or ambulatory-care setting in several ways. They can discuss the surgical procedure with you, and they can answer questions you forgot to ask your doctor or were too embarrassed to ask.

Nurses will explain each step that you will undergo leading up to actual surgery, and they will keep you informed about which doctors you will see before the doctors arrive at your bedside. In addition to teaching nursing students, Dr. Metz specializes in ambulatory care. Two vital aspects of patient education, she says, are helping patients gain a full understanding of the procedure they are about to undergo, and helping them be prepared to cope with postsurgical recovery at home. "Patients want to know how much pain they will have and about pain management," she says. "They want to know about taking showers and exercise. A lot of times they just need someone to talk to, and we're there for that, too. Many times patients have told us their doctors had talked to them, but that they didn't really understand much of what was about to happen until the nurse explained it. We want patients to be well informed, but at the same time we know that it is difficult to absorb a lot of information when you're about to have surgery."

ANESTHESIA

Not long before you are wheeled into surgery, you will meet your anesthesiologist, the physician who administers the medications that will put you to sleep and numb the pain of your surgery. Just as your surgeon asked you some questions, so will your anesthesiologist. He or she will want to know about medications that you may be taking, and whether you smoke, drink, or use drugs. It is vital that you answer those questions as fully as possible because your responses will determine the kinds and combinations of drugs that can be used during your operation.

Your anesthesiologist will explain that the aim at this point in your care is to keep you comfortable during surgery. To do so, your anesthesiologist probably will tell you that a muscle relaxant will be used during your operation to render you immobile while other medications are used to keep you asleep. To aid your breathing, a tube connected to a machine may be inserted through your mouth, down your throat, and into your trachea to provide mechanical respiratory support while you're under anesthesia. Your anesthesiologist will also explain that you will be anesthetized just long enough for the surgery to be done. When you wake up, you will be in recovery.

UNDERGOING SURGERY

In the operating room you will be attended by nurses, technicians, the anesthesiologist, your surgeon, and, if you've elected immediate reconstruction after mastectomy, your plastic surgeon. The operation should take about two hours, plus or minus, depending on how straightforward or difficult your case may be.

The surgical site will be cleaned with an antiseptic, and you will be draped in such a way that only the area to be operated on is exposed. You will be connected to an electrocardiogram—ECG—to monitor your heart; a blood pressure cuff will be placed on your arm; and a clip will be connected to your finger to measure oxygen in your blood and the flow of anesthesia through your body while you're under. You may or may not receive a urinary catheter.

In addition, you will be connected to an intravenous line through which the anesthesia is administered. One of the first medications you will be given is designed to make you drowsy. Usually that drug is Versed, followed by propofol, which will knock you out. Once you're completely under the influence of the anesthesia, the operation begins. If the procedure is more complicated, and thus longer, the anesthesiologist will probably deliver an anesthetic gas to keep you knocked out awhile longer.

RECOVERY

When you come to, you will be in the recovery room, where there will probably be other patients who have had surgery. If you have had a mastectomy, you will have drains connected to your body to eliminate fluids in the chest and armpit. If you've had breast-conserving surgery you may have a drain in the armpit where lymph nodes were removed. For mastectomy patients, your doctor may remove one of the drains within a few days of the operation, but it is not unheard of for a drain to remain in place for up to two weeks. You will be given antibiotics to prevent infection at the drain site. Sutures used to mend the surgical wound usually are absorbed by the body and will not have to be clipped away.

Recovery room nurses will monitor your vital signs, checking your heart activity, blood pressure, and breathing. When you appear to be fully awake and all of your vital signs are stable, then you will be wheeled to your room. At this point, ambulatory-care patients are free to get dressed, sign out, and go home.

Postsurgical Pain

Women interviewed for this book report a mix of responses about pain following surgery. Some say they needed prescription-grade pain medication; others took over-the-counter remedies. Some who underwent mastectomy reported an uncomfortable throbbing sensation, and those who underwent lymph node dissection reported extreme discomfort. Still others said they expected the pain to be more intense than it turned out to be.

Patients are encouraged to report episodes of pain to their surgeon, according to Dr. Metz, so that appropriate measures can be taken. In addition to pain, many mastectomy patients report extreme fatigue after their operations. This is to be expected, say experts such as Dr. Metz. Patients are told to take their recoveries a day at a time, and they soon will begin to feel their energy return.

Reconstructive Surgery and Prosthetics

Among the decisions a mastectomy patient makes is choosing whether to undergo breast reconstruction or deciding instead to use an artificial breast form. Reconstructive surgery can be performed immediately following mastectomy, or it can be put off to some time in the future. Carla D., who is so proud of the decade she has spent without a recurrence of her cancer, had a "tissue expander" implanted at the time of her mastectomy. She chose to have reconstruction more than a year after that. Others, such as Liisa M., the journalist, have chosen to put off reconstructive surgery even longer.

If you are overwhelmed about making medical decisions, this is one that can be put off for a while. This section explores decisions about reconstruction made by some mastectomy patients. There is additional discussion on reconstruction and prosthetics later in the chapter.

Yvonne M. decided to undergo breast reconstruction immediately following her mastectomy. She also chose to have the healthy breast "lifted" to produce what she says is a shapely new contour.

I decided I wanted to do this for two reasons. I didn't want to come out of this and feel disfigured, and I didn't want to look in the mirror—ever—and see the scar. That thought scares me even to think about it. I just didn't want to see anything like that. After the lumpectomy, the mastectomy, chemo, and everything else, I lost thirty-eight pounds. I didn't even try to lose the weight. It was just the stress of the ordeal, and I must say I feel better and I look better.

Lula F. did not undergo reconstructive surgery immediately after her operation because "there was not enough skin there," according to her physician's assessment. Lula also harbored her own concerns about reconstructive surgery. Like some women, she did not want to subject herself to more surgery.

Not too long after I had the mastectomy a friend gave me a magazine article about a company called Bosom Buddies. They make artificial breast forms. I tried their products and found that wearing a breast prosthesis works for me. I never had large breasts, but I didn't want to be out of proportion. I just needed something to correspond with the one I had left. The form is breast-shaped and you just insert it in your bra.

In the three years since her operation, Janice R. has not had reconstructive surgery. Still, she is planning to go ahead with it eventually. She finds that she is more ambivalent about having the operation than she was shortly after her mastectomy. As more time has passed she finds herself growing more accustomed to the absence of the breast.

There's no doubt in my mind that I will have the surgery. This is not a matter of will I do it but when. After I got over the biggest hump (which in my case was the surgery and chemo), I needed a rest. At first I thought I would want reconstruction right away. But none of that seems so urgent any more. We've gone to Hilton Head these past two summers. I go swimming with Dan and the boys. I wear a bathing suit with a breast form. We play tennis. I know I will reach the point of having it done; I just haven't gotten there. At the moment, I'm still looking forward to it. I just have to figure out when it will be. I hope that makes sense.

Geraldine M., who was not immediately notified about the suspicious shadow on her mammogram, chose a prosthesis. Reconstructive surgery never struck her as an option.

When you reach a certain age, some things don't seem to matter like they used to. You know, you get older and your priorities change. Me and this little prosthesis are getting along just fine. At this age I needed to do the least complicated thing and move on. God knows I'm just thankful to still be here. This cancer thing popped up as such a surprise. We weren't ready for it. Like you're supposed to be ready for cancer. But I didn't want to make life too complicated for everybody around me. That was the main thing. That was the main reason why I didn't want another surgery. Burt, my husband, was so broken up. Poor Burt, he thought he was going to lose me. So my job was to just keep everything simple. All of it was just way too much, anyway, especially for him: the chemo, being sick from chemo, wigs, the whole nine yards. So, no, another surgery was way out of the question.

> ### The Law and You
>
> Under the Women's Health and Cancer Rights Act of 1998, patients are protected when they choose to have breast reconstruction after a mastectomy. The law is applicable both to people in group health plans and those with individual coverage. While the law does not require coverage for either mastectomies or reconstruction, its fine print states that if a plan covers mastectomies then the plan is subject to the act's rules. This also means coverage must be provided for physical complications of a mastectomy, which can include lymphedema.

UNDERSTANDING RECONSTRUCTIVE SURGERY

A new breast can be surgically put in place to help restore your looks and your self-confidence. Among plastic surgeons' capabilities is fashioning a nipple. That way your new breast looks as natural as possible.

Preparing for reconstructive surgery requires many of the same steps you have taken regarding other aspects of your care. And again, when seeking a plastic surgeon, ask for recommendations. Your surgical oncologist would be an excellent expert to ask for a recommendation.

Among the things you should know about reconstructive surgery are the ways in which it is performed. It can be done either with an implant or through what is called a "flap" procedure. (You may have heard the term *TRAM/flap*; see below for more about that procedure.) Implant surgery is less extensive than a flap operation.

If you decide to get an implant, you and your plastic surgeon will discuss the structure of the implant itself, which contains saline, a saltwater solution. The implant is put in place through an incision made in the muscle of your chest. Prior to implant surgery you may have to undergo tissue expansion, which is a technique used to stretch the tissues surrounding the breast to create space for the implant itself. A balloon-like expander is placed under the chest wall and is increased in size over a period of several weeks or even a few months. When enough room has been created, then you are ready to undergo the implant procedure.

A flap technique utilizes the patient's own tissues—removed from the back, buttocks, or abdomen—instead of an implant. (The word *flap* simply means that a "flap" of the patient's own tissue is used to help fashion the new breast.) Your plastic surgeon can discuss the merits of taking tissue from your abdomen or buttocks, for example, and using it to fashion a new breast. Yvonne M. underwent a procedure in which some of her abdominal tissue was tunneled under her skin to her chest region to create a new breast. She is very pleased with the outcome of the operation.

Although the most common type of flap surgery is the TRAM/flap, there are others. One such technique is the free flap, a complex surgery in which fat is removed from the buttocks to create a new breast. Another technique involves moving the latissimus dorsi muscle from the back and tunneling it under the skin to use as a foundation for developing a new breast. You will want to discuss all of the procedures with your plastic surgeon, who will be able to explain the benefits and drawbacks of each.

The goal of breast reconstruction is to give you symmetry when wearing a bra. When you are undressed, the "created" breast and the natural one will not look like the pair with which you were endowed by nature, although plastic surgeons say they try to come as close as possible.

BREAST PROSTHESES

Breast prostheses come in a wide range of choices, from the kind mentioned earlier in this chapter by Lula F., which fits in a bra, to a foam form that is made to adhere to the chest. These prostheses are made to look like a breast and come in a range of skin tones. They can be custom-made, or you can buy them ready-made. Custom-made breast prostheses are considered a durable medical device under federal regulations and thus are covered by many private insurers, though some choose not to cover them. Companies that sell prostheses throughout the United States are listed in Resources, at the end of the book.

Chapter 8

Radiation Therapy: Medicine's High-Energy Treatment

At this juncture in your treatment you may want to dispose of the following old saw if you've ever heard it: that cancer care is all about slash, burn, and poison. (Of course, you may have never come across that silly old saying. And if that is the case just forget you ever read it—and don't read the upcoming few sentences, which are an attempt to explain it out of existence.)

The old "slash, burn, and poison" analogy refers to the standard cancer treatments of surgery, radiation, and chemotherapy. There are probably some people who think the saying is funny. Granted, it's kind of catchy. But it has been bandied around a lot recently by people who think a grand revolution is right around the corner wherein patients will simply be able to take a pill and tumors will obediently vanish, possibly even overnight. As it stands, you're living in the here and now, and until that happens—if it happens—you must cope with what medicine has to offer, which is far more sophisticated than what the "s, b, and p" words imply. And there are three other words you may want to ditch regarding radiation therapy: cook, cooking, and cooked. Radiation treatments come nowhere near anything being taught at the French Culinary Institute. They are about disabling cancer cells at the molecular level with high-energy rays.

One of the terms related to cancer treatment that you probably will hear with increasing frequency—often repeated like a mantra—is *local control*. This is not a vague reference to municipal politics. In the parlance of cancer care the term refers to eliminating microscopic traces of cancer in the surgical region after lumpectomy or mastectomy. Surgery is the dominant local treatment. Radiation, for a majority of patients receiving it, is administered to prevent a recurrence.

Radiation therapy is considered a given after breast-conserving surgery, and it is highly recommended to certain groups of mastectomy patients who require beam therapy to the chest wall and to the lymph node region. Whatever your case, the idea is to gain local control. The mission of radiation therapy is to destroy errant cells that may reside anywhere in the vicinity of the former "tumor bed," the site where the cancer once grew. Radiation therapy after lumpectomy or mastectomy is not about treating active disease. Postsurgical treatments such as radiation therapy are defined as adjuvant. That means they are additional strategies designed to provide a measure of assurance that breast cancer does not return.

What You Need to Know

Radiation therapy, also known as radiotherapy, in essence consists of being exposed to high-intensity X rays. Whichever term they use, members of your health-care team are referring to high-energy rays that are focused into a beam. When administered at accelerated levels, X rays have the potency to irrevocably damage cancer cells and substantially reduce the risk that the disease will make a comeback. Healthy cells are damaged too, but because of their normal genetic structure they are able to recover. Cancer cells, which are unstable by nature, have no defenses against the high-energy strike.

Radiation therapy can be a very tedious part of cancer care. It requires a tremendous amount of patience on your part while your physician and those who assist him or her tailor a plan aimed specifically for you. You will have to get treated five days a week for five to seven weeks. The weekend respite is what gives your healthy cells time to bounce back. Each session lasts no more than an hour. Some of that time is spent being positioned and repositioned by the technician. For full benefit, the beam must be directed at slightly different angles throughout the treatment. Your job while being treated is to remain very still.

Once the full course is completed, you will receive a radiation "boost." This final dose is targeted tightly on the site of the former tumor bed. The boost can be given in one of two ways, via either external or internal beam therapy.

The side effects and discomforts from radiation can run an unusual range. You may experience a drop in infection-fighting white cells. Fatigue is another problem that bothers many patients. Still others complain about feeling sunburned, while some report a wide variety of additional skin problems in the treatment area: soreness, itching, peeling, and weepy eruptions.

In addition, the treated breast can become smaller and firmer. Or you might be made uncomfortable by swelling, a condition medically referred to as seroma. Another side effect is a lack of sensation in the treatment area, or the exact opposite: a super-sensitivity in the treated areas of the chest and under the arm. Lymphedema, an abnormal swelling of the arm closest to the treated breast, worsens in some patients. And finally, although more of a serious inconvenience than a side effect, some people point to the amount of time that must be invested to complete the therapy's entire course.

Here are several quick facts you should know about radiation therapy:

❖ The dose of radiation you receive in postsurgical cancer care is significantly higher than that to which you are exposed for other common medical procedures, such as getting X-rayed during a mammogram or a dentist's visit, for example. In external beam radiation, the dose is fractionated. That means the full course is delivered in small doses. Administering more than standard dosages all at once would cause too much damage to normal cells in the treatment area.

❖ As mentioned earlier, local control means eradicating any traces of cancer left behind after your surgery. Radiation is of no help if cancerous cells have already escaped into the bloodstream. That is why mastectomy patients who are being treated for invasive tumors also receive chemotherapy and other systemic medications. Those strategies will be discussed in detail in Chapters 9 and 10.

❖ Radiation therapy is performed by way of a high-energy beam of ionizing radiation, delivered from a machine called a linear accelerator. This primary type of treatment is called external beam radiation. It is conducted as the machine moves above you, targeting predetermined sites in a relatively small range. As mentioned earlier, your job is to remain very still and to assume specific positions as instructed by the technician.

❖ In addition to external beam therapy, there are forms of internal radiation, which can be delivered from radioactive "seeds." While these are usually used to deliver the boost dose—given at the end of therapy—in some instances internal beam radiation is used as the full course. Studies of internal methods are continuing.

❖ Not everyone is a candidate for radiation therapy. Anyone with lupus or scleroderma—two autoimmune diseases in which proteins are produced that cause the body to attack itself—can experience a worsening of those conditions during radiation therapy. In people with scleroderma, a disorder typified by inflammation of the skin, radiation can trigger severe scarring. Scar tissue formation also occurs when people with lupus undergo radiation therapy. Patients with these conditions may have to forgo lumpectomy and radiation and instead have mastectomies to sidestep radiation-induced problems.

❖ Women age seventy and older generally are not candidates for radiation therapy. Patients in this age group tend to have tumors that are less aggressive than those in younger patients. The indolence (lack of aggression) of cancer increases with age because hormone production tends to be much lower. Surgery can adequately treat most of these tumors, followed by the drug tamoxifen or similar therapies, when patients qualify. In addition, elderly women often have other medical problems that can limit their mobility. Radiation therapy requires patients to get onto and off of the treatment bed, which can prove troublesome for some patients. Finally, it is difficult for some elderly women to make daily trips to a center for radiation treatments. Of course, if you are a spry seventy-five- or eighty-year-old and you want the insurance of radiation therapy, don't let anyone talk you out of it.

❖ Decades ago, older radiation techniques were associated with heart and lung damage among patients treated after breast cancer surgery. Radiation oncologists say beams were less well focused than they are now. Those kinds of problems are now very rare. Studies, however, have shown an increased risk of lung cancer in breast cancer patients who are heavy smokers and who are treated with the full course of external beam therapy.

❖ If you are not being treated at a major medical center, cancer center, or breast center, you may want to inquire about the type of device used in your treatment and ask whether it has been properly certified for use.

❖ Radiation therapy is the gold standard of care following a lumpectomy (with exceptions, as noted earlier), and the tinier your tumor, the more effective the treatments. By the same token, the wider the margin of healthy tissue removed around the tumor in a breast-conserving operation, the greater the likelihood of a cure. (As in previous chapters, the terms *breast-conservation surgery* and *lumpectomy* are used here interchangeably.)

❖ The National Surgical Adjuvant Breast and Bowel Project (NSABP) largely influenced standards determining which patients are best served by radiation therapy. Exhaustive NSABP studies have looked at numerous possibilities and have proven that radiation therapy is beneficial. Among the analyses, NSABP scientists have studied the outcomes of lumpectomy alone; lumpectomy and radiation compared with mastectomy; and lumpectomy plus tamoxifen compared with lumpectomy and radiation, to name a few. The upshot: Patients gain a survival edge when radiation therapy is added.

❖ Expect to meet a new group of medical professionals in this phase of your care: a radiation oncologist, a radiation technologist, a radiation department nurse who schedules your appointments, and a physicist. Your radiation oncologist is in charge of your care, the technician operates the machine, and the physicist calibrates the machine and aids in determining the proper dosage.

❖ Your radiation oncologist will supervise a detailed planning session during which time you will be marked with indelible ink or tattooed at the treatment sites. The markings indicate angles where the beam must travel to treat you.

Recalling the Radiation Therapy Experience

Next to chemotherapy, radiation treatment is one of the forms of care patients most identify with cancer treatment, so it's worth clearing up some common misunderstandings about it. Radiation therapy does not make your hair fall out (unless you are a man with a hairy chest, in which case you may experience some hair loss in the treatment area), it does not nauseate you, and it will not cause searing burns on your skin.

Helen S., whose hypertension and diabetes forced a hospital stay for a few days when she had a lumpectomy, admits that the thought of impending radiation treatment sounded daunting.

The first thing they tell you is that you have to be there every day, five days a week. That was going to be a problem for us because I don't drive and my husband's work schedule was changing. The other manager where he works was out with prostate cancer—a lot of cancer going around at that time. I was lucky because my son said he would pitch in and help out on the days my husband couldn't go.

I had heard about radiation before I got cancer—everybody has heard of radiation—but I didn't have any idea what the machine was like until I saw it. Linda, my oncologist's nurse, walked me over to meet the radiation oncologist and the technicians. That's when I saw the machine for the first time.

As far as side effects are concerned, I had a problem with soreness and swelling. Whenever I'd roll over on that side at night I'd wake right up. We have a big leather chair in the den. I started sleeping in there because I could sleep sitting up. That was much more comfortable.

Liisa M., a journalist, recalls having no fear of radiation going into the therapy. After a few treatments, however, the beam had an adverse effect on her skin.

My skin is very sensitive and it felt like a really bad sunburn. They tell you how to treat it, but it takes some getting used to—at least for me it did.

The skin irritation did not deter Liisa from her treatments. She used emollients with aloe vera, as instructed by her nurse. As the mother of three school-age children, she was highly motivated to complete every step of her care and even to find humor in the therapy.

It's like being a supermodel, going in for a shoot and getting your picture taken. You have to hold your arm over your head like this [gesturing]. Then they pose you like this [gesturing again]. And pretty soon you're going like this, and like this [comically gesturing with one arm over her head, then the other]. I was beginning to feel very glamorous—and confused.

How Does Radiation Affect Cancer Cells?

At levels administered in therapy, high-energy radiation not only penetrates your tissue; it possesses an exquisite ability to disable the DNA of unstable cells. Cancer cells are unstable because they replicate in a sloppy fashion whether they are indolent and plodding or dividing at a clip. When hit with a beam of high-energy X rays, cancer cells are destroyed.

Your radiation oncologist knows that it is important to attack cancer cells, because their genes carry instructions that can trigger tumor regrowth. Radiation quite literally targets the molecular structure of cancer cells, forcing tiny molecules that are exposed to the energy to lose the very scaffolding that holds them together. Picture in your mind's eye a spiraling ladder of DNA. Both steps and handrails can be irrevocably broken by radiation.

All of this may sound like the use of *Star Wars* weaponry against cancer, and realizing that nearby healthy cells can be grazed by such powerful rays may be enough to make you feel a bit apprehensive. Certainly, some healthy cells do get scathed. Unlike cancer cells, however, normal ones maintain the ability to repair themselves. Cancer cells, which are faulty from the start, do not possess this ability because they lack a fully stocked "molecular toolkit" that would allow them to repair themselves.

As we shall see later in this chapter, your radiation specialist can adjust the beam in various ways to treat the specific site where your tumor grew. This task can be accomplished by angling the beam, adjusting the amount of radiation released in treatment, and, if deemed necessary, treating you with a "mixed" beam of high-energy X rays and electrons.

Radiation thus provides your physicians with a fast, effective, and relatively painless way of destroying the genetic foundation of cancer cells. (Of course, if your chest feels sunburned you may argue with the word *painless*.) In essence, the basic building blocks of cancer growth can be toppled. Such destabilization prevents cancer cells from reseeding and growing anew. This is a critical job for your radiation specialist to perform in the effort to lower your risk of recurrence.

Why Not Radiation Instead of Surgery?

As mentioned earlier in this chapter, several provocative studies conducted by the NSABP show that local control—ridding the surgical site of cancer cells—is best achieved, particularly in the case of lumpectomy patients, when radiation therapy is added to the treatment regimen. In some instances radiation can be used to shrink a tumor, decreasing its bulk for surgery. Given that radiation has a number of benefits, one of which is a significant survival benefit, some patients may wonder why radiation could not have been used against the entire tumor.

The answer is simple, say experts such as Dr. Beryl McCormick, a radiation oncologist at Memorial Sloan-Kettering Cancer Center in New York City. In breast cancer, radiation therapy works best when used to eradicate only a few scattered cancer cells rather than attempting to rid the breast of an entire tumor. Some radiation oncologists refer to this as sterilizing the surgical area, that is, wiping out all vestiges of a tumor.

Dr. McCormick emphasizes that such limited use of radiotherapy does not apply to all forms of cancer. For men with prostate tumors, for example, external beam radiation is first-line therapy and an option that can be chosen instead of surgery. The fact that radiation can be administered differently from one form of cancer to another again underscores the very differences in the many forms of the disease.

How Radiation Limits Recurrences

A nagging question for some patients is why physicians suspect that errant cancer cells remain behind after surgery. If, after your lumpectomy, for example, the pathologist found negative margins (that is, margins free of cancer cells), why would there be any suspicion of microscopic cells? Are microscopic cells really there?

The short answer to those questions is really quite simple: Doctors don't know with absolute certainty that an errant cell—or cells—wandered from your tumor and remains somewhere in the vicinity of your surgical site. They do have good hunches based on the surgical pathology report—and based on large clinical studies of patients who were treated for breast cancer. After your lumpectomy, if your surgeon removed a small tumor along with a clean margin of healthy tissue and found no traces of cancer in your lymph nodes, then it is likely that all of the cancer was removed during your operation. Again, however, studies have shown that when radiation is added, the likelihood that cancer will not come back is increased. Of course, that is the message from clinical trials. Sometimes individuals have completely different stories that defy the medical literature.

Lula F., the nurse whose mastectomy was performed by a surgeon with whom she worked for many years, did not get follow-up radiation or chemotherapy. Rather, she and her surgeon decided to pursue the most aggressive surgical approach to prevent her cancer from rebounding.

> He offered me the lumpectomy, but I thought at my age it would be safer to have the mastectomy rather than have cancer show up again. This is what I chose. I had a friend who died of breast cancer. I knew what breast cancer could do. I wanted the most thorough operation.

Lula has been cancer-free for nearly fifteen years. She credits undergoing a modified radical mastectomy for a localized cancer with saving her life. (In her own way, she was erring on the side of caution—and making her own bold choices.)

Most physicians also err on the side of caution and recommend the most thorough (to borrow Lula's word) treatment plan for their patients. Radiation oncologist Dr. Frank Vicini of William Beaumont Hospital in Royal Oak, Michigan, points out that numerous studies of women treated for breast cancer show that postsurgical radiation provides a survival advantage. "The evidence is historical," Dr. Vicini says, referring to the long-standing body of scientific literature on radiation therapy, particularly following breast-conservation surgery. "Traditionally, we have seen a substantial reduction in recurrences." Gaining local control, he adds, enhances the likelihood that a patient will not have a recurrence. "There have been studies that looked at patients with all kinds of variables, even patients with negative margins, and the conclusion still has been that these patients benefit from radiation because it reduces the risk of requiring a mastectomy."

Facing Radiation Therapy with Uncertainty

For some patients, additional treatment after surgery can sometimes be viewed as burdensome. These patients cite feeling exhausted and overwhelmed by all they have experienced, from the medical workup leading to their diagnosis, through surgery, and possibly even additional cosmetic surgery after mastectomy. The idea of facing yet another intensive therapy causes a few patients to consider avoiding radiation.

Some patients bargain with their doctors. Ina G., forty-seven, recalls arguing with her physicians about radiation therapy. She wanted to skip the treatments; her two physicians, surgical and medical oncologists, wanted her to undergo the therapy as soon as possible after breast-conserving surgery. They worked out a compromise.

> I was really very tired. Tired of hospitals and doctors. To tell the truth, just tired of being sick. I found out about my breast cancer right after my hysterectomy. I'd had a terrible time with bleeding and fibroids. So I really wasn't prepared, mentally prepared, for breast cancer. They gave me a lot of stuff to read, and in this material was a medical report that said some women do okay without radiation. Sounded good to me. My doctors kept insisting. They said I had Stage I but not textbook Stage I. One of my doctors was a woman, and she said if she were in my shoes, she wouldn't hesitate to get radiation. So we made a deal.

The deal forged between doctor and patient called for Ina's starting radiation therapy after she felt fully recovered from both operations. She says her surgeon and her medical oncologist were so focused on her cancer that she felt they were ignoring her other medical condition. Receiving two serious diagnoses back-to-back was emotionally draining for Ina. Also, as someone who lives alone, she wanted more time to discuss her situation with family and friends and to develop a support network.

For those facing external beam therapy, the thought of undergoing more than a month of treatments can seem like a very large hurdle to scale. Anna K., fifty-four, a homemaker and teacher's aide, started radiation treatments four weeks after her breast-conserving surgery, in 2001. Although Anna would have preferred not having to be treated daily, she is now certain that she made the best choice by going ahead with radiotherapy.

> It's behind me now. That's the good thing. It's hard for me to put in words how wonderful it feels to have such a major hurdle behind me.

Brenda S., thirty-seven, underwent both radiation and chemotherapy following a double mastectomy in 1999. She believes she can help others through her hospital volunteer work and growing activism. She joins marches, walks, and runs to raise money for breast cancer research. She believes her own positive experiences have given her a foundation from which to share her thoughts and to counsel other patients who are as apprehensive about cancer treatment as she once was.

> I tell women—and men, because men get breast cancer too—that if I can get through this, they can too. It's all about focusing on getting healthy. You can't say, gee, this is radiation, this is scary stuff, I might get cancer from it. Hello! You've already had cancer. What you don't want is more cancer. That's why radiation treatments are important. That's what I tell them. I think that message gets across. I sure hope it does.

Radiation Following Lumpectomy

The area or "field" treated with radiation after a lumpectomy roughly corresponds to the area of your surgery and is most keenly focused on the site where your tumor grew. The radiation therapist (who is also called a technician or technologist) is able to angle the beam to avoid striking vital organs, specifically the heart and lungs. The radiation oncologist can order lower doses of radiation if the tumor was small, such as a DCIS. The beam can be narrowed to treat an area as small as one-inch in diameter (see Figure 4).

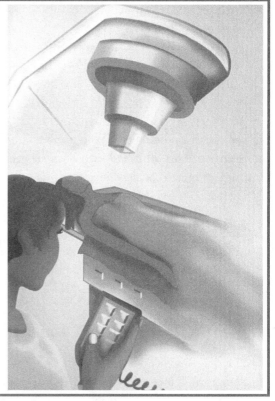

Figure 4. *External radiation is administered during outpatient visits to a treatment center and is delivered using a linear accelerator (as depicted above). Treatments are generally given daily Monday through Friday, allowing the patient to have the weekends off. Your doctor will calculate the dose that will best treat you and then divide that dosage into smaller fractions that will be administered over the course of five to seven weeks. Fractionating the dose this way maximizes the likelihood that any remaining cancer cells are destroyed and limits damage to healthy cells.*
(Credit: Véronique Estiot / Photo Researchers, Inc.)

Although doctors have known for years through anecdotal evidence that some people with tiny tumors, clear margins, and negative lymph nodes can lead healthy lives without radiation therapy, a majority of oncologists will probably encourage their patients to undergo radiation therapy anyway. The exceptions, as mentioned earlier in the chapter, would include women seventy and older and patients who also have autoimmune diseases such as lupus and scleroderma.

Radiation Following Mastectomy

While radiation therapy is offered to almost all patients who have undergone breast-conservation surgery, the therapy is offered only to some patients who have had a mastectomy. If you had a very large tumor, if your tumor grew close to the breastbone, if your cancer invaded chest wall muscles or your skin, or if you had multiple lymph nodes involved (usually four or more), you can expect to undergo radiation treatments.

For patients meeting any of those criteria, studies have shown that postmastectomy radiation can help reduce the risk of local recurrence. Because microscopic cancer cells could have been left behind, there is a possibility of cancer renewing its growth in the mastectomy scar. If you had any of the factors outlined above, your oncologist probably will recommend radiation treatments to be safe. Like patients who had breast-conserving surgery, your exposure to radiation is to achieve local control and to reduce the likelihood of cancer coming back.

As a mastectomy patient, you face a long lineup of treatments, a reality that is certainly trying. Lynette Lee Pack-May, R.N., says optimism is the antidote to the trying nature of cancer therapy. "We always encourage patients to be optimistic," she says. "Optimism is very good medicine and goes a long way."

A Doctor with an Activist's Point of View

Dr. Jack Cuzick, who heads the department of epidemiology at the Imperial Cancer Research Fund in London, reported at a National Institutes of Health conference in the United States that radiation therapy after mastectomy has had a long and complex history around the world.

At the meeting, which focused on adjuvant strategies such as chemotherapy, hormone therapy, and radiation, Dr. Cuzick reported that the use of radiation therapy for mastectomy patients is an issue still very much in debate. Controversy persists despite radiation therapy having been a treatment option for mastectomy patients for more than half a century. Dr. Cuzick believes that many issues involving mastectomy patients and the use of radiation treatments have yet to be fully answered. Here is an excerpt from his speech:

> The first issue in cancer treatment to be addressed by a randomized [clinical] trial was the role of radiotherapy in breast cancer. Although the trial took place in 1948, the question of whether radiotherapy is an appropriate treatment for breast cancer remains controversial.
>
> There is little doubt that radiotherapy is effective in improving local control of the disease. The rate of recurrence with radiotherapy is reduced to about one-third of the rate when surgery alone is used, although the absolute reduction is very much dependent on the extent of the surgery and the nodal status of the patient.

Dr. Cuzick reported, nevertheless, that a majority of clinical trials addressing the use of radiation therapy after mastectomy has demonstrated consistent benefits for patients:

> The relative reduction in local recurrence is substantial in all (clinical) trials.... Slightly better results are seen in larger trials and also in trials employing smaller doses per fraction.

Dr. Cuzick underscored that much remains to be learned about the use of radiation therapy as a form of postmastectomy treatment. Studies are under way in the United States, Europe, and elsewhere to more precisely pinpoint those patients who will benefit most from the procedure:

> It is clear that radiotherapy is of net benefit to patients who are at high risk of local recurrence and inappropriate for others where the risk is low. Much uncertainty still exists about where to draw the dividing line between these groups and the extent to which new techniques have shifted the boundary.[1]

Facts about External Beam Therapy

External beam therapy usually involves a beam of high-energy X rays being directed first at specific sites throughout a specified area, including the axillary lymph node region of the armpit. Then, during the "boost" treatment, the high-energy beam is aimed at the site where the tumor was removed. The total dosage a patient receives is calculated over a period of weeks because, as mentioned earlier, external beam radiation is administered five days a week for five to seven weeks.

High-energy X rays are used in the external beam treatment of breast cancer because this form of ionizing radiation has been found to be the most effective in the destruction of cancer cells. While external beam radiation is a key tool used in efforts to gain local control, radiation treatments, of course, cannot prevent cancer from appearing elsewhere in the body if metastasis has already occurred. If the tumor was very small and localized, it is quite likely that neither metastasis nor local traces of the cancer are present.

Numerous forms of cancer are treated by way of radiation therapy, and to accommodate the treatment doctors need equipment that is precise and versatile. One such device is the linear accelerator, which is widely used in many cancer centers because it can deliver more than one type of beam.

Linear accelerators work by driving electrons along a straight path within the machine, accelerating them to extremely high velocity. This activity produces an electron beam. When the radiation oncologist wants X rays instead, the high-energy electrons can be directed to hit a target inside the machine to produce an X-ray beam.

In addition to delivering a single type of beam or a mixed one, radiation oncologists can adjust a linear accelerator to deliver a beam that penetrates tissue at specific depths. An electron beam does not penetrate very deeply beneath the layers of skin; X rays penetrate deeper.

Internal Forms of Radiation

Another type of radiation treatment goes by the complicated name of brachytherapy (pronounced *BRAY-key-therapy*). It is a still-evolving form of treatment, but it is a choice nevertheless. Brachytherapy can cut treatment time from more than a month to as few as five days. In some instances when patients prefer it, doctors will recommend it as the boost.

The technique can involve placing very slim catheters, called implants, into the breast. At each appointment the doctor will insert tubes into the catheters. The tubes contain radioactive seeds. The treatment takes only minutes to perform. The tubes and radiation are withdrawn when the treatment is finished.

One internal form of radiation therapy, produced by Proxima Therapeutics in Alpharetta, Georgia, promises complete radiation therapy in only five days. The company's website offers a wealth of graphics and testimonials from patients who have opted for the treatment that Proxima has dubbed MammoSite. Unlike other internal radiation therapy techniques, this one does not involve multiple catheters; there is only one. Radiation is produced in a small field within the breast through a protective balloon, which is part of the treatment system.

Preparing for Radiation Therapy

Your radiation oncologist is another specialist who plays a very important role in your postsurgical therapy, and it is vital that they know as much as possible about your cancer in order to be able to provide optimum care. The radiation oncologist must know, for example, where the tumor grew, and whether it was DCIS or an invasive mass. Some breast cancers grow in a complicated way, with tentacles that burrow deep into the tissue. Others grow close to the skin and may even involve the skin. Knowing these variables helps in planning the patient's radiation dose. For these reasons, the pathology report (or reports), a pivotal document in presurgical planning, is also important to the radiation oncologist.

In the following sections, you will get a sense of the tasks the radiation oncologist performs, as well as what to expect during the planning phase of your care. Determining where to deliver a beam of radiation requires precision, and the strategy that best suits one patient may not work for others. Participating in a planning session is a key step that must be taken as you move forward in a type of treatment regimen that is backed by decades of scientific study.

So you can fully grasp the importance of how radiation therapy is performed, we will walk through all of the steps involved, from meeting your radiation oncologist to describing why angles must be precisely plotted before you can be treated with a high-energy beam.

Signing the Consent for Radiotherapy

As part of your preparation for radiation therapy, your radiation oncologist probably will want you to sign a consent form. The document you signed prior to surgery was for your lumpectomy or mastectomy and does not cover all procedures. Additionally, many women receive radiation therapy at facilities that are not connected with the hospital or breast-care center where they underwent surgery. So some of the procedures and even questions your radiation oncologist will pose may seem repetitious, but bear with them. You want the best care you can possibly receive.

Like the consent form for surgery, the one for radiation therapy basically states what the procedure is, how it will be performed, what the risks are, and how long you will have treatment. As with the consent form for surgery, you as a patient have the right to modify it. But have some idea of what you're adding or deleting before you amend the document.

The Therapy-Planning Session

Before you can be treated, you must attend a planning session with your radiation oncologist. This session is important because it involves mapping how your radiation therapy will be conducted. Basically, in order to receive effective doses of radiation, the radiation oncologist must calculate the precise angles at which the beam is to be directed during your treatment.

During the planning session, the doctor will oversee a series of tests and will conduct a run-through of actual therapy, using a harmless beam of light. The tests for the most part require you to lie very still. These dry runs are tedious, not painful. More than anything else, the planning session requires patience on your part.

The idea is for you to be in the best posture for the beam to enter the treatment area. Your arm may be moved above your head, or you may be asked to turn your head to one side. In order to figure out the appropriate angles, the radiation oncologist and a team of highly skilled medical professionals must perform a number of computer-aided calculations. Your part in this is all about being in the proper pose.

In many teaching hospitals, cancer centers, and breast-care centers there are radiation oncologists who specialize in the treatment of breast cancer. Just as you may have sought the expertise of a pathologist who specialized in breast cancer to read your biopsy slides, you may also want to seek radiation treatment from a highly specialized radiation oncologist.

Plotting the Path

During the planning session your doctor will study each position and note the one that best suits your treatment. To help you maintain the best position for each treatment, a mold may be made and put under your arm to make certain that you are in the exact same position for each appointment.

At its most basic, this preparatory phase is about geometry: the angles at which the beam will enter, the volume of tissue to be treated, and the distribution of radiation within the targeted area. Several tasks will be performed to ensure that your radiation therapy proceeds flawlessly. These may include obtaining additional CAT scans, MRIs, and other imaging tests to help calculate the directions in which the beam should be aimed during your therapy. Here are some of the things you can expect:

❖ Your radiation oncologist, aided by a team of supporting medical professionals, will determine the angles at which the radiation will be delivered. A beam is not directed at you without numerous calculations. The radiation oncologist will work closely with a medical physicist who is an expert in beam radiation. Medical physicists are on staff at major teaching hospitals and medical centers. These professionals usually hold a master's or doctorate degree in physics.

❖ You will be measured and marked with either indelible ink or tiny tattoos. The markings are determined from readings of your mammogram and all other pertinent tests and information gathered from your surgery. The markings are the points of entry for the beam of radiation. The beam is delivered at more than one angle to enhance the likelihood that you receive the optimum dose.

❖ A wire mold of your breast will be fashioned, and from that a graphic depiction of the breast will be made. This helps the radiation oncologist determine the volume of tissue to be treated.

❖ Once all of the calculations are complete, a computer-generated therapy plan will be developed. This plan will illustrate the distribution of the dose of radiation within the breast and the armpit.

As you undergo this phase of your care, you may wonder why so many tasks must be performed. The intent behind all of this work, experts say, is to plot the precise "field" in which the radiation can be delivered, while at the same time bypassing such vital organs as your heart and lungs. Bypassing vital organs is one reason why the angling of the beam is so important. In the past, before radiation therapy equipment became as sophisticated as it is now, patients suffered damage to vital organs.

It would seem that once your radiation oncologist has calculated the angles, depths, and volume, you would be finished with this pre-planning phase of your care. Try to bear with it, though, because there is more to come. A harmless beam of natural light is then directed to the ink-marked sites on your chest from a machine called a localizer simulator or radiation simulator. By taking this step, the radiation oncologist knows the path each beam will travel long before you come in for your first treatment.

Undergoing Treatment

Depending on the hospital where you are treated, radiation therapy can begin anywhere from one week to a month after your planning session. The scheduling of your radiation treatments may also depend on whether you underwent breast-conserving surgery or a mastectomy.

Years of research have shown that a large amount of radiation can be delivered safely when the dosage is spread out over several weeks. This is called fractionating the dose, or simply fractionation. It spares healthy tissue from unnecessary damage. When the dosage is fractionated, you have to visit the treatment center daily during the scheduled amount of time to receive the prescribed amount.

Fractionation also means that each dose of radiation lasts only two to four minutes. If you are receiving therapy from several angles (and most patients do receive treatment from more than one angle), each angle may take two to four minutes after the machine is repositioned.

Radiation doses are measured in units called centigrays, and the dose given depends not just on the size to which your tumor has grown, but also on the depth to which your doctor has determined radiotherapy will best help you. In the past doctors used a dosage measurement called a rad, but studies based on centigrays have revealed more precisely how much radiation certain tissues can tolerate (various tissues throughout the body have different levels of radiation tolerance). Again, dividing the dose into small fractions (thus the term fractionated) maximizes the likelihood of destroying errant cancer cells while limiting damage to healthy tissue. All of this information is important, so that you get a sense of why you had to undergo the planning session.

Some patients question why lower doses aren't given over an even longer period of time as a way to further reduce any side effects of treatment, particularly the sensation of a deep sunburn. That's a good question, and one that medical researchers are seriously considering. Teams in this country are also studying the potential benefits of condensing the amount of time a patient may have to devote to external beam radiation.

The Do's and Don'ts of Treatment

When you undergo radiation therapy, you must commit to a new routine—and a new list of do's and don'ts. Even though radiation therapy doesn't take much of your time daily, there are several things you will have to remember in order for the procedure to run smoothly and for you to feel comfortable during this phase of your care:

❖ At each appointment, you will be given a short gown to wear that fastens in the back. You are never to wear necklaces during therapy.

❖ Virtually all roll-on and spray deodorants are out because they contain aluminum, a metal that can adversely interact with ionizing radiation. You will be advised to find an alternative, such as cornstarch or cornstarch-based products.

❖ Soaps and lotions with aloe vera are often recommended because radiation can cause skin irritation. Aloe vera seems to help diminish this reaction in some patients. You're not bound to aloe vera. Feel free to seek out any mild bath soap or lotion.

❖ You will recline on a table that is a lot like an examination table for any other medical procedure. The difference between this table and others is that this one is designed for use with the linear accelerator.

❖ You will be asked to hold your arm in the position determined during your planning session. The linear accelerator is above you. You will be assisted each day in resuming your necessary positions.

❖ When you are posed, the therapist will leave the room to operate the machine from a closed booth. The linear accelerator is not stationary. As its controls are operated to release the beam, the machine's movements will change. Changing the position of the linear accelerator alters the angle of the beam. These changes are in keeping with the angles plotted by your radiation oncologist during your planning session.

❖ If you have questions, the therapist should be able to hear you even if she is in the control room because the rooms are linked by intercom.

❖ You are not allowed to talk, though, while the linear accelerator is running. Aside from the fact that your voice would not be heard above the sound of the machine, your role during radiation treatment is to remain as still as possible. This enables the beam to always reach the appropriate and predetermined sites.

Committing to the Schedule

As mentioned earlier, the treatment sessions are once a day, five days a week, for several weeks. Deborah W., fifty, a buyer for a national chain of department stores, received radiation treatments after breast-conserving surgery. She found the schedule of radiation treatments somewhat daunting, and a daily reminder that reducing one's risk against a recurrence is a process that takes time.

> The tattoos are a big reminder. They never let you put the radiation therapy experience out of your mind. You see them when you're getting dressed or taking a shower. When I would go in for treatment, I tried to focus on something else, like what I was going to accomplish at work that day, or what I'd fix for dinner. I had to postpone all of my out-of-town travel, so I couldn't think about taking a trip. A woman in my support group had said to think about the radiation killing all of the bad cancer cells. But I didn't want to do that; I can't make myself focus on things like that.

Liisa M., who underwent both chemotherapy and radiation after a mastectomy, recalls thinking that she wanted only one thing from radiation therapy: to make certain that all errant cancer cells were, in her words, utterly obliterated. The thought of cancer cells being made harmless because they had been irradiated kept her motivated throughout treatment.

Other patients use different motivators. Dori B., forty-one, a homemaker with four small children, also underwent radiation and chemotherapy. She says she had just one goal in mind.

> I wanted to do everything I could possibly do to make certain that I'm alive. I told the kids that. I said I'm here for you and breast cancer will not take your mommy away. I think they understood that.

Bringing Along a Companion

Having company during this crucial phase of your care is helpful to many patients coping with radiation therapy. Experts suggest having your husband, a friend, or another relative accompany you to any medical appointment that involves a complex form of treatment.

Whoever you choose to accompany you need not come to every treatment session, but having someone come along at least for the first few times, as you get acquainted with the routine, may provide moral support and a boost to your spirits. Dori B. says because her husband was so often away on business, her mother, sister, cousin, and church members each volunteered to accompany her to her appointments.

> Somebody was always with me, all the way through. I never asked for the help, but they babysat and cooked and did some of the grocery shopping. I've got to say this was the most tremendous job of teamwork I had ever seen. It was like they all had a job and they just did it.

Having someone accompany you also helps with remembering things you may want to ask the treatment staff. A companion also can help out with insurance questions and with recalling instructions by your physician and other little details that you may have forgotten. After you have a sense of what radiation therapy is like you may not want or need company. Some patients who go alone sometimes do so before going to work or other appointments.

Getting a Boost

The last week of your therapy probably will be devoted to the radiation boost. The practice is common in many hospitals and breast-treatment centers throughout the United States. In a study reported in *The New England Journal of Medicine,* researchers in the Netherlands discovered benefits for patients under the age of forty who received a booster dose. Dr. Harry Bartelink, of the Netherlands Cancer Institute, examined the cases of 5,569 patients from the Netherlands, Belgium, and France, all of whom received five weeks of whole-breast radiation. Afterward, 2,261 of the patients received a second, shorter series of treatments directed at the area where the tumor had grown.[2]

Dr. Bartelink found that when considering all of the age groups, 7.3 percent of the women in the standard treatment group developed new tumors, compared with only 4.3 percent of women who received a boost of additional radiation. The scientists also found that because women under forty have a higher risk of developing new tumors, they had a greater benefit after receiving the boost. When looking only at women under forty, Dr. Bartelink found that among younger patients, only 10.2 percent developed new tumors, compared with 19.5 percent of those who did not receive additional radiation.

Whereas adding the extra dose of radiation at the end of therapy has been standard at most treatment centers in the United States, giving a boost had not been as widely practiced in Europe before Dr. Bartelink's study. The study's compelling results were expected to make the final boost of radiation standard practice globally.

Locating More Information on Radiation Therapy

There are several places to turn to for more information on radiation therapy. First, the obvious: your radiation oncologist. If you want to talk to someone besides your physician, the folks who staff the phone lines at the National Cancer Institute's hotline, (800) 4-CANCER (800-422-6237), are always helpful, on this and other subjects. For reading material, try the National Cancer Institute's brochure *Radiation Therapy and You,* which can be downloaded from the NCI website and printed out (see Recommended Reading). If you don't have a computer, ask a friend or relative to print the brochure for you.

Chapter 9

Chemotherapy

After surgery, the sole reason for treatment is to destroy cancer cells that may have escaped the tumor. Cancer patients often ask why this additional therapy is needed. The surgeon plainly stated that all of the cancer was removed, patients say, so why continue? The short answer is that your surgeon undoubtedly removed all of the cancer that could be seen. There remains a possibility of microscopic cancer cells being left behind, cells that may still reside near the former tumor site or those that may have hitched a ride aboard the bloodstream, destined for parts unknown. Cancer is a cunning disease, typified by stealth and bearing the potential to recur. Escaped cancer cells are capable of establishing new tumors in distant sites, and because of their microscopic size there is no immediate way of telling where they may be. They're too small to show up on an X ray or bone scan—and certainly far too microscopic for you to sense their whereabouts. It is mostly for those reasons that treatment after surgery is strongly urged.

Unlike radiation, which is local therapy, "chemo" is systemic—that is, it impacts the entire body. Hormone therapy, another systemic treatment, will be discussed in the next chapter. Chemotherapy can be broad-spectrum, killing all rapidly dividing cells, even the healthy ones on the scalp (that's why it can lead to hair loss). Or it can be targeted, deactivating a specific site inside cancer cells or on their surfaces. Chemotherapy usually is given as a combination of drugs to maximize their cancer-killing effects.

This chapter opens with an exploration of "adjuvant" chemotherapy: outpatient treatment given to prevent a recurrence. We also examine side effects that can occur as a result of treatment, and how you can cope with the most rigorous drug regimen you will probably ever receive.

Chemo and You

Of all postsurgical treatments, chemotherapy is the one most identified with cancer care. You may have even skipped earlier chapters in the book and flipped directly to this one to learn more about chemo. There is no escaping the fact that everyone has heard negative stories about chemotherapy.

Yes, you will probably lose your hair, but it will grow back. Yes, you will probably feel more fatigued than usual, but there are medications to combat the anemia that leads to tiredness. There are also medications to combat the nausea that will likely result from your treatment. Still, you probably won't feel like leaping tall buildings in a single bound, and you probably will have some very valid questions about the short- and long-term effects involved with taking such powerful drugs.

Advocates, as we will learn in this chapter, would like to see lower chemotherapy doses and drugs with less toxicity. Chances are, though, you are more likely to feel better than you thought you would while undergoing treatment—despite the potency of the medications. The first several sections of this chapter are aimed at helping you feel more comfortable about chemotherapy by giving you the lay of the land: what chemotherapy is about, what the drugs are and how they work, what you can expect, and how you can cope.

Chemotherapy isn't offered to everyone who has been treated surgically for breast cancer. If your tumor was invasive, if it was two centimeters or larger, or if you had lymph node involvement, then you probably will be a candidate for chemotherapy. If your tumor was smaller but there are other unfavorable factors, such as the lack of hormone receptors or evidence in your pathology report of an aggressive tumor, then you, too, will probably be a candidate. In any of these cases, the patient receives what oncologists call adjuvant chemotherapy. *Adjuvant* means additional. That means the drugs are not being used to treat active disease, but rather are being given as an added measure to ensure that cancer does not come back.

Although timing varies depending on circumstances, expect chemotherapy to begin about a month after surgery. Of course, if you are receiving neoadjuvant chemotherapy, which is drug treatment *before* surgery, then that timetable does not apply. The treatments are given in cycles over periods ranging anywhere from three months to six months, depending on the characteristics of the patient's cancer. The more extensive the cancer, the more likely it is the treatment will last longer. For early breast cancer, rarely does chemotherapy extend beyond six months.

The drugs used in treatment fall into several broad categories, some of which are used only for breast cancer. Generally, these drugs are administered in what is called combination therapy. That means more than one type of drug is delivered as a way to attack errant cancer cells in various phases of reproduction.

Summarizing the Experience

Let's hear from a few breast cancer survivors about what chemotherapy was like for them:

Ann H.
I exercised, I went to work—I had a marvelous experience.

Ann says she did not have a marvelous experience *because* of chemotherapy, but rather *in spite of* it. Shortly after her treatment began, she traveled out of town to hear her daughter, an artist, deliver a lecture. Ann never missed a day of work (she is an editor) and even managed all of her usual routines, like grocery shopping and running errands. When her hair began to thin because of the medications, her daughter shaved her head. To Ann's surprise, when she arrived at work after her chemo began, everyone in the newsroom was wearing a hat as a show of support. Furthermore, her straight, silvery mane afforded her a surprise when it grew back.

My hair came back thick and curly—very, very beautiful. I couldn't believe it. It eventually went back to the way it was. But this shows you that chemo is not as bad as people think. The hair loss certainly is not permanent.

Maryanne B.

I got a lot of hats. I wanted to go into this with a positive attitude because I knew it was going to be a challenge based on what it was like for my sister-in-law when she had breast cancer. I wanted to be prepared. I decided before I even started my treatment that I was going to be happy and keep my positive attitude. I kept saying to myself that chemo would not get me down. The hats really helped. I got every kind of hat you could think of.

Liisa M.

At my last appointment before chemo, I talked with Jean, the head oncology nurse. She gave me a flu shot and asked me about my thoughts on chemo. I told her I knew it wasn't as bad as it had been in years past, but that I thought it varied from person to person. She stared straight into my eyes and said, "Most people don't have severe reactions anymore. I promise you that your worst night will be the night before." She was right.

Rob P.

The nurses were so upbeat it was hard to be depressed about it even though I knew I had had surgery for a Stage III cancer and that people probably wouldn't fault me too much if I got depressed. I got depressed, but I tried to be upbeat, too. One nurse who did my blood work said that while I was getting my infusions would be a good time to listen to tapes or get caught up on any reading I wanted to do. I would put the headphones on, but soon I'd be out like a light. I had some of my most pleasant dreams while getting chemo.

Edna N.

I can't say I relished the thought of my hair falling out or making a choice between hats or wigs. What I can say to anyone facing this is that you have to put your best foot forward. You have to put everything else in your life aside while you concentrate on what you have to do to get better.

Seems easy to say that now. When I first heard I had to have chemo I was frightened to death. Most of what I had heard about chemo was bad news. Your hair falls out, you're sick as a dog, and it's your chemo doing this to you, not your cancer. But I found ways to deal with the hair loss, and I never really had a problem with nausea.

The worst thing was memory and concentration issues, and that's something you're confronted with every minute you're awake. At one point I was trying to make oatmeal cookies but my concentration was so bad I couldn't even follow the instructions on a Quaker Oats box.

Barbara C.
I had an infiltrating ductal carcinoma. It was grade 3, Stage IIA, and 2.8 centimeters. I lost all of my hair. Even my eyebrows fell off. I had to draw them on every morning in this elaborate makeup job. One of the chemo drugs I was taking was responsible for the total loss of body hair. It also caused some other really bad side effects, like joint pain and weakness. My knees were in pain. My legs hurt, too. But all of that was a small price to pay to get my life back. I have been cancer-free for four years.

Cassandra Y.
My doctor offered me a choice right off the bat. She said I could go with standard chemo or try an experimental drug combination. I was only thirty-six and had a mastectomy for a very aggressive cancer. Believe me, there weren't a lot of options. I was all over the National Cancer Institute's website looking for something my doctor might have missed or didn't know about, looking for options, but couldn't find a thing. I decided to go with the experimental chemo because I thought that would probably be my best shot. I really think in retrospect it was. I know I'm not 100 percent out of the woods yet, because I haven't reached that five-year mark. That's golden and I'm almost there. About the chemo choice, my dad always said you get to make maybe three or four really huge decisions in life, and I know without a doubt that was definitely one of mine.

Adjuvant Chemo Improves Prognosis

For anyone who had invasive breast cancer—no matter what size the tumor—adjuvant chemotherapy is designed to wipe out cancer cells that may be hiding or dormant. The stickler with most patients about adjuvant chemotherapy is that it is recommended even when there is no visible trace of cancer to be found. Many patients wonder why that is the case. The answer: Randomized clinical trials have shown that patients who undergo chemotherapy receive years of benefits by having a reduced risk of recurrence when compared with patients who do not receive chemotherapy.

If your tumor was relatively large, you may also have undergone a round of radiation therapy, or you may expect to get radiation after your course of chemo. You may be wondering why both radiation and chemo are necessary. Again, randomized clinical trials have shown a survival benefit. Experts in the treatment of breast cancer generally agree that adjuvant chemotherapy has been one of the best innovations for treating invasive breast cancer, because far fewer patients today go on to develop advanced disease. Having chemo is not a guarantee that you will remain recurrence-free later on, but it is your best bet that you will have done everything in your power to prevent breast cancer from coming back.

When Should Adjuvant Chemo Start?

As stated throughout the book, no two cases of breast cancer are alike because the characteristics of each individual's cancer are based on the types of cells that composed the tumor. Still, your oncologist probably will inform you that chemotherapy best serves you when it is administered as soon as possible after your surgery.

There is no time for dawdling. Starting chemotherapy as soon as possible—usually about a month after surgery—allows the medications to attack cancer cells that may remain and are capable of establishing new tumors elsewhere. For patients receiving adjuvant chemotherapy doctors are trying to eradicate what are known as micrometastases. If your tumor was at least two centimeters, then the likelihood of micrometastases being present is fairly high.

Weary after enduring diagnosis, a biopsy, surgery, multiple rounds of tests, and possibly radiotherapy, you may question the value of treatments that induce side effects and last for months. Yet doctors know that when a breast cancer patient begins chemotherapy as soon as possible after surgery, she or he stands the strongest chance of having the best prognosis—and that, simply put, is to remain cancer-free.

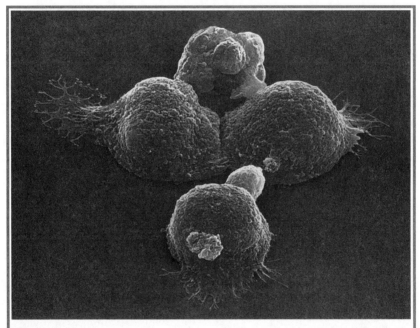

Figure 5. *A scanning electron micrograph of breast cancer cells magnified more than 5,000 times, which shows the cells' uneven surfaces and projections. Cancerous cells originate from a single normal cell that carried one or more mutations. Malignant cells proliferate and grow in an uncontrolled manner retaining those mutations in each new generation of cells. Millions of malignant cells, such as these, form tumors capable of infiltrating and destroying surrounding healthy tissue and traveling to distant sites in the body to seed secondary tumors. Cells spread to different parts of the body through the blood and lymphatic systems. A major reason for chemotherapy is to destroy cells that have broken away from the primary tumor. Doctors now know that cancer cells can escape the primary tumor very early in the cancer's evolution, which provides strong reason for the systemic treatment.*
(Credit: SPL / Photo Researchers, Inc.)

Here is another reason for not wasting time. While medical scientists are aware that breast cancer often first spreads to the lymph nodes, they also know that cancer is unpredictable. By the time you are diagnosed, escaped cells may be well on their way to developing a new tumor—or tumors—in your bones, liver, or lungs. For that reason alone, adjuvant chemotherapy can prove to be of far more benefit than harm (see Figure 5, previous page).

Debating the Pros and Cons of Chemo

From time to time arguments have surfaced in the medical community over whether current standards are too rigid; perhaps fewer women need to undergo chemotherapy. Another viewpoint asks whether it wouldn't be better to develop tests to determine who would fare best on the treatments. The facts currently are this: Rates of recurrences are declining, and there are no tests at the moment that are capable of screening vast numbers of patients to determine who would be best served by chemo. Most doctors tend to err on the side of caution, however, so a majority of patients in the United States who had surgery for invasive primary breast cancer are offered adjuvant chemotherapy.

Ultimately, the decision to have the treatments rests with you. You must weigh all that you have been told about your cancer and the likelihood of it appearing again. The decision to have chemotherapy will be one of the biggest decisions you will make in the course of your treatment for breast cancer.

Adjuvant chemotherapy, therefore, is administered to be on the safe side—just in case breakaway cancer cells are present. Oncolo-

> ### A Quick Memo on Chemo
>
> Chemotherapy evolved as an adjuvant treatment because doctors found that even when tumors appeared to invade local breast tissue to only a small degree, cancer cells still escaped into the blood and established new tumors elsewhere. If you would like additional information on chemotherapy, several major pharmaceutical companies operate websites about their drugs and about chemotherapy in general. Siemens runs one of the best Internet sites on issues involving breast cancer, chemo, and related topics. The Siemens site can be found at www.imaginis.com.

gists know, for example, that a patient who is node negative and who had a very small noninvasive tumor is unlikely to have a recurrence of breast cancer. In cases such as that, adjuvant chemotherapy may not be worth the risk of side effects.

There remain several groups of patients for whom adjuvant chemotherapy is strongly recommended, based on data culled from large clinical trials. Studies have shown that people meeting certain criteria (such as small high-grade tumors or large invasive ones) are more likely to have a recurrence. That means the benefits of chemotherapy outweigh the risks of side effects and possible adverse effects.

Here is a list of reasons outlining why adjuvant chemotherapy may be recommended:

1. *Unfavorable pathology.* High-grade tumor that is ER/PR negative, which means the cancer lacks hormone receptors and thus the patient would not be eligible for hormone treatment. A high-grade tumor—regardless of size—would be one consisting of very poorly differentiated cells, which suggests an aggressive tumor whose breakaway cells may have begun to seed tumors elsewhere.

2. *Presence of multiple affected lymph nodes.* When several lymph nodes are affected, the possibility that cancer is elsewhere in the body is higher, even if the tumor detected in breast tissue is considered to be relatively small.

3. *The cancer invaded surrounding muscle or other local structures.*

What Doctors Think about Adjuvant Therapy

Until adjuvant chemotherapy came along as a standard method of care in the 1980s, there was far more uncertainty about the fate of patients with invasive breast cancers. Adjuvant therapy offered more than local treatment because its systemic nature allowed treatment beyond the field that a surgeon could effectively reach with a scalpel. (*Systemic* means the drugs travel everywhere in the body.) This is not to say adjuvant chemotherapy solved all patients' problems; re-currences do happen. But doctors now know as a result of large com-prehensive studies that for patients who live in countries where adjuvant chemotherapy is widely utilized, survival is significantly longer than for those who live in nations where the practice is un-derutilized. A group of British doctors admitted as much in 1997, when comparing the success of American patients to those in the United Kingdom.

The British doctors, members of a team calling itself the Early Breast Cancer Trialists Collaborative Group, in a study of forty-seven thousand women, found a stunning difference between patients with early breast cancer who received adjuvant chemotherapy and those who did not. "The under utilisation of chemotherapy," the sci-entists wrote, "is one of the explanations for poorer breast cancer survival in the United Kingdom," compared with countries such as the United States. The study itself served as an argument in favor of adjuvant chemotherapy because of increased survival benefits afforded women who had undergone about six months of chemo-therapy.[1]

Commenting on the treatment of breast cancer over the last half century, Dr. Frank Arena, an oncologist and breast cancer spe-cialist in Great Neck, New York, says adjuvant chemotherapy is a relatively new innovation when viewed historically. Its emergence and refinement in the United States, however, has helped change invasive early breast cancer from being viewed as a potentially fatal disease. "Twenty-five, thirty years ago, there was no such thing as adjuvant chemotherapy [for early breast cancer]," he says. "But we knew that chemotherapy worked for women with metastatic disease, and gradually we saw results for patients treated for primary breast cancer. Now we're in a new age of treatment because we know that adjuvant chemotherapy works."

Dr. Neal Rosen, who heads a laboratory focused on developing new breast cancer treatments at Memorial Sloan-Kettering Cancer Center in New York City, believes adjuvant chemotherapy is impor-tant because it reduces the likelihood of a recurrence. He says, "Ad-juvant chemotherapy is used when there may be tumor around but you can't see it. The idea of adjuvant therapy is to render [patients] tumor-free. With adjuvant chemotherapy we know that we can lower the possibility of a recurrence, and because we know we are able to do that, we know there is a benefit."

Reporting his research findings at the National Institutes of Health's Consensus Development Conference in 2000, Dr. Jonas Bergh said adjuvant chemotherapy for early breast cancer without question saves lives. The conference focused on all of the adjuvant therapies for early breast cancer: chemotherapy, radiation, and hormone therapy, such as tamoxifen, which will be discussed in the next chapter.

Conclusions drawn at consensus conferences usually influence breast cancer care for at least a decade. Dr. Bergh, a professor of molecular oncology at the Karolinska Institute and Hospital in Stockholm, Sweden, believes, however, that patients must be carefully selected for chemotherapy. He reported, "Adjuvant chemotherapy and tamoxifen probably save more lives than any other therap[ies] for cancer. Despite this major achievement, the principal problem with adjuvant chemotherapy is selecting patient subgroups to receive any particular therapy.... In the future we hope to have a bio-molecular 'fingerprint' of cancer that will allow us to tailor an optimal approach for each patient. The most critical issue today is to find the optimal balance between patients who should be offered adjuvant therapy and those who are at sufficiently low risk not to be offered such therapy."[2]

In adjuvant chemotherapy, recurrences are prevented through the destruction of cancer cells that may be indolent (nonaggressive), in a dormant phase, or hiding. Because chemo goes everywhere in the body, the added (adjuvant) treatment has a better chance of reaching those cells. Without chemo, there is a greater chance of recurrence.

Neoadjuvant Chemotherapy

If your tumor was large, or if you have inflammatory breast cancer, your doctors may recommend neoadjuvant chemotherapy. We touched on this form of treatment earlier in the book. The prefix *neo-* in no way implies a different kind of therapy. It simply means that the order of surgery and chemotherapy is reversed, with chemo coming first. The chemotherapy drug combinations remain the same, unless, of course, the patient is participating in a clinical trial and something new is being tested. Neoadjuvant chemotherapy is also referred to as pretreatment, induction, or primary chemotherapy. Regardless of what term is used they all mean the same thing: The order of surgery and chemotherapy is reversed.

Dr. Lisa Newman, director of the breast center at the University of Michigan in Ann Arbor, explains that the object of neoadjuvant chemotherapy is to substantially reduce a tumor's size. For patients with notably large tumors, delivering chemo prior to surgery can make the cancer more amenable to surgery. You may also recall that Dr. Rajiv Datta mentioned in Chapter 7 that neoadjuvant chemotherapy can be administered to shrink a tumor with the expectation that afterward the patient would be a candidate for breast-conserving surgery. Large-scale studies are reinforcing the theory that preoperative chemotherapy is advantageous for a growing number of patients with advanced primary tumors.

"Chemo Brain"

For decades women being treated for breast cancer have complained about a phenomenon called "chemo brain." They describe it as impaired cognitive function that at times can seem overwhelming. Chemo brain began, they say, not long after they started their cycles of chemotherapy.

Edna N., a mother of three grown children, says that sometime around her third cycle of chemotherapy her ability to concentrate and her memory—both short-term and long-term—seemed to fail her. "Not being able to follow a simple recipe was one thing," Edna says. "But it got worse. I was filling out a form that needed my mother's maiden name and I couldn't remember it. That's when I got scared. I thought I was losing it for sure." She says her oncologist suggested counseling.

I was offended by the counseling recommendation. I thought I needed to be off chemo for a while. But I think he was picking up on other cues because I was crying as I was trying to explain this issue of not being able to remember my mom's maiden name. I'm telling him my ability to concentrate was shot, and there were some other things I threw in as part of the discussion. I must have come across as a real basket case. I told him I kept losing my keys. He said that's normal. I said, yeah, well even when I know where they are I can't remember which one's for the front and which one's for the back. I used to know by just glancing at them. Now it was like a friggin' calculus problem trying to figure out which one goes where. He kept saying, "If you just make an appointment to see Jan, she can help."

Jan's a psychologist. She sat in on a few of the support-group sessions. She was way too perky for my tastes, the kind who wears a sweater like a scarf, a bubbly type. I just wanted my concentration back. Plus, I don't think I was explaining the situation very well. I was just making bad matters worse.

Edna eventually talked to the psychologist, who helped her understand that although she was having some concentration and memory problems—not unusual during breast cancer treatments—much of what she was experiencing was panic and stress. Cancer treatment is very stressful, and when Edna couldn't recall something right away, her psychologist theorized that panic overwhelmed her.

But this in no way implies that women are not experiencing the condition widely known as chemo brain. Indeed, it is believed to be fairly common, affecting large numbers of women of all ages who are undergoing chemotherapy for breast cancer. The disorder is also believed to affect men and women being treated for other malignancies. Most studies, however, have concentrated on breast cancer patients.

Some estimates suggest that as many as 40 percent of women receiving chemotherapy for breast cancer may be affected by the condition, but other estimates put the figure as low as only 15 percent. For years doctors explained away chemo brain as patients' anxieties seeming to get the best of them. In other words, chemo brain was "in their heads," and thus not a problem associated with cancer treatments. But research from several quarters now suggests that chemo brain may be caused by a multitude of factors. For one thing, chemotherapy can induce changes in hormones, and the chemical alterations may have a profound effect on brain function. Questions nevertheless persist as researchers attempt to explain why some patients develop cognitive deficits and others do not. Could it be that chemotherapy somehow has a direct, toxic effect on the brain? Perhaps chemo drugs are attacking neurons, the cells that comprise the brain's billions of tiny building blocks.

Many researchers argue against those possibilities because most molecules that make up chemo drugs are too big to squeeze through nature's filter: the blood-brain barrier, a protective sheath that keeps most substances that are circulating in the bloodstream out of the brain. There are exceptions to that rule. Methotrexate, a major drug used in cancer therapy, can make its way into the brain when delivered in high enough doses. But not everyone treated for breast cancer is given methotrexate.

A study conducted in 1998 by researchers at the Netherlands Cancer Institute found that cognitive impairment occurred whether women treated for breast cancer received high or standard doses of chemotherapy.[3] But a team at M.D. Anderson Cancer Center in Houston suggested in a June 2004 analysis that some cognitive deficits may exist before chemo even begins. The study also questioned whether chemo brain has been overestimated. The best way to get a handle on the problem, the researchers said, is to study women as they had done: before chemo begins, and again afterward.[4]

Researchers at Princess Margaret Hospital and the University of Toronto found that chemo brain can be mild to moderate and that the condition tends to diminish when chemo ceases.[5] Edna says her memory problems persisted for months after she finished her cycles of chemotherapy. Now that cancer treatments are nine years behind her, she believes that her concentration and memory are "okay now."

What Kinds of Drugs Are Used in Chemotherapy?

Oncologists rely on a growing stable of medications for adjuvant treatment. Each drug found its way into therapy for early breast cancer because of success in the treatment of metastatic disease. In some instances an oncologist may rely on a single agent for treatment, but for the most part adjuvant therapy involves a combination of drugs.

Drugs that are used to eradicate cancer cells have different missions. Some medications attack the very mechanisms of cell division; these drugs can disable components of cancer-cell DNA. Others interfere with the ways in which cancer cells metabolize nutrients. Still others force cancer cells to commit suicide.

Basically, several broad categories of drugs can be used in chemotherapy. Each category has a specific way of attacking cancer cells:

1. *Alkylating agents.* These drugs, which include cyclophosphamide (Cytoxan), damage the DNA in charge of a tumor's cell growth. In chemotherapy this drug is usually abbreviated as C. Epirubicin (Ellence) is another alkylator used routinely in adjuvant chemotherapy, and it is usually designated as E.

2. *Antimetabolites.* Drugs in this category interfere with the division of cancer cells, causing the cells to die as they attempt to reproduce. The names of drugs in this class are methotrexate and 5-fluorouracil (5-FU). This pair is usually designated as M and F.

3. *Antibiotics.* An anticancer antibiotic is a very different kind of medication from the kind of drug that kills bacteria. This kind of antibiotic stops tumor growth by inhibiting the reproduction of cancer cells. The term *biotic* means growth. So, breaking the word apart, it would mean antigrowth of

cancer cells. A major drug in the class is Adriamycin (doxorubicin). Adriamycin is designated as A.

4. *Antimiotic agents.* Drugs in this group stop the genes in cancer cells from replicating. Three major drugs in this category were originally drawn from a natural source, the periwinkle plant. These medications include Oncovin (vincristine), Navelbine (vinorelbine), and Velban (vinblastine). All are chemically different.

5. *Antimicrotuble agents.* Drugs in this category also have a history in nature. They originally were based on compounds found in the bark of the Pacific and European yew trees. These drugs interfere with a process that most kids learn about in high school biology: mitosis. They prevent cancer-cell division. The two drugs in this class are Taxol (paclitaxel) and Taxotere (docetaxel). Both are designated as *T.*

6. *Targeted therapy.* An evolving form of cancer therapy zeroes in on the very mechanism causing the cancer cell to proliferate. A targeted therapy is one in which the drug's activity is specific to a certain site or chemical activity of a cancer cell. The specificity is so keen the drug has no effect on other cells or other parts of the tumor. Herceptin, a major drug for metastatic breast cancer, was the first such medication in this class. It blocks the activity of the HER-2 oncogene (see Chapter 5). Herceptin is what is known as a monoclonal antibody, and while it is used primarily for patients with advanced breast cancer, clinical trials are being conducted to test its use in the adjuvant setting. Although many in the scientific community acknowledge that Herceptin was the first targeted therapy, others argue that tamoxifen, which has been around since the 1960s, actually should hold that distinction. Tamoxifen zeroes in on the estrogen receptors of cancer cells that possess them, blocking the receptors and preventing estrogen from entering the cell's inner domain. Tamoxifen is discussed in detail in Chapter 10.

Combination Chemotherapy

Oncologists administer several combinations of chemotherapy to achieve different objectives in the prevention of a recurrence. Two or three drugs can be given during the period of treatment. The choice of drugs is deliberate and based on the characteristics of the tumor, its size, and whether lymph nodes were involved. The drug Cytoxan is one of the most widely used in combination therapy. Dr. Larry Norton, physician-in-chief at Memorial Sloan-Kettering Cancer Center in New York City, was one of the world's pioneers investigating combination chemotherapy for breast cancer. He and his colleagues found that the use of multiple drugs in adjuvant care and for advanced disease have helped to improve the prognosis for patients.

Here are some of the combinations of medications that are used in the adjuvant treatment of breast cancer:

1. Adriamycin and Cytoxan (AC)

2. Cytoxan, Adriamycin, and fluorouracil (CAF)

3. Cytoxan, methotrexate, and fluorouracil (CMF)

4. Cytoxan, Ellence, and fluorouracil (CEF)

5. Taxotere, Adriamycin, and Cytoxan (TAC)

Preparing for Chemotherapy: The Workup

Just as you have had to prepare for other important milestones in your care, so it is with chemotherapy. In many ways, however, there may be more preparatory steps for chemotherapy than for other aspects of your care because of the potent nature of the medications that are used. You will undergo "reference blood tests" so that the blood samples taken throughout your treatment can be compared to the reference set. You will get another physical examination, and you will be asked to complete a consent form for chemotherapy.

Chemotherapy can be administered in many ways: through an IV, through a port, or in pill form. A port is a semipermanent device that allows medications to be infused into the vein without the nurse having to find a vein each time in which to place an IV needle. The port is inserted into the chest and into a blood vessel. A catheter linked to the port is accessible outside of the body. It is the device through which a nurse can infuse a precisely measured drug dose from a syringe. Yet another consent form is required for the surgical placement of the port, if that is how your chemo will be delivered. A simpler form of therapy comes in pill form. Hormone therapy, as you will learn in Chapter 10, comes mostly in pill form.

Keep in mind that chemotherapy is all about chemistry: your body chemistry and how it will respond to the drugs that are designed to beat back cancer. For that reason, oncologists require very detailed information about their patients before starting adjuvant chemotherapy. The physical examination and blood work you will undergo prior to treatment are very extensive. Again, your pathology report (or reports) is vital, and your oncologist will review all documents and slides before recommending the types of drugs to be used. Your surgical report will be reviewed, as will all of your X rays and previous laboratory reports.

Here are some of the tests you can expect prior to beginning your treatments:

1. *Complete physical.* During the examination the doctor will take note of how well your surgical scar is healing. If you did not have a port put in place during surgery, your doctor may discuss port placement with you.

2. *CBC, or complete blood count.* This is a blood test that focuses on three things: red blood cells (RBCs), hemoglobin (the oxygen-carrying component of red blood cells), and the hematocrit. The latter is the percentage of your blood that contains RBCs. The percentage differs between men and women. Women have a lower hematocrit.

3. *White-cell count.* This is a measurement of the many cellular components that fight infection, such as neutrophils, monocytes, lymphocytes, basophils, and eosinophils. A particularly low white-cell count may mean that the patient has an infection. An extremely low white-cell count can be

brought on by chemotherapy, a condition called *neutro-penia*. This is a serious situation because the chemotherapy may have to be postponed or the dose lowered while the patient's white cells replenish. Medications are available to treat neutropenia.

4. *Blood chemistry*. This measurement analyzes blood plasma. Plasma is the fluid portion of the blood and contains the electrolytes sodium, chloride, calcium, and magnesium, all of which are needed to help the body function normally.

5. *Platelet analysis*. This measurement examines the "sticky" cells in blood that cause clotting. Platelets help you stop bleeding after a cut or scrape.

6. A *complete medical history*. The doctor will take note of illnesses, including infections, you have had in the past. Chemotherapy depresses the immune system; therefore, it is important for your doctors to have a sense of what has affected you in the past. Your doctor will also ask about all medications, vitamins, and other supplements you are taking, because they could have a bearing on chemotherapy.

The workup probably will be conducted within two weeks prior to chemotherapy. Blood tests and other exams, such as scans and X rays, will continue throughout the entire period of your treatment. Your doctor especially wants to take note of your blood profile as chemotherapy continues. This will provide a sense of how well your bone marrow is functioning, whether you have developed an infection, and whether anemia or neutropenia has developed.

You should bring a list of questions, which can be posed during the appointment when your medical history is taken. You are probably very curious about chemotherapy, and this may be a good opportunity to ask questions that can dispel some of the mysteries about treatment. In addition, ask your doctor to recommend another patient who has completed chemo and might be willing to discuss the procedure with someone just beginning the process. Those who have already undergone chemotherapy inevitably have insights into the nuances of treatment that doctors and nurses may be unaware of.

Registered nurses Judith McKay and Nancee Hirano in their book *The Chemotherapy Survival Guide* say there are several things you should know when receiving chemotherapy. For instance, "During chemotherapy you should feel no pain or burning. Pain or burning from the IV indicates that the needle or catheter is not positioned properly in the vein and that it should be checked or changed. You should not feel nauseated because you will probably be given medicines to prevent nausea. Most people get through their chemotherapy treatments without any discomforts."[6]

The Treatment

Mental health experts have long emphasized that undergoing chemotherapy is an anxiety-inducing experience, and patients have voiced that concern as well. Your first day of chemo is like your first day of any new encounter and will probably make you nervous and anxious no matter how hard you try to feel like your old self.

You may want to bring along a companion to your first few chemotherapy treatments. Judith McKay and Nancee Hirano advise in their book that it is important to incorporate a few coping mechanisms. Such measures will minimize your anxiousness as you embark upon this new avenue of care. They write:

> Get comfortable. Because chemotherapy patients often have to sit for an extended period of time, most clinics have comfortable recliner chairs for them. Loosen tight waistbands, ties or collars. Bring a sweater or shawl or ask your nurse for a warm blanket if you get cold. Try to position the arm that has the IV comfortably. Some chemotherapy medicines leave a metallic taste in your mouth (or your mouth may feel dry from the anti-nausea drugs or from anxiety), sucking on hard candy or chewing gum can be a help. The anti-nausea drugs that you may get before your chemotherapy can also make you sleepy. If you feel that way, you may want to doze or listen to music on tape.[7]

A Patient's Diary

In Orlando, Florida, WESH-TV news anchor Wendy Chioji, an athlete who has run the Boston Marathon, discovered in 2001 that she had breast cancer. To help her viewers better understand breast cancer and its treatment, Wendy maintained a diary on the station's website. The following is an excerpt from her experiences: "I had my first chemotherapy treatment Tuesday and it was a doozy. The actual medical procedure was a piece of cake. The nurse gave me an antinausea drug through an IV, then Adriamycin and Cytoxan, the two chemo drugs.

"I felt great and even planned to go to work Tuesday night. Silly me. I think I missed the window of opportunity to take the anti-nausea drug I had at home, because I felt awful. You may have noticed I wasn't at work this week. It has been like the worst hangover you've ever had (of course I don't know what that feels like, ha, ha). But today I am beginning to feel better. One down, three to go of the AC cycles."[8]

Wendy faced down cancer treatment valiantly, logging her experiences in the growing diary she shared with viewers:

> I plan to return to work soon, and things will be a little different, not just for me, but for my coworkers, too. The chemo drugs destroy healthy cells as well as sick cells. That means my white blood cell count drops, and I could get very, very sick if I'm around sick people. And if I get sick it'll delay my chemo treatments.
>
> That means I'll be working with antibacterial wipes and Lysol. I won't even share a phone—lots of germs there. Right about now, I feel exhausted and a little stiff from lying around my house for two days, but things are looking up. It was a two-Smoothie day!! How could it be all bad?

In an interview for this book, Wendy said she began her chemo experience armed with information. As a major part of her education, she consulted a friend who had also undergone chemotherapy. Wendy wanted to get a sense of what the experience would be like from someone who had gotten the treatment recently and who would be honest about the effects of the drugs. That friend, Ann Hellmuth, the deputy managing editor of a Florida newspaper, told Wendy that chemo was not like stories she may have heard. Chemo, Ann emphasized, would not impair Wendy's ability to work and enjoy life.

During chemotherapy, Wendy took a trip to visit friends in Chicago. She also found a new and encouraging role model in Lance Armstrong, the Tour de France champion cyclist who survived cancer. Wendy says she asked lots of questions prior to chemo—not because she feared the impending experience but because she wanted to be empowered as she began a new and trying aspect of cancer treatment. "Ann is a great friend," she says. "I learned a lot from her, and for me knowledge is power. People are afraid of what they don't know. To others [who are facing chemotherapy] I say try to get as much information as you can about it, and that way you can make intelligent and informed decisions. One thing I really learned was that you have to take charge of your own health care."

Common Side Effects and Ways to Cope

Side effects differ from one patient to another because they depend on the medications administered, drug dosages, and length of time on chemotherapy. Generally, problems are temporary. This section outlines the primary problems that can occur as a result of chemotherapy. The next section discusses medications administered to abate these side effects.

Here are several problems patients may encounter while receiving chemotherapy.

Depression: Chemotherapy is one of the most intensive forms of medical care. Studies have documented that it can lead to depression and anxiety. Experts suggest taking part in leisure activities and having fun. Antidepression medications are available.

Fatigue: This common side effect can be alleviated through regular exercise. If blood tests reveal anemia, medication can bolster red blood cell counts.

Hair loss: Of all side effects involving treatment, this one is faced with the most dread and can lead to depression. Doctors have tested some wild ideas to keep hair on peoples' scalps, such as applying ice to patients' heads during chemo treatments to slow blood flow to the scalp. Theory holds that the icy temperature should preserve hair follicles. Results remain inconclusive. The good news is that hair loss is temporary. Hair can grow back thicker and shinier than before. Drug companies, meanwhile, are working on medications to preserve hair.

Increased risk of infection: Chemo can have a harsh effect on the bone marrow where blood cells form. When the number of infection-fighting white cells is low, the patient is at risk of infection. Patients are cautioned to avoid raw foods and to maintain proper hygiene, especially by washing their hands thoroughly and regularly. Medications are available to boost white cells.

Menopause: Chemotherapy can induce a temporary menopause in young women. For those near menopause but who are still menstruating before chemotherapy, the treatment probably will produce an irreversible cessation of periods.

Mouth sores: Some medications can cause bleeding gums and sores in the mouth and throat. The American Cancer Society recommends paying strict attention to oral hygiene and informing your physician as soon as oral problems occur. If sores erupt, the American Cancer Society suggests a diet of soft foods and liquids. Patients should avoid salty, acidic, and rough-textured foods until sores heal. Medications can be prescribed to alleviate discomforts.

Nausea: Chemotherapy causes nausea by activating the chemoreceptor trigger zone (CTZ) in the brain. This spurs the release of neurotransmitters, chemical messengers in the brain that cause the feeling of nausea in the stomach. Eating smaller meals helps control nausea. Several medications are available to relieve nausea in chemotherapy patients.

Combating Side Effects with Medication or Meditation

One of the most delicate balancing acts in all of medicine is the management of medications taken during the course of chemotherapy. It is not just the complex drugs used against cancer that require your physician's constant vigilance but also the accompanying medications that minimize the side effects of treatment. Now that you are a cancer patient, one of the first rules of self-advocacy is to make certain that you are prescribed the medications vital to your care. In other words, you don't have to suffer through intense side effects without any relief. Don't be afraid to speak up and ask your health-care team if there are medications that can help with depression or anxiety, for example. Another important option you may want to consider as you help yourself cope with treatment is to ask about your center's complementary and alternative therapies.

Many cancer and breast-care centers offer sessions either for individuals or for small groups of patients on various forms of relaxation therapy and low-impact exercise. The list at many major cancer centers is long and can run the gamut from yoga, meditation, and t'ai chi to music and art therapy. Inquire at your center to find which among its offerings of complementary and alternative therapies would best suit you. Some centers refer to these types of therapies as *integrative medicine*. Whatever the title, you may open a new window onto an intriguing experience. Mind/body medicine, for example, was once considered offbeat but now has a role in helping cancer patients cope with chemotherapy and manage pain or other side effects. One major cancer center, in the description of its classes on guided imagery, explains that the technique "has many of the benefits of meditation, but uses our imagination and virtually all of our senses to create a deep sense of comfort."

If, however, you feel that medication will best help you cope with the effects of chemotherapy, then it is important that you learn some of the details about the medicines you're seeking. You should have a discussion with your physician about prescription and over-the-counter drugs. Your talk should include what the drug is, what it interacts with, and how vital it is to your care.

Any of the medications from the following list may be prescribed, administered, or recommended during chemo:

1. *Anemia:* **Epogen** and **Procrit** both stimulate the bone marrow to produce the progenitor (precursor) cells that mature into healthy red blood cells. Anemia can cause fatigue, dizziness, and shortness of breath. These drugs alleviate those problems by triggering the growth of the very cells that feed all tissues with oxygen.

2. *Nausea:* **Compazine, Reglan, Kytril,** and **Zofran** are all antinausea drugs that come in a variety of preparations, from pills to IV formulations to rectal suppositories. Compazine and Reglan block the neurotransmitter dopamine. You are advised against driving after taking either of them because they can make you drowsy. Zofran can be administered by IV drip just before your chemo. Both Zofran and Kytril block another transmitter known as serotonin. Neither causes drowsiness.

3. *Infections:* **Antibiotics** are the drugs used to combat infection. Your doctor may choose any from a number of antibiotics. Infections are most likely to occur when white cell counts are low.

4. *Depression:* Antidepressants come in a wide variety of choices. Some doctors have chosen to prescribe **Paxil.** Still others may choose **Prozac** or another medication in its class.

5. *Lack of appetite:* **Decadron,** a steroid medication, can be used to stimulate appetite and improve the patient's sense of well-being. The drug is also prescribed in combination with Kytril and Zofran to control chemotherapy-induced nausea and vomiting. **Marinol,** a prescription medication that mimics the appetite-increasing feature of marijuana, is another choice.

6. *Low platelet count:* **Neumega** is a drug containing the growth factor that stimulates the bone marrow to produce platelets, which aid in blood clotting.

7. *Neutropenia (low white cell count):* Granulocyte-colony stimulating factor (**G-CSF**) and granulocyte macrophage-colony stimulating factor (**GM-CSF**) are proteins produced by the body to boost infection-fighting white cells. Growth-factor medications are critial, especially if you develop an infection while on chemotherapy. In three-quaters of patients who take either G-CSF (Neupogen) or GM-CSF (Leukine), white cell counts increase. **Neulasta** is an updated version of a drug known as **Neupogen.** Both drugs boost white-cell populations. Neulasta is a pegylated formulation, which means it remains in the body longer performing its job.

In addition to the above medications, which must be prescribed by a doctor, there are also several over-the-counter drugs that can help with chemotherapy's side effects. One of them is **milk of magnesia,** an old standby used to treat constipation and dating to the nineteenth century. It works by forcing water into the large intestine to soften stools for easier elimination. **Magnesium citrate (Senokot)** is another drug used to treat constipation. It works differently from milk of magnesia.

Additional Tests

Blood tests, physical examinations, scans, and questions from your health-care providers will continue throughout your months of chemotherapy. Of the tests, however, blood tests will be of the utmost importance because they determine how the treatments are affecting you. Are your red blood cells in particularly low supply? What about your white-cell count? During chemotherapy your doctor will order the same panel of blood tests that you underwent in your initial workup. Repeat tests will analyze your RBCs, hemoglobin, and hematocrit, your plasma, platelets, and family of white blood cells.

The tests tell a story that may not be obvious in a simple physical examination. A low hemoglobin count, for example, may explain your fatigue or dizziness; an extremely low white-cell count may be evidence of neutropenia, which could lead to hospitalization. Do not miss any of your scheduled lab appointments, even as bothersome as they may seem, because monitoring the effects that chemotherapy is having on your healthy cells is the only way your doctor will know whether to continue your treatments as they have been planned.

More on Chemo from the Patient's Perspective

People who have undergone chemotherapy for breast cancer have a wide range of responses about how they felt during treatment. Maryanne B. says she was pleased to reach such a milestone in her care, because "that meant I had succeeded. I was glad to get to that point because I knew that I was saving my life." Maryanne continued to work and care for her family during chemotherapy.

Liisa M. says her experience was not as debilitating as she had expected, but there were some surprises.

> I started chemo on a Monday after Thanksgiving. The previous week I had ten medical appointments in five days. It was, to put it mildly, overwhelming. My mastectomy scar was still fresh and I had not yet regained my full strength from the surgery.

Given all that she had heard about chemotherapy, she knew she would have to experience it before she could fully form an opinion about treatments that a great many people fear.

> My first three doses (given three weeks apart) were Adriamycin and Cytoxan. Other than the obvious—hair falling out, tiredness—I had very few side effects. I must say there is that lovely moment in the bathroom when you discover that the beautiful red color in the Cytoxan has flowed right through you, turning your urine red.

Also, I discovered within hours that the peppermint tea that I love made me queasy. For about three days, I couldn't bear the smell of cooking. I bore up well, thanks probably to the Paxil and my determination to get through the treatments.

Rob P., fifty-eight, a former lineman for an electrical utility, was haunted by the thought that he was being treated for "a woman's cancer." Though he took medication to treat his depression, it really wasn't sadness about going through chemotherapy that he experienced. In his mind, the form of cancer he developed was not one that men usually got. As for chemo, Rob says he decided to face down chemotherapy with the same courage he summoned when he had to repair fallen electrical cables on dark, rainy nights.

I got through the mastectomy okay. It was when I got my workup for chemo that it really hit me, that this was treatment for cancer, and not just any cancer, but breast cancer. Being a man that's difficult, because you think of it as a woman's cancer.

They told me to forget everything I had ever heard about chemo because I wouldn't get nauseous, and I didn't. I didn't have to worry about my hair, because as you can see there isn't any. They put me on AC [Adriamycin and Cytoxan]. I got through it, no problem.

Activists Want More Treatment Options

Gentler treatments are high on the list of developments activists would like to see for people undergoing adjuvant treatment for breast cancer. Medical science has worked diligently to reduce many of the difficult side effects of chemotherapy. The Susan G. Komen Breast Cancer Foundation, a patient-advocacy organization, is funding studies at major universities that are developing new drugs to treat the disease. The organization is also funding studies that will answer questions about the basic biology of breast cancer. You can peruse the kinds of studies the organization is funding by logging on to its website at www.susangkomen.org.

Musa Mayer, author and advocate for people with breast cancer, also supports the development of new drugs. Ms. Mayer, a breast cancer survivor, has written extensively about the disease and is kept busy with speaking engagements that take her all over the United States. "Of course advocates would love to see something other than chemotherapy in use in adjuvant treatment," she says. "Or at least we'd like to see the possibility of lower doses with less toxicity. But I think it's unrealistic to imagine that within the foreseeable future we will be able to dispense with chemo altogether, especially for the 25 percent to 30 percent of women whose tumors are ER/PR negative."

Ms. Mayer adds that those who advocate for people with breast cancer also would like to see researchers investigate more precise methods of choosing patients for chemo. Currently, patients meet a general set of standards, even though some, based on the characteristics of their cancer, may not need months of chemotherapy. "In my view the ideal is not to banish certain kinds of drugs but to do the research that enables us to use them intelligently, and only with patients who are likely to benefit. As it is today, we treat a great many women in the adjuvant setting because we don't know who is likely to recur. It is time—past time—for the hit-and-miss treatments to end."

On her wish list of futuristic developments, Ms. Mayer would like to see scientists produce forms of screening that could reveal when tumor cells are present after breast cancer surgery. Such screenings would immediately inform oncologists which patients would benefit most from chemotherapy. "The problem isn't with the chemo and the side effects," she says. "It's that we don't have the biomarkers to indicate which cancers are indolent and unlikely to recur, and which are aggressive and would benefit most from strong chemo combinations. I believe that being able to use the drugs we have in a more targeted fashion may ultimately be more effective (and more feasible) than new drugs we may discover. But, of course, we ought to do both kinds of research."

As Ms. Mayer points out, science moves forward in small, incremental steps, which means years are consumed before huge changes occur and revolutionary new approaches are available to patients.

Investigating New Approaches:
Clinical Trials

Sometimes you can get a hint of what cancer treatment will be like years from now by joining a clinical trial where doctors are testing new therapies. Dozens of new approaches are being researched for adjuvant treatment, many of them offered through clinical trials.

As registered nurse and breast cancer survivor Bettye Green explains, a common misconception about clinical trials is that people commonly think they are designed to test drugs that lack a track record. Ms. Green made her pitch for clinical trials to a group of breast cancer survivors while addressing a conference in New York City sponsored by *MAMM* magazine. To the surprise of many patients, she said, clinical trials involve new uses and combinations of existing drugs. As the head of two local patient-advocacy groups in South Bend, Indiana, she often explains this nuance to people leery of new approaches. Only through human testing, she points out, can new treatment strategies find their way into the various regimens doctors refer to as standard therapy. Drugs never before tried in the adjuvant setting, Ms. Green said, can be tested in combination with medications used successfully for years in the treatment of patients with advanced breast cancer. Tamoxifen, for example, has been studied in clinical trials for more than thirty years.[9]

Your oncologist or nurses should be able to help you find a clinical trial if you are interested in joining one. There are several questions you need to learn the answers to in advance: Would the research drugs be significantly better than the ones offered by my physicians? Are there any costs that I will have to bear? What is the true aim of this study?

Looking at an Old Drug in a New Way

Dr. Dennis Slamon, director of the Revlon/UCLA Women's Cancer Research Program, believes that by employing a strategy normally used for patients with advanced disease, doctors may be able to prevent recurrences in women prone to an especially aggressive form of breast cancer.

As the developer of Herceptin, the breakthrough breast cancer drug designed to treat cases of the disease when the HER-2 onco-gene is present, Dr. Slamon brought a stronger degree of hope to pa-tients with metastatic breast cancer. Herceptin received U.S. Food and Drug Administration approval in 1998. After several years of the medication being used against late-stage disease, Dr. Slamon began organizing studies in 2001 to test a simple but powerful principle: Perhaps Herceptin might be able to help patients earlier. In 2005, Dr. Slamon's hypothesis was proven to be correct.

Following exhaustive clinical trials, the National Cancer Insti-tute announced that Herceptin, when given in combination with chemotherapy, reduces the risk of recurrences among those with early-stage breast cancer that is marked by the gene aberration. Two clinical trials that ran simultaneously and that involved more than 5,000 volunteers demonstrated that early-stage patients who re-ceived Herceptin were 52 percent less likely to have recurrences than those who did not receive the drug. Dr. Slamon says clinical trials have produced invaluable information on treating one of the most aggressive forms of breast cancer:

> The Herceptin-chemotherapy combinations have been shown to decrease breast cancer deaths by 27 percent in women whose metastatic [advanced] breast cancer is char-acterized by an alteration in the HER-2 gene. This is significant because the life expectancy of patients who have the genetic alteration can be as low as half the life expectancy of patients who don't have it. By giving Herceptin and chemotherapy at an earlier stage we hope to help patients who have the ge-netic alteration live longer and ultimately have the best chance of being cured.... We believe that Herceptin holds significant promise to help women who are newly diagnosed with aggressive breast cancer.[10]

Furthering Your Research on Adjuvant Chemotherapy

You can learn more about clinical trials by logging on to the National Institute of Health's website at www.clinicaltrials.gov. There, you can find information explaining how clinical trials work as well as a listing of which trials are enrolling patients. As mentioned earlier, you can also call the National Cancer Institute to ask a question about cancer by dialing (800) 4-CANCER (800-422-6237). The help line is operated Monday through Friday, 9:00 A.M. to 5:00 P.M.

Another good source for clinical trial information is the American Cancer Society's website: www.cancer.org. Or you can call the cancer society at (800) ACS-2345 (800-227-2345).

Finally, another excellent site where you can learn about clinical trials and adjuvant chemotherapy is the National Comprehensive Cancer Network. You can find that organization on the web at www.nccn.org, or you can call (888) 909-NCCN (888-909-6226).

10

Hormone Therapy: Counteracting Estrogen

At this point in your medical odyssey you may feel as if you know as much about breast cancer as your physicians, and in many ways you just might know more. You probably have had surgery; you may have also finished six or more weeks of radiation treatments and possibly even chemotherapy. Despite all that you have experienced and learned since your diagnosis, now maybe your doctor is offering something extra, a drug you may have to take for the next five years.

Hormone therapy is an adjuvant treatment. It probably should be known more precisely as "antihormone therapy," because the drugs involved mostly inhibit estrogen's cancer-driving activity. Hormone therapy targets and inhibits progesterone's activity as well. But as you have probably now guessed, estrogen is a dominant and domineering hormone with the ability to change the course of a cell's fate.

Decades ago, before doctors had an array of medications to usurp the power of hormones, they resorted to surgery to eliminate patients' natural sources of these compounds. In premenopausal women, surgeons would perform an oophorectomy—removal of the ovaries. In postmenopausal women, they would remove the adrenal glands, which aid in estrogen's production after the ovaries are no longer functioning. Taking away these hormone sources provided some level of assurance that a woman's natural hormones could no longer fuel cancer growth.

But while surgery is still performed on occasion, estrogen production now can be eliminated—or at the very least its concentration lowered—without the patient having to face an operation. Different medications can counteract estrogen in different ways. And a flurry of studies over the years has shown that drug therapy, often with just a pill a day, can substantially lower the risk of recurrence.

Patients who successfully complete one of the most common forms of hormone therapy are said to have literally added years free of breast cancer to their lives. This is not to imply that hormone treatments are without side effects or that every patient is successfully treated with them. What the studies of these pills have offered is a strong measure of hope for a vast number of people.

In this chapter we explore an array of medications used to prevent natural hormones from causing a recurrence of breast cancer. First among the drug classes are medications known as SERMs, selective estrogen receptor modulators. The drug tamoxifen was the first SERM and is the prototype for medications in this class.

An additional—and very important—class is known as the aromatase inhibitors. Aromatase is an enzyme distributed throughout a variety of tissues in the body, particularly fat. It is also found to some extent in muscle and bone tissue. Aromatase is capable of converting androgens, produced by the adrenal glands, into estrogen. This method of estrogen production is the primary route through which estrogen is manufactured after menopause.

Estrogen's "Big" and "Little" Faucets

Dr. Silvana Martino, of the John Wayne Cancer Center in Santa Monica and the University of Southern California in Los Angeles, believes the best way to understand how antiestrogen drugs work is to first understand how the body makes its hormones. Each of the drug classes prescribed to thwart estrogen goes about doing so in a different way. The methods of counteracting estrogen are based precisely on how estrogen is produced in the body. As she explains it:

> Basically in the female body there are two main origins of estrogen. The primary sources are the ovaries, which produce 80 percent of a woman's estrogen, and the remaining sources are the adrenal glands. One [adrenal gland] sits on each kidney, and they make prohormones (androgens) that are converted into estrogens. There is a very important enzyme that also has a role here. It converts prohormones into estrogen and it is called aromatase. So when a woman is premenopausal, she has two sources of estrogen, a big faucet and a little faucet. When she is postmenopausal she then has only one, the adrenal glands. The adrenals are essentially the small faucet because the big faucet has already been turned off.

Dr. Martino, who has been a lead investigator in numerous clinical studies, particularly those examining how safely and how well certain classes of drugs work, emphasizes that some antihormone medications can be taken by both pre- and postmenopausal women. Other drug classes are aimed primarily at postmenopausal patients. Most drugs designed only for postmenopausal women, she says, zero in on the enzyme aromatase, which plays a prominent role in the "little faucet" production of estrogen.

A Primer on Hormone Receptors

You may recall from your pathology report that doctors made note of your hormone-receptor status (see Chapters 4 and 5). This is a key bit of information you've probably been mulling in the back of your mind. If you're one of the many women who is said to be hormone-receptor positive, now is the time to give more thought to what that designation really means. About two-thirds of women diagnosed with breast cancer are hormone-receptor positive, which means they had the kind of cancer whose growth was stimulated by the hormones estrogen and/or progesterone. If the cancer was hormone-receptor positive, then the pathologist further indicated in the report that the tumor was estrogen-receptor positive and/or progesterone-receptor positive, a finding that made these patients candidates for antiestrogen drugs. (The antiestrogen drugs are also used against progesterone.)

On your pathology report your hormone-receptor status was written simply as ER+ (only estrogen receptors were found), PR+ (only progesterone receptors were found), or ER+/PR+ (both estrogen and progesterone receptors were found). The plus sign is shorthand for *positive*. If you are hormone-receptor negative then your report would have indicated that fact with a minus sign, as in ER–.

Receptors are proteins to which hormones bind on the surface of many types of cells—not just cancerous ones. If you went on a hunt for receptors you'd primarily find them (mostly estrogen receptors because nature endowed estrogen with a dominant role) on the surface of cells in tissues that estrogen influences: For instance, cells that make up breast tissue, cells comprising structures of the female reproductive tract, cells of the skeletal system and brain. Think of hormone receptors as the front porch and doorway of a cell. They are where the natural hormones arrive and then proceed into the cell's inner sanctum, where they drive cell growth. SERMs very effectively block that entrance.

Perhaps now you can see with more clarity that the results of your hormone-receptor test tell your doctors a very complex story, and the most likely plot is that estrogen drove the growth of your tumor.

A Basic Guide to Hormone Therapy

Tamoxifen (sold under the brand name **Nolvadex**) was the first drug that medical scientists found capable of preventing breast cancer in women who did not have the disease but who were at high risk as a result of either genetics or having had the disease in the past. It is used as adjuvant therapy (you may recall from previous chapters that *adjuvant* means additional treatment after surgery), or it can be used as a treatment for those whose cancer has spread. You can read more about tamoxifen later in this chapter.

Raloxifene (sold as **Evista**), an osteoporosis drug, has not been approved for the treatment of breast cancer by the Food and Drug Administration, but medical scientists have been documenting an impressive amount of data about it. The most extensive data involving raloxifene focus on its ability to prevent breast cancer in women at high risk but who have not been diagnosed with the disease. Until more data are available it is not recommended as hormonal therapy for those who have already been diagnosed with the cancer. (You can read more about raloxifene later in this chapter.) Tamoxifen and raloxifene belong to the class of drugs known as SERMs. SERMs can act like estrogens in some tissues and antiestrogens in others.

Toremifene (sold as **Fareston**), also a SERM, is another close relative to tamoxifen, but it can only be prescribed to postmenopausal women, and among them primarily those with metastatic disease. Tests are being conducted to determine whether it can be more widely used in postmenopausal women who cannot tolerate tamoxifen. Toremifene is mostly prescribed to patients who have tested hormone-receptor positive. However, it also has been prescribed successfully to women whose hormone-receptor status is unknown.

Fulvestrant (sold as **Faslodex**) is a drug that can home in on the estrogen receptor and then eliminate it. The drug can be used when tamoxifen is no longer effective or is not well tolerated by the patient. Key side effects are hot flashes and nausea.

Drugs known as aromatase inhibitors target what Dr. Martino referred to as estrogen's "small faucet" of production. The inhibitors zero in on and bind to the aromatase enzyme. When the enzyme is inactivated, estrogen can no longer be produced in postmenopausal women. Three aromatase inhibitors have been approved by the FDA: **exemestane (Aromasin), letrozole (Femara),** and **anastrozole (Arimidex).** All three were first designed to treat advanced breast cancer, but studies have found a strong role for these medications in adjuvant therapy and in posttamoxifen therapy. Osteoporosis and fractures can be a side effect of these drugs. Read more about aromatase inhibitors later in this chapter.

Eliminating ovarian hormones by using drugs to chemically halt hormone production or by surgically removing the two organs (ovarian ablation) is still an option for some premenopausal women. Ovarian ablation is a proven way to control hormone-dependent breast cancer. When drug therapy is chosen, doctors use drugs such as **Leuprolide,** but there are others. This kind of therapy now is being tested as an adjuvant treatment. Side effects can include the range of menopausal symptoms, particularly hot flashes.

Megestrol acetate (sold as **Megace**) is a progesterone-like drug prescribed for advanced breast cancer that is most often prescribed when cancers do not respond to other hormone therapies. A major consequence of the drug is weight gain. It is sometimes given to breast cancer patients who have lost a significant amount of weight.

Goserelin (sold as **Zoladex**) is another medication for premenopausal women. It is a synthetic version of a natural hormone known as gonadotropin-releasing hormone. If you take this drug you will block all hormone production by the ovaries. Goserelin can be taken by patients with early or metastatic disease.

Tamoxifen

Of all the medications used in hormone therapy for breast cancer, tamoxifen (see Figure 6) and its generics are the most widely prescribed globally. It is prescribed at 20 milligrams a day, which can be taken as a single 20-mg tablet or as two 10-mg tablets, one in the morning and the other in the evening. The drug is covered by insurance for those with a prescription drug plan.

Tamoxifen is backed by decades of research, which has shown that as an adjuvant treatment for early-stage breast cancer (primary disease), the medication not only helps prevent a recurrence but also helps ward off the emergence of new cancers in the opposite breast.

As the first SERM, it is the yardstick by which other drugs in the class are measured. Prime among the many roles played by tamoxifen is its ability to reduce the risk of breast cancer recurrence by interfering with estrogen's ability to penetrate cells.

You can undergo tamoxifen therapy whether you had radiation treatments, chemotherapy, or both. You can be pre- or post-menopausal; your surgery could have been breast-conserving or mastectomy. You can even be a man. None of these variables matter. The outcome of your estrogen-receptor test is the key. Tamoxifen is the medication that many physicians say single-handedly helped ensure

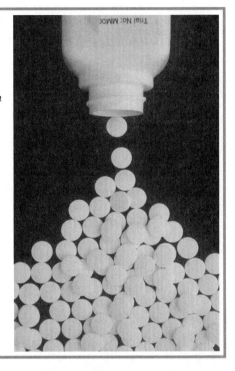

Figure 6. *Tamoxifen has long been a mainstay for patients being treated for early-stage, hormonally sensitive breast cancer. It belongs to the class of drugs known as selective estrogen receptor modulators, or SERMs, which block estrogen's ability to activate cancer cells. Doctors now know that there is a significant survival advantage for postmenopausal women who take tamoxifen for five years and then undergo an additional two-and-a-half years of treatment with a type of medication known as an aromatase inhibitor. Unlike tamoxifen, aromatase inhibitors do not block estrogen. They prevent androgen hormones from being converted into estrogen in women whose ovaries no longer produce the hormone. (Credit: James King-Holmes / Photo Researchers, Inc.)*

a bright prognosis for scores of estrogen-receptor-positive women around the world. As wondrous as that may seem, tamoxifen is not a miracle drug, nor is it completely problem-free.

Although chances are low, one side effect of tamoxifen is endometrial cancer in some postmenopausal women. (The endometrium is the lining of the uterus.) Oncologists always tell women who are taking tamoxifen to report any unusual vaginal bleeding. Vaginal bleeding would be an instant signal of concern to postmenopausal women because menstruation has ceased. However, the chances of endometrial cancer are so low that you should not be dissuaded from taking tamoxifen if it is prescribed. Doctors insist—and studies demonstrate—that the benefits of the drug far outweigh its risks.

Another tamoxifen side effect can be DVT (deep vein thrombosis): clotting in the deep blood vessels of the legs. The condition can be dangerous because a clot can travel to a lung and lodge there, an event that can prove fatal. The clotting problem also poses a risk for stroke. These problems are also rare, but they are side effects that you should be aware of. Other side effects of tamoxifen include nausea, hot flashes, and cataracts.

Despite the medication's drawbacks, oncologists point to a long list of its benefits, underscoring the very favorable outlook for the hundreds of thousands of women who have not had recurrences. If your oncologist is recommending tamoxifen, you might want to have a frank discussion about the drug and its side effects. Try to bear in mind that the endometrial cancer risks are extremely low. If you're very worried, you might want to gather a sampling of opinions about tamoxifen and other types of hormone-based medications from several oncologists.

The Cost of Your Medication

Tamoxifen is not inexpensive. Nolvadex, the brand-name version, runs more than two hundred dollars a month. Even a generic form of the drug can cost a hundred dollars monthly. If you find that in addition to your other medical expenses, the drug remains out of reach, do not cut corners and resort to splitting pills or missing a dose to save money. When this drug is prescribed, it is very important to your survival. As mentioned in Chapter 2, pharmaceutical companies offer programs to help patients who cannot afford their medications. AstraZeneca, tamoxifen's maker, offers such programs for a variety of their drugs. If you cannot afford tamoxifen, AstraZeneca offers a special program that provides it for free. You can find out more by calling (800) 424-3727.

WHAT PATIENTS SAY ABOUT TAMOXIFEN

Having gone through three surgeries for breast cancer—a lumpectomy, a mastectomy, and reconstructive surgery—Yvonne M. says when she takes her tamoxifen, she feels that she has in her hand the best weapon possible to prevent the cancer from coming back.

> I gladly would not have gone through this ordeal. But when the doctor said to me, "You no longer have cancer," that was very encouraging. I'm taking tamoxifen and I'm pretty optimistic, and I just say thank God it wasn't worse.

Some women who tested hormone-receptor negative, such as Liisa M., say they wish they could take tamoxifen or one of the other hormone therapies.

> No, I didn't qualify for it. Is that the right word, qualify? Meet the criterion? Whatever, I didn't get it. And I really wish I could have, because it offers that extra little measure of protection that I wish I had.

At a New York oncologist's practice, several women who take tamoxifen or who had taken it in the past offered their thoughts on the drug, which, despite its drawbacks, has been hailed by doctors as having served an enormous public health benefit.

This woman has had no side effects from the medication:

> It'll be two years in June and I have no complaints. I had a lumpectomy and didn't need chemo or anything like that. I'm on tamoxifen, and nothing else. I know it has side effects but I've been on it for two years. And no—I've had no problems, knock on wood.

No complaints from this woman, either:

> A little queasiness when I first started taking it, but nothing to speak of.

Nor this woman:

> I'm doing great.

A former tamoxifen taker did not like the medication:

> Nolvadex didn't settle well with me.... I was nauseated the whole time I took it, which wasn't very long.

ACTIVISM AND TAMOXIFEN

Barbara Brenner, executive director and founder of Breast Cancer Action, the San Francisco–based advocacy organization, was among the first activists to speak out against using too many superlatives when discussing tamoxifen. She is especially wary of using the word *preventive* when describing how the drug staves off breast cancer in people who take it.

Ms. Brenner, herself a breast cancer survivor, contends that tamoxifen should be regarded only as a drug that helps reduce breast cancer risk. Some people who take tamoxifen, Ms. Brenner points out, develop breast cancer despite the drug. Scientists, she adds, have yet to develop a problem-free method for what she calls primary prevention: inhibiting cells from becoming cancerous in the first place. "If this drug had no side effects," she says, "we wouldn't complain, but tamoxifen is a known carcinogen. And it not only causes endometrial cancer; it also causes blood clots and a lot of other medical problems. When activists like us started asking [medical scientists] for prevention, we were talking about primary prevention."

For Ms. Brenner, primary prevention means stopping cancer before it even starts. As she puts it, "In the medical field and the public health field, prevention means something completely different than it does to the general population. To most people prevention means that the disease will never occur if you follow this or that step. But in the medical field there is primary, secondary, and tertiary prevention. These pill trials [clinical studies of tamoxifen and similar medications] are in the nature of secondary prevention because there is no guarantee here. There is no guarantee that you are ever home free."

TAMOXIFEN: THE GOOD, THE BAD, AND THE UGLY

There are several facts about tamoxifen with respect to its benefits and its drawbacks that you may want to think about if your oncologist believes you are a good candidate for the therapy:

❖ Tamoxifen has an unusual mechanism of action as a SERM. It can block estrogen activity that can lead to cancer-cell growth, but it also has the ability to halt the activity of cells that are on the path to becoming cancerous—those that are not quite malignant. It is believed that tamoxifen can trigger precancerous cells to undergo apoptosis, or programmed cell death. These cells can be forced to die before they have a chance to evolve into full-blown tumors.

❖ Tamoxifen enhances skeletal strength because in the bones it acts like natural estrogen, serving to stave off osteoporosis. In the liver, where cholesterol is metabolized, the drug weakly helps to reduce low-density lipoproteins, the so-called bad form of cholesterol. By comparison, natural estrogen plays a stronger cholesterol-lowering role.

❖ With respect to the risk of endometrial cancer, researchers are analyzing predisposing factors, such as whether, for example, previous hormone replacement therapy taken to abate menopausal symptoms could be a contributor to the growth of endometrial tumors in some patients.

Raloxifene: The First "Designer" Antiestrogen

The story of raloxifene is conveyed here not because this medication is one your doctor will prescribe to prevent a recurrence, but because the saga of raloxifene's emergence is an illustration of how treacherously long it takes to develop a compound into a cancer drug. Raloxifene remains under study, and the only way to be prescribed the medication as of this writing is to participate in a clinical trial where it is being tested.

Raloxifene is the first "designer" antiestrogen because its developers chemically configured it to sidestep the problems associated with tamoxifen. Foremost, it was designed to avoid adversely affecting the uterus. Raloxifene was meticulously developed to possess tamoxifen's good points and to bypass most of its bad ones. Tamoxifen, on the other hand, emerged on the scene three decades before raloxifene as the result of a chance discovery. It was originally developed as a fertility drug in the 1960s, but it didn't work well in that capacity. It sat on the shelf for years before it was resurrected for tests as a potential anticancer medication. Raloxifene's much shorter history is far different.

Sold as Evista, raloxifene is a product of Eli Lilly & Co. It began its pharmaceutical life as a drug aimed at increasing bone density in postmenopausal women at risk of osteoporosis. It has been under extensive investigation for more than a decade as a medication capable of decreasing the risk of breast cancer in postmenopausal women who have never had the disease.

With tamoxifen's start as a fertility drug and raloxifene's as an osteoporosis medication, you might think SERMs must first begin in another role before being tested as a treatment against breast cancer. While that may seem to be the case, it tells only a small part of a larger story.

The first public inkling that raloxifene might serve in a capacity similar to tamoxifen came after results of an Eli Lilly–sponsored study of women with osteoporosis. In that analysis, which ran between 1994 and 1998, researchers found that in addition to bone protection, raloxifene could reduce the risk of invasive breast cancer by 76 percent. A large-scale study of 7,705 women conducted at centers in this country and Europe (dubbed the MORE trial) took up the mantle from there.[1]

Participants in MORE, whose average age was 66.5, were studied at 180 clinical centers in twenty-five countries for four years. All of the women took raloxifene as a two-pill-a-day regimen for four years. Results from the trial paved the way for raloxifene's approval in 1997 as an osteoporosis medication.[2] (A criticism of the trial by some in the activist community was that MORE may have been conducted as an osteoporosis project but breast cancer prevention was the study's true aim. While there is nothing really wrong with a study having more than one objective, critics saw duplicity and charged that other osteoporosis drugs were already on the market that protected bones better.)

Even though it is a SERM, raloxifene is chemically distinct from tamoxifen. Like tamoxifen, raloxifene can latch onto estrogen receptors and block them, preventing the natural hormone from pene-trating cells in selective tissues. Raloxifene acts as an antiestrogen in the breast and uterus. It also has natural estrogen's bone-strengthening capability in the skeletal system.

Still, the MORE trial not only answered key questions; it served as the study that got raloxifene on the market with the hope of eventually using it as an anticancer agent. The MORE trial showed that in healthy women, the drug appears to prevent invasive breast cancers by 72 percent, just slightly less than what the smaller company-sponsored study had demonstrated.[3]

Researchers then turned their attention to more fully investigating raloxifene's anticancer effects in healthy postmenopausal women at high risk for the disease. The National Surgical Adjuvant Breast and Bowel Project, in collaboration with the National Cancer Institute, began the STAR (Study of Tamoxifen and Raloxifene) trial, one of the largest clinical studies of breast cancer prevention in history. From the start, the plan was to study the two drugs in twenty-two thousand women across the United States, Canada, and Puerto Rico.

Some of the enthusiasm driving the STAR investigation was derived from the Breast Cancer Prevention Trial, the large-scale study in the 1990s that found tamoxifen could prevent breast cancer in women at high risk, but who had never had the disease. As a toe-to-toe analysis between raloxifene and tamoxifen, the STAR research project was designed to see how the two medications compare. Researchers also hope to determine whether raloxifene offers benefits that tamoxifen lacks. The study began in 1999 and was scheduled to run five years, and then was to be followed by seven additional years of follow-up study.

The randomized, double-blind trial enrolled women at least age thirty-five who are at increased risk of breast cancer due to inheritance or other factors. Participants received physicals, mammograms, and pelvic examinations as part of the study. While only postmenopausal women were to receive raloxifene, both pre- and postmenopausal women were enrolled in the tamoxifen arm. Along with STAR, additional studies of raloxifene are bound to occur over the next several decades, researchers predict, given the three decades worth of tamoxifen studies.

FROM MORE TO CORE

The STAR trial is not the only scientific investigation seeking more answers from raloxifene. USC's Dr. Silvana Martino, who has been one of the nation's leading scientific investigators examining the effects of the drug, says that results of the MORE trial were so exciting that a decision was made to continue it in as many participants as possible. Thus, the CORE trial embarked on another four years of raloxifene research. In the CORE trial, 3,510 women continued taking raloxifene, and 1,703 women took a placebo.

Reporting final results in 2004 at a meeting of the American Association of Clinical Oncology, Dr. Martino and her colleagues found that after eight years on the drug, participants' breast cancer risk was reduced by 66 percent. What CORE proved, Dr. Martino said, is that raloxifene has a potent ability to block estrogen's ability to fuel breast cancers. "Whether one looks at the MORE trial, the CORE trial, or the two combined," she said, "the same biology is observed, and, yes, this agent does have the ability to reduce the risk and incidence of breast cancer."[4]

SIDE EFFECTS EVEN WITH A DESIGNER DRUG

Despite raloxifene's distinction as the first designer SERM, it is not free of side effects. While Dr. Martino reported that no new toxicities were discovered in the CORE trial, she did underscore that a serious but rare blood-clotting problem discovered during MORE continued in the CORE study. As mentioned earlier in the chapter, there is a similar risk of abnormal clotting with tamoxifen.

While the likelihood of someone developing a dangerous clot while taking either drug is extremely low, the risk is not zero. One woman in the MORE study died of a pulmonary embolus. Patients who have taken raloxifene have complained of hot flashes, abdominal bloating, and water retention. During the MORE trial more women in the raloxifene group than in the placebo arm of the study reported new or worsening cases of diabetes compared with participants taking placebos. The diabetes cases were extremely rare.

Aromatase Inhibitors

Exactly how the "small faucet" of estrogen production occurs is one of the wonders of human biology. Although this secondary source of estrogen is not as complex as the cycles involved in ovarian hormone production, its estrogen production can still be robust. In fact, experts say it can pose a threat to those who have developed hormone-dependent breast cancer after menopause.

For postmenopausal women, estrogen is produced in a catalytic process involving the enzyme aromatase, which is prevalent in fat, muscle, and bone tissues, including the fat tissue of the breast. The enzyme is capable of converting adrenal hormones—androgens, the prohormones mentioned earlier by Dr. Martino—into estrogen. (Premenopausal women produce some estrogen through this manner, but for them ovarian hormone production is far more powerful.) An aromatase inhibitor is a type of drug that halts the activity of aromatase and shuts down postmenopausal estrogen production. For postmenopausal women treated for hormone-dependent cancers, these medications can eliminate estrogen from the body.

As Dr. Martino explains, the small faucet does not switch on at menopause; it functions throughout a woman's life: "When women are premenopausal they have two sources of estrogen production. When a woman becomes postmenopausal she has only one, and that source originates from the adrenal glands. Aromatase inhibitors have the ability to interfere with the enzyme. They have a very straightforward way of interfering with the biology of estrogen production."

The Food and Drug Administration has approved three aromatase inhibitors. The drugs are for patients whose pathology report found their cancers to be hormone-receptor positive: ER+, PR+, or ER+/PR+. You may find the drugs to have tongue-twisting names. They are: anastrozole (sold as Arimidex), exemestane (sold as Aromasin), and letrozole (sold as Femara). All of the drugs were first approved as treatments for advanced breast cancer. Initial studies showed aromatase inhibitors to be effective in patients whose cancer had spread and in whom tamoxifen was no longer effective.

In 2002, Arimidex became the first aromatase inhibitor to gain an FDA okay for use in adjuvant therapy. Since then, doctors have found a prominent role for aromatase inhibitors in the treatment of *early* breast cancer. An expert panel from the American Society of Clinical Oncology announced at the San Antonio Breast Cancer Symposium, in December 2004, that five years of tamoxifen is no longer the optimal treatment choice for postmenopausal women and recommended that an aromatase inhibitor be offered as initial therapy or after treatment with tamoxifen to reduce the risk of a recurrence.

Aromatase inhibitors differ in the way they act in the body. Arimidex and Femara are known as nonsteroidal aromatase inhibitors. When the drugs are stopped, aromatase again catalyzes adrenal hormones in fat and muscle tissue, causing estrogen to be produced. Aromasin is an irreversible steroidal antiaromatase medication. It acts as a false substrate for the aromatase enzyme. In short, it chemically confuses the enzyme, making it impossible for aromatase to convert androgens into estrogen. Although Aromasin dramatically lowers circulating estrogens in postmenopausal women, it has no discernable effect on other adrenal hormones.

Other aromatase inhibitors are in the pipeline. Vorozole is an aromatase inhibitor under intense study in the U.S. and Europe. This drug, which has the commercial name Rivisor, is what is known as a third-generation aromatase inhibitor, having been developed long after others in the class. It has had success in clinical studies conducted in Germany and France. As of this writing it has not been approved for use in the United States.

CAN YOUNGER WOMEN TAKE AN AROMATASE INHIBITOR?

Generally, the answer to that question is no. As Dr. Martino pointed out, younger women receive most of their estrogen from their "big faucet" of production: the ovaries. Taking an aromatase inhibitor would eliminate only the 20 percent coming from the "small faucet," the conversion of androgens into estrogen. In a scenario such as this, the patient would still have the majority of her estrogen supply, which would produce more than enough hormone to stimulate cancer-cell growth.

Therefore, prescribing an aromatase inhibitor alone to a patient with functioning ovaries would not be in the patient's best interest, doctors say, because the amount of estrogen produced by the ovaries is overwhelming. The amount produced by the conversion of androgens into estrogen is minuscule by comparison.

However, studies in Europe are changing how doctors are using aromatase inhibitors. Doctors are eliminating ovarian hormone production through either drug therapy or surgery, then prescribing an aromatase inhibitor to eliminate any remaining estrogen production through the conversion of adrenal hormones. In some European studies doctors first prescribed Zolodex (see "A Basic Guide to Hormone Therapy," earlier in this chapter) to premenopausal patients before prescribing an aromatase inhibitor.

ARE AROMATASE INHIBITORS FREE OF SIDE EFFECTS?

Medical researchers are still investigating what the long-term side effects of aromatase inhibitors may be. They already know there is an increased risk for bone thinning and osteoporosis due to the total-body elimination of estrogen. Some patients who have taken the medications report hot flashes, perspiration, fatigue, headaches, and nausea. The risk for dangerous blood clots appears to be lower than it is for tamoxifen. The good news is there is no increased risk for endometrial cancer, because the drugs do not work like tamoxifen.

If you would like more information on hormone therapy in the treatment of breast cancer, log on to www.breastcancer.org, which carries several discussions on the topic, including information about the benefits and drawbacks of aromatase inhibitors.

11

Recurrence: If Breast Cancer Comes Back

Once you've had breast cancer, it's hard to believe you can
get anything else. Every cold is metastasis to the lungs;
every headache is metastasis to the brain.
— *Bev Parker, Y-Me National Breast Cancer Organization*

Nothing quite prepares you for the possibility of a recurrence. Nothing your doctors say, nothing the members of your support group say, nothing you might have thought—until it happens. Rachel W. remembers what helped to set her on the path to a more optimistic outlook after she was told her cancer had returned:

The second cancer showed up on a mammogram almost seven years after I had cancer the first time. It wasn't a good time. In fact—and I say this with emphasis—it was the worst thing that could happen. I know breast cancer recurs. I just didn't want it to come back when it did. I had just gotten married for the first time at age forty-three, and even at that age I was still thinking about motherhood. I wanted to have a baby. We had moved to the East Coast, where my husband had gotten a new job. My first doctor here was not very encouraging. He had a way of speaking in general terms. He would preface everything he said with "Studies tell us," or "According to the medical literature." He didn't make much eye contact, and I found that quite off-putting. Did this mean he thought my case was hopeless and he couldn't look me eye to eye? He also wasn't dealing with my emotional reaction. I was visibly upset and he wasn't dealing with that.

I missed my doctors who got me through this the first time. I missed the nurses. I especially missed my family-practice doctor. He had been through cancer himself. He's an older gentleman, in his late sixties, and a good friend. I called him and he understood right away. He told me not to let anyone extinguish my hope. He said his grandfather was a doctor who made house calls. Out of all the items in his grandfather's black bag, the thing that worked the most miracles was a poem he read at the end of each visit. He said it was about hope. I remembered then that I had seen the poem framed on the wall in my doctor's office with his medical degrees. He recited it to me over the phone, and that's when everything for me became crystal clear.

Understanding Recurrences

Fewer patients treated for breast cancer today will have a recurrence. But while that may be comforting news to some, the words ring hollow for those who are confronted with a new diagnosis of the disease. Unfortunately, few, if any, issues involving breast cancer come with easy answers—or ways to prepare you when the disease rebounds.

A recurrence has an impact on multiple levels. True, it is a cancer and as such must be dealt with in much the same way as an initial cancer is treated. But the emotional impact is greater. There is a stronger sense, survivors say, of cancer seeming to want to play its trump card.

Lynette Lee Pack-May, R.N., says that at many major centers, but certainly not at all, there are separate support groups for patients diagnosed with recurrent breast cancer. She says having access to support groups that are separate from those geared toward the newly diagnosed is important because the issues are different and the emotional stakes are higher. "Most patients try to keep a positive attitude," she says, "but as you probably can guess this is very difficult. It is very difficult for patients to hear that cancer has come back. We let them know that there is treatment and there is hope. We work very closely with these patients to help them in every way possible, including the emotional issues."

Ms. Pack-May encourages patients to become well informed about what their doctor means when he or she says that cancer has returned. A new diagnosis of breast cancer does not necessarily mean the first cancer has recurred. With breast cancer there are distinct differences in *how* cancer can come back. In short, she says, being diagnosed with cancer a second time does not have the same meaning to all patients.

Here are some of the ways in which cancer can return. You may want to discuss each of these with your physicians and ask for in-depth explanations:

Second primary: According to cancer experts, having a primary cancer diagnosed a second time is not, by definition, a recurrence of cancer, because a second primary generally occurs in a different location. It also may have pathologic features that make it different from the first cancer.

Local recurrence: This type of recurrence is either in the same breast or in the scar tissue remaining from the breast that was removed in a mastectomy.

Regional recurrence: This type of recurrence usually refers to a return of cancer in the lymph nodes, particularly those nearest the breast that was treated previously.

Distant recurrence: When cancer is detected in a site such as the bones, liver, or elsewhere, it is considered a distant metastasis of the original cancer.

Even though there is an ongoing debate in medicine over how much tissue should be taken in a lumpectomy, Ms. Pack-May says patients should not rush to judgment and assume a cancer recurrence is the result of inadequate surgery. Cancer comes back for many reasons, some of which have yet to be fully defined. She says, "Who has a recurrence and who does not have one is not based on surgical error; it's the way cancer works. I think most patients who are treated for breast cancer are aware that cancer can return. In fact, when patients are diagnosed we never say, 'Your cancer will never come back.' I assist the doctor on consults. We always say, 'We can't say your cancer will not return. But your chances for survival are excellent.' One of the roles of the health-care professional is to help patients with some very difficult issues. This is one of them."

Here are more thoughts from Rachel W. about breast cancer and experiencing a recurrence:

> I was never naïve about breast cancer. I knew it could return. My mother had breast cancer and I lived through what she endured. Once you have had breast cancer you know that you are never really free. I said as much in a support group before I had the recurrence; others there said they knew exactly what I meant. It came up after a woman broke into tears as she was explaining that she had just been told of her recurrence.
>
> The discussion quickly turned to how we all felt vulnerable, even when everything was going well. I said, "To me it's like a pot on low boil. You know it's there. You know it can be a problem. It doesn't have to be, but when you least expect it, it boils over and you get burned." As I write about that day and recall how that woman sobbed so inconsolably, I realize how cavalier we as newly diagnosed women must have sounded to someone just handed a devastating diagnosis. Our smugness must have been unbearable. Me, with that lame metaphor. When cancer returns there are no words for your grief. No matter how much you pray for cancer not to recur, in the end, you feel that you have been betrayed by God.

An Activist Who Has Been There

Bev Parker, director of information services at Y-Me National Breast Cancer Organization, knows intimately of what she speaks when she counsels hotline callers seeking information about breast cancer recurrence. Bev experienced a recurrence when she was well on her way toward twenty years being cancer-free. "There are more women who call the hotline when they are first diagnosed than when they have a recurrence," she says. "We do get callers with recurrences, and they prefer to speak to somebody who has had a recurrence, or someone who has had mets [a metastasis of their cancer]."

As someone who likes to help others, Bev would take calls from patients frightened about news of their recurrence and would try to help in any way she could, even before she had a recurrence. Often, the calls about a cancer recurrence are the most difficult ones handled by Y-Me's hotline. Still, the skills Bev had honed to help counsel others fell short when she needed words of comfort and advice herself. "Usually, whenever somebody called and asked to speak to a volunteer about a recurrence, I would take the call, and I would say this and I would say that. I knew exactly what to say. But when I found out about my own recurrence I called the Y-Me hotline, even though I was a volunteer there. I needed to talk to somebody about it. When I found out about my recurrence I didn't know what to say to myself. What could I say? It makes a difference when it's you."

Despite having been through cancer twice, Bev says she and other Y-Me counselors do not make many recommendations to those who call.

> We mostly listen to the callers. We don't make decisions for them. We'll say, "Have you considered getting another opinion?" We recommend that they go to a breast surgeon, and we encourage them to go to cancer centers because that's where they'll find the latest techniques. Some may want to see their general practitioner, or they want to go to the doctor who delivered their babies. A lot of people say, "I had breast cancer in my left breast and now it has metastasized to the right breast." And we'll tell them it's a new primary, not a metastasis, and that you have your best chance for a cure with a new primary. Of course, there are no guarantees of a cure unless you live to be very, very old and die of something else—only then will you have been cured of breast cancer.

I asked if Bev recommends support groups to those experiencing a recurrence. "Some people will find a lot of hope in support groups the second time around; others will say they don't find much help in the groups, and that they'd rather go it alone. Then there are the ones who say, 'I went to a support group and there were people there who were dying.' And they'll leave because they don't want to be around them. Then, of course, there are others on the opposite end, who have advanced disease, who say they're involved with end-of-life issues and that the support groups are not very helpful."

Bev says she always tries to encourage a sense of hope among those who call the hotline.

> A lot of times when people call, they'll ask, "How long has it been since you were first diagnosed?" and I'll tell them nineteen years. And they'll get so excited and say that's great. I don't have the heart to say after sixteen years I had a recurrence. Generally, I don't tell people I've had a recurrence; I just say nineteen years since the first diagnosis, because it gives them hope. I thought I was fine all those sixteen years. The first time, my treatment was rather unconventional. Now I'm on tamoxifen and being watched very carefully. But, as I tell people on the phone, there is no guarantee with this.

Becoming a Patient Again

Lee N. has received a clean bill of health after a recurrence.

> Ever since I started dealing with this, eleven years ago, I've tried not to dwell on the question of what-am-I-going-to-do-if-it-comes-back-again. What will my life be like? I don't go there. I have to do what's best for me psychologically. I just know what I won't do, and those are the things I am very definite about. I know there are certain chemo combinations I don't want again. Those drugs make you awfully sick. It was torture. I'm sounding a bit pessimistic. I think my sense of humor was damaged by the chemo [laughing]. But I am grateful—grateful for a lot of things. I thank God for my doctors.
>
> The other thing I want to mention that isn't very inspiring is that I was surprised to find that I had so many fly-by-night friends. I suppose I should say so-called friends. Cancer, I've discovered the very hard way, lets you know who your

friends are. When people find out you're sick and you're being treated for cancer, especially for a second time, some stop calling. Poof! They're gone, just like that. They just stop. It's amazing. Or they find excuses not to visit, or they'll e-mail you silly get-well cards. You get the impression they're thinking, If I get too close I'll catch it.

Julie H. was treated for a second primary in the opposite breast, which was diagnosed five years after she was treated by lumpectomy the first time.

At the time of my first diagnosis I thought it was the hardest thing I had to get through; it was like my will was being tested. Well, surprise, it wasn't the hardest thing. When you hear about it the second time your index of fear goes from code yellow to code red.

Fran D. cried uncontrollably when she was diagnosed the first time. The second diagnosis, which came a few years later, left her numb.

I wish I had better news. Someone had said in my support group years ago that ER+ tumors don't recur, or are less likely to recur. I don't remember exactly how it went, but that was the gist of it, and I liked the sound of it because it said, essentially, that luck was on my side, and maybe I didn't have to worry so much. I never mentioned it to my oncologist, never asked him about it. It's just one of those things that kind of sounds like if a doctor started to explain it, it would turn out to be something absolutely different. I didn't want anybody to burst the bubble. As long as I could believe it, it could be true.

A Doctor Makes a Clarification

Dr. Paul Peter Rosen, breast cancer pathologist and author of textbooks on breast cancer, says patients facing a recurrence should not believe that one type of breast cancer is more likely to recur than another. There are too many variables. While far fewer women with ER+ breast cancers experience a recurrence now than they did in the past, having one estrogen-receptor status over another does not automatically mean you are protected.

> There are different circumstances, so it is not—it never could be—a rule. Someone may have a big cancer that is ER+; there may be positive lymph nodes. Another person may have a small cancer that is ER–. The big cancer, even though it is ER+, is more likely to recur. So you can't rely only on estrogen-receptor status. There are multiple factors. There are a lot of reasons a cancer is more likely to recur—or not recur. A medullary carcinoma that is ER– has a low probability of recurring. So you can see that it is not ER status alone. You will want to consider tumor size, nodal status, and type of breast cancer, along with other factors.

Dr. Rosen also emphasized that conducting well-organized studies is the best way to answer questions about susceptibility to recurrence. "If you were comparing invasive lobular carcinomas, you wouldn't be able to say that only the ER– cancers were more likely to recur than ones that were ER+. You would have to stratify individuals so they all were equal. They all would have to have the same-size tumors and same nodal status, and other factors. Only after you studied them could you say what the differences are between ER+ and ER– cancers. Again, ER status is one of many factors that influence recurrence."

"For the sake of argument," I asked Dr. Rosen, "isn't it true that people who had ER+ cancers were able to take advantage of more treatment strategies, and wouldn't that, in turn, lower the number of patients with ER+ cancers who experience a recurrence?" He replied, "The matter of treatment is another issue. People with ER+ cancers are more likely to be treated effectively with tamoxifen and other drugs. But treatment has nothing to do with the intrinsic nature of recurrence."

Regardless of ER status, Dr. Rosen believes that patients can get a better perspective on what their doctors are saying about recurrence if they get a second opinion on their new set of specimens and other tests. "Women who have a diagnosis—whatever it is, malignancy or abnormal biopsy—should seriously consider a second opinion from an expert," he says. "I am not trying to encourage more business. I have more work than I can handle. But there are plenty of people around the country who can fill that need and give women answers to their questions."

Selecting an Oncologist and Surgeon

Just as you had to choose physicians when you were first diagnosed, the same holds true for a recurrence. It's likely that you might want to see the physicians who treated you when you were first diagnosed. But as both Bev Parker and Dr. Rosen point out, you may want to seek a second opinion.

Experts underscore that because women who have had breast cancer in the past are considered at high risk and usually are monitored much more closely, many recurrent cancers can be discovered when they are quite small. Your chances of recovery are excellent. Certainly, there are instances when the disease may be discovered at an advanced stage. Even then, you have options, and you will want to talk to your oncologists about strategies to enhance and maintain your quality of life.

Your doctor may offer choices with which you are quite familiar: surgery, radiation, chemo, and hormone therapy. As reported in Chapter 10, aromatase inhibitors are being used successfully in postmenopausal women diagnosed with ER+ cancers. If you were first treated years ago, these drugs didn't exist. Additionally, strategies involving new drug combinations are helping those whose tumors were ER–. Another important point is to remember clinical trials, no matter what your estrogen-receptor status happens to be. Your oncologist may suggest that you participate in one to take advantage of a promising treatment option that otherwise may be years from becoming standard therapy.

Of course, by signing up for a trial you may wind up receiving a placebo or may simply be administered standard treatment, which is the regimen the one under study is being compared to. The only way researchers can determine if new treatments are better than old ones is to test them against the standard of care. Nevertheless, most oncologists think it's worth the effort to enroll in a trial if you are strongly interested in one.

Ms. Pack-May, the nurse practitioner, emphasizes the importance of working closely with your medical team. Regardless of where along the spectrum of possibilities your recurrent cancer is found, never forget that you can talk to your doctors, nurses, support-group members, and others about your concerns, fears, and anxieties. Empathy from the health-care team is very helpful to patients. As Ms. Pack-May says, "We know that sometimes just listening can be more important than all of the other things we do."

The Poem That Inspired Rachel

Rachel W., who earlier remarked about a poem read to her by her family-practice physician, says it was a simple set of words that helped her feel better about the new medical challenge that lay ahead. For others it may be spending time in the company of family or friends, a note, a quiet moment with your spouse or partner, perhaps even talking to a stranger who lends an ear. Rachel's doctor said his grandfather, who practiced in Ohio during the early twentieth century, rode a horse from one patient's house to another and read these words to sick and worried patients:

Hope

It comes to you when least expected
like a beacon breaking fog upon the void,
signaling its source of light.
Beckoning, harkening, assuring
that day whether filled with clouds or sunshine
always follows night.

— Anonymous

Chapter 12

A Final Word: Life Beyond the Odyssey

I can spot the sisterhood now. We're everywhere.

— *Liisa M., breast cancer survivor*

What happens after being treated for breast cancer? Can you ever forget the experience? Many who have been there and see it through a lens made clearer by time say the disease invariably transforms an ordinary life into one forever shaped by an extraordinary challenge. And though that challenge is behind you, as you move onward it dominates your sense of self and your sense of the world.

Whether you had a lumpectomy or reconstructive surgery, or you wear a prosthesis, you can appear to the world as if nothing quite so life-altering ever occurred. While most women will say a breast comes nowhere near defining who they are as a person, there is no escaping the fact that cancer affected a part of the body that is emblematic of many milestones in life: your having come of age, your sexuality, and, certainly for a vast number, motherhood.

Many who have experienced breast cancer look back on it and say the disease forced them to regroup emotionally and build a stronger sense of who they are. Most find a deeper meaning in life itself: sometimes more humor, a greater desire to explore the world, or a deeper wish to give back through advocacy. In this final chapter, people who have traveled the odyssey share their thoughts on resuming intimate relationships or starting new ones, on how they interact with friends and relatives after breast cancer, and, finally, on how they have dealt with a new sense of the gift of life.

Your Sexuality

Resuming sexual intimacy is something many who have been treated for breast cancer will have to consider. Though no two relationships are the same, having been treated for breast cancer puts many survivors on common ground. Each cancer survivor must ask herself—or himself—how much the disease and its treatment have affected her or his self-image, sense of self, and self-esteem, all of which are elements of one's sense of sexuality. If you feel as if breast cancer has robbed you, then it may be more difficult to respond sexually, regardless of how sympathetic your partner is. Yvonne M. describes how she dealt with her sense of self while embarking upon a new intimate relationship.

> With breast cancer I was dealing with an accumulation of losses. The loss of my breast, and along with that the loss of a major part of what I thought made me a woman. I was divorced when all of this happened. But when you find out that you have breast cancer, one of the first thoughts that goes shooting through your mind is that you will never be attractive again.
>
> There's this part of me that always says don't make big changes when you are in a crisis, but I did. I had always been a little bit overweight, but after breast cancer I lost the weight. When I had my reconstruction, the doctor lifted the other breast. Now I have two uplifted breasts. So I looked better than I did before the operation.
>
> Physically, I've had the biggest scare of my life, but I am paying more attention to myself now. I cut my hair. I am taking better care of myself. I had to do something different with my life to feel better about myself and to feel more feminine, because cancer seems to take that part of you away. I'm

dating. I never thought that would happen in my fifties. But I told him about my cancer and what I went through, and he understands. Right now, everything is okay.

Women such as Yvonne found that breast cancer left them feeling less feminine at first, but later the road to recovery turned out, in many ways, to be a path of self-discovery. Part of Yvonne's self-discovery began with accepting her new reality that breast cancer changed her both emotionally and physically.

In the chapter on surgery, you may recall that Yvonne mentioned that she never wanted to see her chest with the mastectomy scar. In the same chapter, Lula F. shared her trepidations about looking in the mirror at her chest after the mastectomy. She says it was one of her most difficult moments.

Yet just as breast cancer can leave you troubled about your sexuality and how you feel about yourself, it can exacerbate fears of abandonment—fears that your husband/boyfriend/partner will leave you because the surgery has produced a physical change. Though Carla D. recovered promptly after her surgery, she says her operation left her with psychological scars, the deepest of which manifested as a fear that her husband would leave her.

Not too long before I found out I had breast cancer, we were in counseling for difficulties in our marriage. We had been separated for about a year. Before breast cancer we never talked much about sex. I mean, we had sex; we just didn't talk about it. After breast cancer, I wanted to know if he would still love me, but I didn't know how to ask that question. I also didn't initiate intimacy because I didn't know if I would be rejected. Nobody wants to be rejected, especially after having gone through what I had gone through.

This is my point: I didn't say anything about sex, and frankly, neither did he. He told me years later that breast cancer made me seem fragile. It took us a very, very long time to work through all of those issues.

Did we go back to counseling? No. Going back to a counselor was out of the question because, for me at least, it would have been too much of a reminder. It would have re-

minded me of the time when we were working through his in-
fidelity, and I didn't want to think of him that way any more.

Additional Notes on Sexuality after Breast Cancer

If discussing sexual issues was difficult before breast cancer, as Carla
found, then having that kind of heart-to-heart talk will remain so afterward. Breast cancer by itself does not open new channels of communication unless you are ready to open them.

There are several other issues about sex that you may want to
take note of:

1. If you are premenopausal, pregnancy may still be possible.
   You will want to discuss this issue—as well as an appropriate
   method of birth control—with your physician and your
   partner, especially if taking tamoxifen is part of your treatment regimen. Tamoxifen can lead to birth defects.
   Radiation therapy also can produce birth defects.

2. You may want to talk with your partner about how your
   surgery has made you feel about yourself. The discussion
   may lead to pleasant surprises. You may find that your partner was waiting for you to discuss sexual matters when you
   were ready.

3. Studies have shown that many women who have undergone
   chemotherapy experience pain and discomfort during inter-
   course. You may want to return slowly to sexual activity.
   Medications prescribed for years after treatment, such as
   tamoxifen and aromatase inhibitors, dramatically lower (if
   not totally eliminate) the estrogens that normally circulate
   in the body. That means vaginal lubrication may be difficult. For those who believe they are ready for sexual activity,
   water-based vaginal lubricants, such as KY Jelly, may be
   helpful.

Painting Life with a Broad Brush

What did the experience of being treated for breast cancer mean for those who lived it? Does the word *survivor* take on special meaning to those who have been through the odyssey?

The word *survivor*, many say, has multiple meanings. It can mean surviving with one's emotions intact after the shock of diagnosis. Surviving also means having triumphed through major losses: the loss of a breast (or sometimes both breasts), of one's hair (during chemotherapy), and of one's previous sense of self. Yet having been through the odyssey is also about discovering anew the deep wells in life: the well of laughter, the well of the spirit, the well of life's preciousness, and the well of wonder—the need to explore the world and its innumerable possibilities.

For many breast cancer survivors, the disease, its treatment, and the emotional roller-coaster involved with the experience produce countless memories—good ones as well as bad. Some survivors say breast cancer and its treatment helped deepen their appreciation for humor. Liisa M., a mother with a busy career, is a survivor who found humor at virtually every turn, even during various phases of her treatment.

> The radiation unit is a place where people are pretty dignified and keep to themselves. I had great hopes for my radiation experience. I wore a dress and had just gotten my prosthesis. But the first thing they do is throw a hospital gown at you. It never occurred to me what to do with my prosthesis. It just so happened that I was wearing a baseball cap, so I put the prosthesis in there. A man came and sat down next me. And there was this really awkward moment when he saw it. What do you do? So I said to him, "When in your life did you ever think you would sit down next to a bald woman with her breast in her hand?" It was just one of those ludicrous situations you find yourself in. He was laughing so hard he was crying. Every time he saw me after that he would burst into laughter.

In addition to finding humor during treatment, Liisa also found it during her follow-up care. After her mastectomy, when she went in for a mammogram of her healthy breast, she jokingly asked about pricing.

> I asked them, "Do I get a discount now? Because the reality here is this: There's only one." I was just being funny. Medical costs being what they are, I thought the charge would be the same. But they said no. The cost would be 50 percent less—and they were serious.

Liisa believes her experience with breast cancer has made her far more vigilant when it comes to certain aspects of the health-care system. The facility where she received her mammograms prior to diagnosis is part of a large corporation that performs numerous radiological procedures. She blames the company and its doctors for improper diagnosis and had considered suing. Her husband talked her out of taking such action. Nevertheless, memories have not faded.

> I feel that I have to stay on top of the radiation people. They missed the tumor the year before. The only things they caught were the calcifications. My children very nearly lost a mother and inherited a radiation company.

But while survivors such as Liisa find humor throughout their experiences, others describe their treatment and life thereafter in philosophical terms. Retired nurse Lula F., who once cared for high-risk obstetric patients, says breast cancer helped her see life differently.

> I think of life as a blessing, and I really think that I was blessed because I didn't have to have radiation or chemo, but it still took a toll on me. For three or four years I was afraid it would come back. But that was something I just had to live with. The worst thing about breast cancer, for me, was the mastectomy. In the beginning, when I first suspected that something might be wrong, I really didn't want to tell anyone. I thought I'd save it until after Thanksgiving; I didn't want to ruin the holiday for my family. I didn't want anyone thinking, Mom is sick; Mom has breast cancer. But my daughter found out. She heard the message from the doctor's office on the phone answering machine. And getting back to the point I was trying to make,

yes, I do think of life as precious. I understand it as a gift, even more so now.

Breast cancer helped Yvonne M. better appreciate her son's hopes and plan.

> I made a commitment to myself that I would not be critical of my son. That's what I decided after going through everything involved with breast cancer. He had been saying he wanted to be a policeman or join the Marines. I was always very much opposed to those ideas. But now, after breast cancer, I say if he wants to be a policeman or join the Marines, that's okay. I don't want to keep pushing him and pushing him. That's how I am different. It's his life and he has to do what makes him happy, not what makes me happy. He has to make choices that are important to him.
>
> When I look back on breast cancer, I think the hardest thing for me was going in for the reconstructive surgery. I felt really scared then. I was in the intensive care ward after the mastectomy and reconstruction. There was a woman in there who was much younger than I am. She had stomach cancer and she was dying. Things can turn out so differently. I now believe that you always have to be prepared for what life hands you; you never know what it will be. Maybe I talk too much about cancer, but in a way that might be my therapy. Once you've had it, it really makes a big impact. You can't forget it the way you can forget other medical problems.

Barbara G., a high school math teacher and the mother of a son in his twenties, says breast cancer helped her develop a different perspective on life.

> I definitely have a positive outlook. You just have to grab hold of life and do everything you can, while you can. Some people wait until they retire. I don't want to take that chance. I like to travel. I've been all over. I've been to Maui. I am on sabbatical now. I'm going to Miami. I've been to Paris and to Australia. During Easter vacation I'm going back to France, this time to the Loire Valley. I'm having so much fun picking out all of the chateaux I am going to see.

Although Barbara found ways to inject more levity into her life, there were a few times during and after breast cancer treatment when she found herself holding her breath, wondering what would happen next. Even though she was diagnosed with DCIS, there was evidence of calcifications in various parts of her breast, a discovery that necessitated a mastectomy. "He was very emphatic that I had to have a mastectomy," she says of her oncologist. At first Barbara did not want reconstruction, but later she changed her mind.

Yet the reconstruction did not proceed as smoothly as her surgeon had expected it would. Barbara had to have a second surgery because the initial graft did not take. Ultimately the reconstruction worked out well. The experience also helped her move beyond the denial that had flooded her after she first learned of her diagnosis and the need for a mastectomy. "I am really glad I did it," she says, "and I feel spared." Still, she had more experiences to come with doctors and hospitals.

> After breast cancer I had a hysterectomy, for several reasons. I had been getting severe pains and cramping. And when I got my blood work done, the Ca-125 [blood test for ovarian cancer] was very high. It could have been ovarian cancer, but it turned out to be very bad endometriosis. That was a huge worry.

Preceding breast cancer, Barbara had to cope with another life-changing event.

> I am divorced. In a way I am glad the divorce had already happened before the two diagnoses. I had close friends around. If I'd had those problems at the time I was going through the divorce, it would have been different. But I am pleased about the order of things. We're still friends. He's my son's father. We're certainly not enemies.

Life after breast cancer has prompted Cassandra E. to take up sports and other activities she never considered prior to her diagnosis; she's teaching herself how to write haiku, a form of Japanese poetry. But her experience with breast cancer is never far from her mind.

In some ways I live for the next blood test, and I'm on pins and needles waiting for the results from my MRI. But I don't let that hold me back. I've learned to ski and play golf. I've taken up haiku. The man I lived with for fourteen years finally said, "I do." Did breast cancer make him do it? Girl, I don't know. But I'm not complaining.

Having accumulated thousands of frequent-flyer miles, Cassandra, a teacher, is using them to see the world.

I travel a lot, because I realized I had been out of the state twice—in my whole life. Now, when school's out I'm on the road or in the air. Some of the travel hasn't been about fun. My grandmother died and we went to Louisiana for the funeral. She lived to be ninety-seven; she was never sick a day in her life.

One afternoon she told my aunt she was going to take a little nap, and she just passed away—just like that. Freaked my aunt out when she couldn't wake her up, but after the shock we all realized what a beautiful life she'd had, and to have lived so long. She had seven children and outlived four of them, but always had a couple of them close by.

I want to be just like that, with that kind of longevity. I don't have any children of my own, but I've been like a mother to my stepson and stepdaughter, so I hope they'll come around when I'm old. I still plan to be on the planet living and breathing in 2061. That's when I'll be ninety-seven.

Being with friends and family is important for Rob P., who also is indulging his wanderlust.

I'm having fun learning new things. I've taken up carpentry. This is one of my prized projects [points to a small grandfather clock that was hand-painted by his wife]. We're hardly home anymore. Actually, we're thinking about selling the house; we've lived here thirty-two years. Our son and his family live in Germany, and he's invited us to come stay with them. But that'll be a rest stop. I'd like to see Poland, Russia— you name it. Audrey [his wife] wanted to see China, but now she's afraid of catching SARS. Maybe we'll go to Japan instead.

Mind/Body Medicine

Rob, like many other breast cancer survivors, has become deeply interested in mind/body medicine. Every day, he sits in a quiet place for about an hour and directs his thoughts and energy to his immune system, helping it, he says, to boost white blood cells that can fight and destroy fledgling cancer cells.

> Audrey's got me into visualization therapy, nothing formal. We do it here at home. I started doing it while on chemo and just kept it up. It's like meditation. I'm always using visualization therapy to keep any new cancer cells away.

Maryanne B., who struggled to receive a proper diagnosis and respect from those she entrusted with her medical care, says she is also interested in using the power of her mind to keep cancer away in the future.

> More than anything, I believe in the power of positive thinking. No one has taught me anything about this. But I just believe that if I keep focused on not getting cancer again, it won't come back.

Moving Back into Routines

Just as some survivors found new reasons for extensive travel and pursuit of new goals, still others move seamlessly into vital roles that were very much a part of their lives before breast cancer. Catherine B., who had several family members in the United States and Ireland who were diagnosed with breast cancer, moved effortlessly back into her role as matriarch over a large family of five children and six grandchildren.

During chemotherapy, Ann H. was hardly away from her position as an assistant managing editor for a major Florida newspaper. She continued in that position after breast cancer. Ann is a woman with attitude; she says emphatically that she did not want to allow cancer to get in her way.

Never Shying Away

Many survivors who were in the public eye remain so years after treatment. Orlando television news anchor Wendy Chioji, who helped viewers learn about the disease by reporting on her own treatment, has continued her prominent role on television, reporting on a wide range of issues. Judy B. continues to inform millions about all forms of cancer through her family's online site. Zora K. Brown is continuing her advocacy work for patients and has written a book about breast cancer. She is starting research on yet another one, which will focus more on the psychological issues affecting people with the disease. Geri Barish still maintains a very public role by calling attention to breast cancer and working with patients affected by the condition. Geri believes it is important for those in the activist community to continue working closely with scientists who are searching for new treatments and for answers about the basic biology of breast cancer.

Many people who have survived breast cancer, like Liisa M., say the experience has helped make them stronger. Liisa adds that she is strengthened now by a vast army of survivors she never before recognized.

> I can spot the sisterhood now. We're everywhere, and they are recognizing me as a survivor. The American Cancer Society sells hats and shirts, all sorts of things with the little rosettes on them. I was at the mall wearing a plaid shirt with the rosette. And women would come up to me and say, "I had it eight years ago," or, "I had it ten years ago." They recognized the rosette. They ask me how I am doing and when I had breast cancer. It's amazing. Really amazing—and very sustaining.

Some call the experience character building. Others say they managed to flourish in spite of challenges, overcoming scars both physical and emotional. And just as cancer survivors recognize the visible symbols of the emblematic rosette and the pink ribbon, there is something less tangible—even mystical—they can see in one another. They recognize the depth in others who like themselves have known suffering, who like themselves have weathered a devastating diagnosis and yet have prevailed, flexing like a willow in a gale but ultimately, again, standing whole and strong.

Appendix

Researching Breast Cancer and Finding Support via the Web

A generation ago, in the old paternalistic era of medical care, a physician would be your primary source of breast cancer information—and there was precious little he thought you would understand. Now, your doctors—men and women—may direct you to certain websites to help you broaden your knowledge about the disease and perhaps to help you learn something about the center where you're being treated.

Naturally, some newly diagnosed people are neither willing nor eager to seek information about cancer. Many shy away from delving into too much information about a matter they find emotionally difficult. But if you are among those who make a beeline to the Internet to clarify any number of medical issues, there are some ideas you may want to consider as you begin exploring breast cancer data on the World Wide Web.

With the emergence of Google and other search engines, unbelievable amounts of medical information appear with just a few keystrokes. Plug in the words *breast cancer* and a Google search returns nearly five million "hits." Two questions nevertheless arise: How much of that information is useful, and how would you go about paring down so much data to investigate exactly what you want to learn?

A simple response answers both questions. Such an overwhelming amount of information is useless. Conducting a broad Google search produces links to thousands of legitimate medical research papers. Also appearing are entries from purveyors of breast cancer myths and people after a fast buck—those who prey on the vulnerability of cancer patients. Hucksters, it turns out, have websites, too.

Dr. Ian Smith, whose medical advice is aired regularly on the ABC television-network program *The View*, suggests refining your search by using Google or other search engines to lead you to the websites of major cancer organizations, sites you can be assured will carry current information to answer a broad range of questions.

ASCO's website People Living with Cancer (www.plwc.org) is designed in an easy-to-read format aimed at a spectrum of patients from the newly diagnosed to those with advanced disease. People with virtually any form of cancer are invited to visit the site. Breastcancer.org, on the other hand, is focused only on information about breast cancer. Visitors to the site can join chat rooms, read breaking news about breast cancer, and see graphics about breast and lymph node anatomy. These sites are just two examples of the kind Dr. Smith says have their content reviewed by experts before it is posted for the public.

Dr. Smith, a Harvard graduate who trained at Dartmouth Medical College and the University of Chicago's Pritzker School of Medicine, authored the book *Dr. Ian Smith's Guide to Medical Websites*. It tells how to effectively navigate the World Wide Web for medical information. In an interview for this book, Dr. Smith said information culled from medical websites is not a substitute for advice given to you by your physicians. But data gleaned from the web, he believes, can better inform the questions you ask your doctors. Indeed, web-based resources also can add to your team of supporters through listservs and chat rooms, plugging you into a support network that circles the globe. The Internet, Dr. Smith said, is an instant gateway into the communities of advocates and survivors. Once you've mapped where on the Internet you would like to go, be prepared for a vast kingdom of medical information, and for the potential to meet patients like yourself.

He thinks several rules of thumb should guide any web-based medical research. Paramount among them is to seek information on sites that maintain the highest standards. Another is making certain that data you believe to be relevant to your case are accurate and current. He says:

Dr. Smith's Rules for Navigating the Web

1. Be aware of who produces the website you're reviewing.
2. Become familiar with the websites of organizations devoted to cancer treatment and patient advocacy.
3. Analyze the information you are reviewing. Is it useful for your particular needs? Can the information help advance your care?
4. Shun information by Internet advertisers offering treatments not recommended by your physicians.
5. Be wary of information that is not current. Web pages generally carry dates indicating when they were last updated.

Before you start researching information on the Internet, it is important to understand that the World Wide Web is a reservoir of entirely unregulated information, so you must enter it with caution. That being said, the Internet is a wonderful source to find whatever it is you want to know. The first thing I always tell people is to go to the most credible portals as their entry sites into the Internet. I recommend going to the major government, academic, and advocacy sites, for example, the National Cancer Institute, the Mayo Clinic, or the American Cancer Society. All of these sites, whether government, academic, or advocacy group, are updated regularly, and the information is vetted through experts. This is where you will find information about the most relevant research.

You can find the National Cancer Institute at www.cancer.gov; the Mayo Clinic at www.mayoclinic.org; and the American Cancer Society at www.cancer.org.

Advocacy sites not only offer news about breast cancer research but also provide useful information to both the newly diagnosed and breast cancer survivors. Topics can run the gamut from insurance issues to concerns about sexuality following breast cancer surgery. Noted advocacy groups include Breast Cancer Action (www.breastcanceraction.org), the Susan G. Komen Breast Cancer Foundation (www.komen.org), and Y-Me (www.yme.org), to name a few. A complete list of government research institutions, academic medical centers, and advocacy organizations is in the Resources section at the end of the book.

Dr. Smith further emphasizes that the most credible websites provide access into other excellent sites, linking you to additional information on a particular topic. "You'll know when you're on the most credible sites," he says, "because major websites are very particular about who they link you to."

A prime example is the American Cancer Society's website. On the society's web page informing visitors about the National Breast and Cervical Cancer Early Detection Program, for example, you can be linked directly to the Centers for Disease Control and Prevention (CDC), the government agency that oversees the program for low-income and uninsured women. You will find that links from one major site to another abound as you investigate specific questions about breast cancer.

You should be aware that some medical websites sell space to earn money, which suggests to Dr. Smith that you can double-click into a domain more interested in your wallet than your health:

> **Cancer Research on the Web**
>
> If you would like to find certain medical research papers, you can do so through several sites:
>
> 1. The American Society of Clinical Oncologists (www.asco.org) — Provides news and abstracts of research presented at its meetings
> 2. CANCERLIT (www.cancer.gov/search/cancer_literature) — A database of the National Cancer Institute
> 3. Medscape (www.medscape.com) — Registration required; great source for current medical research
> 4. PubMed (www.nlm.nih.gov/hinfo.html) — Database of the National Library of Medicine

My feeling is that you need to know the structure of a website. Of course the content is important, but even some of the most credible websites sell advertising. Banners running alongside the page may provide links to information the [hosting] site cannot be held accountable for. But there are certain standards of validation, ways of certifying that a health site carries credible information and meets standards of quality and integrity, and I think this is very important to know.

[An organization called] HON is one of the big ones when it comes to certifying information on a medical website. Look for it at the very bottom of the homepage of the most credible health websites. The American Cancer Society has a HON insignia at the bottom of its homepage. This is like the Good Housekeeping Seal of Approval for the World Wide Web. It usually reads, "We subscribe to the HONcode principles of the Health On the Net Foundation."

The National Cancer Institute is not a HON website, but as the premier federal cancer research center in the United States, the NCI's web ethics are clearly spelled out when you click on "Policies" at the bottom of the homepage. Other excellent sites have similar ways of conveying their ethics, even when they do not carry a special insignia.

Joining a Thread

Thanks to the Internet, new words are quickly being added to the English lexicon, and new definitions are becoming attached to old words. Take the word *thread*, for example. Once upon a time it was simply something guided through a needle. Now the word *thread* defines the comment-and-response formats of web-based discussion groups known as web logs, or blogs. Blogs devoted to breast cancer are growing rapidly, and patients find these outlets helpful to understanding themselves as patients and understanding how the experiences of others can add dimension and context to their own medical therapy.

Another communication format that has attracted breast cancer patients and survivors for more than a decade is the listserv, which operates through a central e-mail server. Listserv messages can be sent to hundreds of registrants at once. Someone may pose a question about the effects of radiation therapy on the skin, and a dozen or more people on a listserv might post responses spelling out their experiences. If you are interested in finding a very understanding group of people, then a listserv may be what you're looking for. Such a community is not entirely about hand-holding, however. Heated discussions have been known to erupt over various topics. The beauty of a listserv is its 24/7 availability. Just log on and you're in a global support group.

Gilles Frydman, of New York City, is one of the world's experts on listservs for people with cancer. He founded the Association of Cancer Online Resources—www.acor.org—in the early 1990s after his wife developed breast cancer. In the beginning, when Frydman was debating how best to help his wife, he knew a support group would be great. One with boundless reach into cyberspace, he thought, would be even better. His ingenuity led to one of the earliest breast cancer listservs in the United States. Only now, he says, have academics begun to study the impact of listservs on the emotional well-being of those with cancer.

The number of ACOR.org's lists has grown tremendously over the years. Now when visitors log on to the site, they can register for one or more of the two hundred–plus listservs sponsored by the organization. The lists are aimed at virtually every form of cancer, including many rare ones. Frydman estimates that nearly two million e-mails are sent among registrants weekly. Although numerous, ACOR.org's lists now exist among thousands of others, including many devoted to breast cancer.

Chat rooms, another option for those seeking support and information on the web, can have a variety of sponsors, ranging from the websites of newspapers to those of major medical centers and patient-advocacy groups. In some formats, cancer specialists may be invited to answer questions from the public. In other formats, particularly on sites devoted only to breast cancer, chatting is conducted in a less structured pattern.

Finally, joining any discussion on the web gives you an opportunity to ask questions (even silly ones) or air concerns that may be considered controversial—all with the comfort of knowing that you can do so while remaining totally anonymous.

Notes

❧ ❧ ❧

CHAPTER 1: DIAGNOSIS

1. N.H. Lauersen, M.D., Ph.D., and E. Stukane, *The Complete Book of Breast Care* (New York: Fawcett Columbine, 1998), 68–69.

2. D. Smith, S.C. Lester, and J.E. Meyer, "Large-Core Needle Biopsy of Nonpalpable Breast Lesions," *Journal of the American Medical Association* 281 (1999): 1638–41.

CHAPTER 2: A POSTDIAGNOSIS CHECKLIST

1. Jami Bernard, Cancer Girl column, "Telling Everyone," *MAMM* 3, no. 1 (October 2000): 72.

2. N. Keene, *Working with Your Doctor: Getting the Healthcare You Deserve* (Sebastopol, CA: O'Reilly and Associates, 1998), 25.

3. "Legal and Financial Concerns," Web page of the National Coalition for Cancer Survivorship: www.canceradvocacy.org/resources/essential/caregiving/legal.aspx. Posted Dec. 18, 2003.

4. Ibid.

5. Web page of the Omni Choice Prescription Drug Plan: www.omnichoicerx.com.

CHAPTER 3: FACTS, FICTION, AND URBAN LEGENDS

1. Laurie Tarkan, "As a Hormone Substitute, Soy Is Ever More Popular, but Is It Safe?" *The New York Times*, Aug. 29, 2004, Section F, 5.

2. References to sulforaphane, a compound in broccoli, as a possible substance to prevent breast cancer are condensed from the author's notes taken during the 224th annual meeting of the American Chemical Society, Aug. 19, 2002, Boston, MA.

3. J. Higdon, "Soy Isoflavones," Web page of the Linus Pauling Institute Micronutrient Information Center of the Oregon State University: www.lpi.oregonstate.edu/infocenter/phytochemicals/soyiso. Updated Aug. 16, 2004.

4. C.M. Velicer, et al., "Antibiotic Use in Relation to the Risk of Breast Cancer," *Journal of the American Medical Association* 291 (2004): 827–83.

5. M.C. Leske, et al., "Electromagnetic Fields and Breast Cancer on Long Island: A Case-Control Study," *American Journal of Epidemiology* 158, no. 1 (2003): 47–58.

6. "Fact Sheet: Cancer Clusters," Web page, Cancer Facts of the National Cancer Institute: http://cis.nci.nih.gov/fact/3_58.htm. Updated Feb. 24, 2004.

CHAPTER 4: TYPES OF BREAST CANCER

1. C.J.F. Van Noorden, L.C. Meade-Tollin, and F. Bosnan, "Metastasis," *The American Scientist* 86, no. 2 (March–April 1998): 13.

2. From the author's notes taken during the 90th annual meeting of the American Association for Cancer Research, April 10–14, 1999, Philadelphia, PA. Dr. Folkman was the plenary session speaker.

CHAPTER 5: A PRIMER ON RISKS, PART I: AGE, GENES, AND ETHNICITY

1. M.C. King, et al., "Breast and Ovarian Cancer Risks Due to Inherited Mutations in BRCA1 and BRCA2," *Science* (October 24, 2003): 643–46.

2. F. Collins, "Scientists Pinpoint Location of Possible Third Gene Involved in Hereditary Breast Cancer to Chromosome 13," National Human Genome Research Institute news release Aug. 2000. News release archives 1999–2000.

3. E. Warner, et al., "Surveillance of BRCA1 and BRCA2 Mutation Carriers with Magnetic Resonance Imaging, Ultrasound, Mammography, and Clinical Breast Examination," *Journal of the American Medical Association* 292 (2004): 1317–25.

4. S.H. Ahn, et al., "Prevalence of BRCA1 and BRCA2 Mutations in Korean Breast Cancer Patients," *Journal of Korean Medical Science* (April 19, 2004): 269–74.

5. K.C. Chu, C.A. Lamar, H.P. Freeman, "Racial Disparities in Breast Carcinoma Survival Rates: Separating Factors That Affect Diagnosis from Factors That Affect Treatment," *Cancer* (June 1, 2003): 2853–60.

CHAPTER 6: A PRIMER ON RISKS, PART II: OBESITY, HORMONE REPLACEMENT THERAPY, AND OTHER EXPOSURES

1. T.J. Key, et al., "Body Mass Index, Serum Sex Hormones and Breast Cancer Risk in Postmenopausal Women," *Journal of the National Cancer Institute* 95 (August 20, 2003): 1218–26.

2. C.C. Wee, et al., "Screening for Cervical and Breast Cancer: Is Obesity an Unrecognized Barrier to Preventive Care?" *Annals of Internal Medicine* 132 (May 2, 2000): 697–704.

3. Heather Bell, R.D., M.P.H., "Yes, but Is Weight Loss the Be-All and the End-All? Take a Look at These Four Questions," *Health and Nutrition Newsletter* (July 2004). A Publication of Tufts University, Friedman School of Nutrition, Science, and Policy.

4. The Writing Group for the Women's Health Initiative, "Risks and Benefits of Estrogen Plus Progestin in Healthy Postmenopausal Women: Principal Results from the Women's Health Initiative Randomized Controlled Trial," *Journal of the American Medical Association* 288 (2002): 321–23.

5. S.A. Smith-Warner, et al., "Alcohol and Breast Cancer in Women: A Pooled Anaysis of Cohort Studies," *Journal of the American Medical Association* 279 (1998): 535–40.

6. R. Sinha, et al., "2-Amino-1-methyl-6-phenylimidazo[4,5-b]pyridine, a Carcinogen in High-Temperature-Cooked Meat, and Breast Cancer Risk," *Journal of the National Cancer Institute* 92 (August 16, 2000): 1352–54. Also information from the author's notes taken during Dr. Sinha's presentation at the 91st annual meeting of the American Association for Cancer Research, April 6–10, 2000, San Francisco, CA.

7. References to Dr. Kala Visvanathan's work on carcinogenic compounds in cooked meats are from the author's notes taken during the 91st annual meeting of the American Association for Cancer Research, April 6–10, 2000, San Francisco, CA.

CHAPTER 7: SURGERY

1. B.H. Lerner, M.D., *The Breast Cancer Wars: Hope, Fear, and the Pursuit of a Cure in Twentieth-Century America* (New York: Oxford University Press, 2003).

2. M. Mayer, *Advanced Breast Cancer: A Guide to Living with Metastatic Disease* (Sebastopol, CA: O'Reilly and Associates, 1998).

3. The article and editorial on the subject of surgical margins appear in the *Journal of the National Cancer Institute* 92, no. 4 (Feb. 16, 2000).

4. F.A. Vicini, et al., "Impact of Young Age on Outcome in Patients with Ductal Carcinoma-in-Situ Treated with Breast Conserving Therapy," *Journal of Clinical Oncology* 18, no. 2 (Jan. 2000): 296–306.

5. "Almanac Study Shows Significantly Better Quality of Life After Sentinel Node Biopsy Compared with Axillary Node Dissection," *PRNewswire*, Dec. 10, 2004.

CHAPTER 8: RADIATION THERAPY: MEDICINE'S HIGH-ENERGY TREATMENT

1. J. Cuzick, Consensus Conference Question: *For Which Patients Should Post-Mastectomy Radiotherapy Be Recommended?* National Institutes of Health Consensus Development Conference, Nov. 1–3, 2000, Bethesda, MD.

2. H. Bartelink, et al., "Recurrence Rates after Treatment of Breast Cancer with Standard Radiotherapy with or without Additional Radiation," *New England Journal of Medicine* 345 (2001): 1378–87.

CHAPTER 9: CHEMOTHERAPY

1. J. Ragaz, et al., "Adjuvant Radiotherapy and Chemotherapy in Node-Positive Pre-Menopausal Women with Breast Cancer," *New England Journal of Medicine* 337 (1997): 956–62.

2. J. Bergh, Consensus Conference Question: *Who Should Not Receive Chemotherapy?* National Institutes of Health Consensus Development Conference, Nov. 1–3, 2000, Bethesda, MD.

3. F.S. Van Dam, et al., "Impairment of Cognitive Function in Women Receiving Adjuvant Treatment for High-Risk Breast Cancer: High-Dose vs. Standard-Dose Chemotherapy," *Journal of the National Cancer Institute* 90 (1998): 210–18.

4. C.A. Meyers, et al., " 'Chemobrain' in Breast Carcinoma? A Prologue," *Cancer* 101, no. 3 (June 1, 2004): 466–75.

5. I.F. Tannock, et al., "Cognitive Impairment Associated with Chemotherapy for Cancer: Report of a Workshop," *Journal of Clinical Oncology* 22, no. 11 (June 1, 2004): 2233–39.

6. J. McKay, and N. Hirano, *The Chemotherapy Survival Guide* (Oakland, CA: New Harbinger Publications, 1993).

7. Ibid.

8. Excerpts from Wendy Chioji's diary as carried on the Channel 2 WESH.com website in July 2002. Permission granted to use excerpts in July 2002.

9. From the author's notes taken during *MAMM* magazine's national conference on breast cancer June 21–22, 2002, Sheraton New York Hotel Towers in New York City. Bettye Green, R.N., delivered a lecture on June 22 on the importance of joining clinical trials.

10. Dennis Slamon, M.D., Ph.D., "New Studies of First Successful Targeted Therapy for Breast Cancer Launched; Thousands of Volunteers Sought," press release June 20, 2001, University of California, Los Angeles, Geffen School of Medicine.

CHAPTER 10: HORMONE THERAPY: COUNTERACTING ESTROGEN

1. S. Cummings, et al., "The Effect of Raloxifene on Risk of Breast Cancer in Postmenopausal Women: Results from the MORE Randomized Trial," *Journal of the American Medical Association* 281 (1999): 2189–97.

2. P.D. Delmas, et al., "Effects of Raloxifene on Bone Mineral Density, Serum Cholesterol Concentrations, and Uterine Endometrium in Postmenopausal Women," *New England Journal of Medicine* 337 (1997): 1641–47.

3. M. Lippman, et al., "Indicators of Lifetime Estrogen Exposure: Effect on Breast Cancer Incidence and Interaction with Raloxifene Therapy in the Multiple Outcomes of Raloxifene Evaluation (MORE) Study Participants," *Journal of Clinical Oncology* (June 2001): 3111–16.

4. From the author's notes taken during the 40th annual meeting of the American Society of Clinical Oncology, June 5–8, 2004, New Orleans, LA.

Suggested Reading

1. *The Breast Cancer Wars: Hope, Fear and the Pursuit of a Cure in 20th Century America* (New York: Oxford University Press, 2003), by Barron H. Lerner, M.D., Ph.D. Dr. Lerner is an associate professor of medicine and public health at Columbia University's College of Physicians and Surgeons. He has written a sweeping story that explores a wide range of issues, including controversies surrounding the Halsted, a disfiguring surgery that was widely accepted for three-quarters of the twentieth century.

2. *Bathsheba's Breast: Women, Cancer and History* (Baltimore, MD: Johns Hopkins University Press, 2002), by James Stuart Olson. This book documents the heartbreak of breast cancer since the time of the pharaohs. It is an intriguing look into the history of the disease. Olson highlights several prominent women who battled breast cancer, including Mary Washington (mother of the first U.S. president), Hitler's mother, former First Lady Betty Ford, and Happy Rockefeller, among others.

3. *Dr. Susan Love's Breast Book* (New York: Perseus Books, 2000), by Susan M. Love, M.D., et al. This six-hundred-page, illustrated tome provides a detailed examination of the breast in health and disease. It examines benign conditions as well as breast cancer. The book has been a mainstay in the library of women diagnosed with breast cancer ever since its first edition was published in 1990.

4. *Women's Cancers: How to Prevent Them, How to Treat Them, How to Beat Them*, 3rd ed. (Alameda, CA: Hunter House Publishers, 2003), by Kerry A McGinn, R.N., N.P., and Pamela J. Haylock, R.N., M.A. This comprehensive book includes four chapters containing information solely on breast cancer written by a nurse practitioner who is also a breast cancer survivor.

5. *Examining Myself: One Woman's Story of Breast Cancer Treatment and Recovery* (London: Faber and Faber, 1993) by Musa Mayer. A personal account of breast cancer by an activist and writer who in-

vites the reader into her life as she copes with breast cancer and the realities that follow. Former network news reporter Linda Ellerbee, herself a breast cancer survivor, describes the book on its cover as "the very best book anybody has ever written about what it is like to have breast cancer." Although written in the 1990s, the book is still available through Internet booksellers.

6. *100 Questions & Answers About Breast Cancer* (Boston, MA: Jones and Bartlett Publishers, 2003) by Zora Brown and LaSalle D. Leffall, Jr., M.D., with Elizabeth Platt. An excellent book that provides answers to a wide range of questions anyone who is newly diagnosed may ask. The book is written entirely in a question-and-answer format by breast cancer survivor Zora Brown, founder of breast cancer support groups for African American women; Dr. Leffall, a professor of surgery at Howard University and a former president of the American Cancer Society; and Elizabeth Platt, a science writer and daughter of a breast cancer survivor.

7. *Recovering from Breast Surgery: Exercises to Strengthen Your Body and Relieve Pain* (Alameda, CA: Hunter House Publishers, 1995), by Diana Stumm, P.T. Through words and illustrations the author describes the best stretches, massage techniques, and exercises for recovery from the pain and loss of mobility that can follow mastectomy, lumpectomy, radiation, reconstruction, and lymphedema.

8. *Her-2: The Making of Herceptin, a Revolutionary Treatment for Breast Cancer* (New York: Random House, 1998), by Robert Bazell. This riveting account explores the scientific work on the molecule Her-2 and the development of the drug Herceptin. The book also examines many of the larger-than-life personalities involved in the scientific work, especially Dr. Dennis Slamon of UCLA, who played a critical role in understanding the molecule and developing the drug.

9. *Living Beyond Breast Cancer: A Survivor's Guide for When Treatment Ends and the Rest of Your Life Begins,* (New York: Times Books, 1998), by Marisa C. Weiss, M.D., and Ellen Weiss. A comprehensive book about what to expect after treatment for breast cancer.

10. *Lymphedema: A Breast Cancer Patient's Guide to Prevention and Healing,* 2nd ed. (Alameda, CA: Hunter House Publishers, 2005), by Jeannie Burt and Gwen White, P.T. This book, which is ap-

proved by the National Lymphedema Network, explains the many things women can do to prevent or minimize the condition.

11. *Living Through Breast Cancer: What A Harvard Doctor Wants You To Know About Getting the Best Care While Preserving Your Self-Image* (New York: McGraw Hill, 2005), by Carolyn M. Kaelin, M.D., MPH. In 2003, while training for a 190-mile bike ride to raise money for breast cancer, Carolyn Kaelin, a respected breast cancer surgeon at Brigham and Women's Hospital in Boston, discovered at the age of 42 that she had the disease. Her story is perhaps one of the most unusual in that it describes how one of the country's top experts in breast cancer suddenly had to face the reality of the disease herself.

12. *No Less a Woman: Femininity, Sexuality & Breast Cancer*, 2nd ed. (Alameda, CA: Hunter House Publishers, 1995), by Deborah Hobler, MSW. Ten women describe how they coped with cancer. The author, a breast cancer survivor herself, draws on these stories to discuss how to talk with family and friends, retain intimacy with a partner, and adjust to a new body image.

13. *Why I Wore Lipstick: To My Mastectomy* (New York: St. Martin's Press, 2004), by Geralyn Lucas. A producer for television's newsmagazine, 20/20, Lucas discovered at the age of 27 that she had breast cancer and was thrust into a world of aggressive medical treatment that few women her age experience. The story is compelling for a variety of reasons and especially because it reveals that breast cancer knows few boundaries.

14. *The Breast Cancer Survival Manual* (New York: Owl Books, 2003), by John S. Link, M.D. A California breast cancer specialist, Dr. John Link has answered numerous questions for the newly diagnosed in this comprehensive guide.

BOOKS ABOUT CANCER TREATMENT

1. *Chemotherapy and Radiation Therapy Survivor's Guide* (Oakland, CA: New Harbinger Press, 1998) by Judith McKay and Nancee Hirano. This book is written by two nurses who are well aware of the questions patients have and the fears they harbor about these two major forms of cancer treatment. The chapters touch on several key issues: understanding cancer, side effects, relaxation techniques, and the need for good nutrition during cancer treatment.

2. *Choices: The Most Comprehensive Sourcebook for Cancer Information* (New York: HarperResource, 2003), by Marion Morra and Eve Potts. A hefty tome. This book runs more than 1,000 pages and is written in a question-and-answer format that covers every major form of cancer. Breast cancer is discussed in Chapter 13. The authors provide questions and answers on a range of issues, including breast cancer symptoms, surgery, chemotherapy, radiation, etc.

BOOKS ABOUT THE MOLECULAR ASPECTS OF CANCER

1. *One Renegade Cell: How Cancer Begins* (New York: Basic Books, 1999), by Robert A. Weinberg. From one of the world's most highly regarded authorities on cancer biology, Dr. Weinberg of the Whitehead Institute at the Massachusetts Institute of Technology explains in very reader-friendly and elegant language how a single cell sets off the series of ill-fated events that lead to cancer.

2. *Dr. Folkman's War: Angiogenesis and the Struggle to Defeat Cancer* (New York: Random House, 2001), by Robert Cooke. This book offers a detailed look into the work of Harvard University scientist Dr. Judah Folkman, who was the first to theorize that cancers grow by creating their own blood supply, a process called angiogenesis. This book, by a veteran science writer, recounts the resistance Folkman met from doubtful colleagues. Folkman's discoveries formed the research foundation for targeted drugs aimed at destroying tumor blood vessels.

BOOKS ABOUT NAVIGATING THE HEALTH-CARE SYSTEM

1. *Cancer Clinical Trials* (Sebastopol, CA: O'Reilly and Associates, 1999), by Robert Finn. A comprehensive guide on how clinical trials can effectively aid patients with all forms of cancer.

2. *Making Informed Medical Decisions* (Sebastopol, CA: O'Reilly and Associates, 2000), by Nancy Oster, et al. A guide to getting the most out of the health-care system by knowing how to find medical information and learning the language of doctors in order to get the kind of care you deserve.

BOOKS ABOUT THE ENVIRONMENT AND CANCER

1. *Living Downstream: A Scientist's Personal Investigation of Cancer and the Environment* (New York: Vintage Reprint Edition, 1998), by Sandra Steingraber. Written by a biologist and cancer survivor, this book tells of cancer developing in members of Steingraber's

adoptive family. She traces the cancers to concentrations of deadly toxins in her rural region of Illinois. She draws additional environmental links to cancers that have occurred in Massachusetts and on Long Island in New York.

2. *Silent Spring* (Boston, MA: Mariner Books, 1962), by Rachel Carson. This is the book that opened America's eyes to the potential of environmental causes of disease. Written by a marine biologist who died of breast cancer two years after her book's publication, *Silent Spring* is still widely read and can be purchased from online booksellers and in bookstores.

EXPLAINING CANCER TO CHILDREN

1. *What Is Cancer Anyway? Explaining Cancer to Children of All Ages* (Wethersfield, CT: Dragonfly Publishers, 1998), by Karen L. Carney. This book is one in a special series and is designed to provide clear information for children when someone in their family is diagnosed with cancer. Two characters, Barklay and Eve, explain details about cancer and offer explanations on why people lose their hair.

2. *Michael's Mommy Has Breast Cancer* (Coral Springs, FL: Hibiscus Press, 1999), by Lisa Torrey and Barbara W. Watler. Aimed at children between the ages of five and ten. The story is designed to encourage a broader family discussion about breast cancer when mom is diagnosed with the disease.

BOOKLETS

The American Cancer Society offers *Breast Cancer: Treatment Guidelines for Patients*. The publication covers many aspects of breast cancer treatment from diagnosis through chemotherapy. It is aimed at the patient who has been diagnosed for the first time but is useful for those who have had recurrences. You can download a copy if you have Internet access by logging on to www.nccn.org. The booklet runs about sixty-eight pages and provides information on a wide range of topics.

Another booklet, *Taking Time: Support for People with Cancer and the People Who Care about Them,* is a publication of the National Cancer Institute. This sixty-eight-page booklet addresses a range of concerns. You can obtain it free by calling the NCI's toll-free line, (800) 4-CANCER (800-422-6237). Ask for booklet #92-2059.

The NCI's booklet, *Radiation Therapy and You,* can be downloaded from the Internet at www.nci.nih.gov/cancertopics/radiation -therapy-and-you. This publication examines how radiation therapy is performed and explains that treatments do not make you radioactive. It also offers tips on treatment when skin becomes sensitive during treatments.

PAMPHLETS

The following pamphlets are available from the National Cancer Institute, which you can obtain free by calling the NCI's toll-free line (see above) or print out from the NCI's website:

Chemotherapy and You: A Guide To Self Help During Treatment (www.nci.nih.gov/cancertopics/chemotherapy-and-you)

Taking Part in Clinical Trials: What Cancer Patients Need to Know (www.nci.nih.gov/clinicaltrials/resources/taking-part-treatment -trials)

Taking Time: Support for People With Cancer and the People Who Care About Them (www.cancer.gov/cancerinfo/takingtime)

Resources

❦ ❦ ❦

This portion of the book provides resources to help you research a range of issues pertinent to your care. The first three sections list resources associated with treatment. Finding a cancer center or breast-care center is likely to be your first matter of concern. Institutions listed here are not intended as recommendations but rather as sources from which to start your own research. The third section lists resources dealing with complementary and alternative medicine, including a source aimed at helping patients be aware of medical quackery and quacks.

Later sections list various advocacy groups, organizations that provide information on cancer, information on symptom-control as it relates to chemotherapy, and where to buy wigs, hats, and breast prostheses. The last sections delve into financial issues associated with breast cancer and addresses topics such as what your insurance should cover, where to seek financial assistance if your medications are unaffordable, and help with workplace issues.

Selecting a Cancer-Care Center

In this section, you will find a list of all of the major cancer centers that have been designated by the National Cancer Institute as comprehensive cancer centers. These institutions are marked with an asterisk (*). The benefits of treatment at a comprehensive cancer center are wide-ranging and include access to clinical trials, information on basic cancer research, and access to a full range of cancer services, including psychosocial care.

The National Cancer Institute has a second designation: clinical cancer center. These are noted in the list below by a double asterisk (**). Clinical cancer centers provide many of the same services as comprehensive cancer centers but may not conduct as wide a range of research projects as comprehensive centers. A final designation is community cancer center. These institutions usually are found in smaller cities. The Association of Community Cancer Centers is a national organization of 650 cancer centers, group practices, and cancer clinics.

Alabama
University of Alabama at Birmingham Comprehensive Cancer Center*
1824 Sixth Ave. South
Birmingham AL 35294   (800) 822-0933 (800-UAB-0933)
(205) 975-8222
Website: www.ccc.uab.edu

Alaska
Providence Alaska Medical Center
Cancer Program
3200 Providence Dr.
P.O. Box 196604
Anchorage AK 99519   (907) 562-2211
Website: www.providence.org

Arizona
Arizona Cancer Center
The University of Arizona
1515 North Campbell Ave.
P.O. Box 245024
Tucson AZ 85724   (800) 622-2673 (800-622-COPE)
(520) 626-2900
Website: www.azcc.arizona.edu

Arkansas
University of Arkansas for Medical Sciences
Arkansas Cancer Research Center
4301 West Markham St.
Little Rock AR 72205   (501) 686-6000
Website: www.acrc.uams.edu

California
City of Hope National Medical Center*
1500 East Duarte Rd.
Duarte CA 91010   (800) 826-4673 (800-826-HOPE)

(626) 359-8111
E-mail: becomingapatient@coh.org
Website: www.cityofhope.org

Chao Family Comprehensive Cancer Center*
University of California, Irvine
101 The City Dr.
Orange CA 92868   (714) 456-8200
Website: www.ucihs.uci.edu/cancer

Jonsson Comprehensive Cancer Center*
University of California, Los Angeles (UCLA)
8684 Factor Building UCLA Box 951781
Los Angeles CA 90095   (310) 825-5268
Website: www.cancer.mednet.ucla.edu

Norris Comprehensive Cancer Center and Hospital*
University of Southern California
1441 Eastlake Ave.
Los Angeles CA 90033   (800) USC-CARE (800-872-2273)
(323) 865-3000
Website: http://ccnt.hsc.usc.edu

University of California, Davis*
Comprehensive Cancer Center
4501 X St.
Sacramento CA 95817
(800) 362-5566 (general information)
(916) 734-5900 (patient referral)
Website: http://cancer.ucdmc.ucdavis.edu

University of California, San Diego*
Comprehensive Cancer Center
9500 Gilman Dr.
La Jolla CA 92093   (858) 534-7600
Website: http://cancer.ucsd.edu

University of California, San Francisco*
Comprehensive Cancer Center
P.O. Box 0128 UCSF

2340 Sutter St.
San Francisco CA 94143   (800) 888-8664
(415) 476-2201
Website: http://cc.ucsf.edu

Colorado
University of Colorado Cancer Center*
1665 North Ursula St.
Aurora CO 80010   (800) 473-2288 (referral line)
(720) 848-0300
Website: www.uccc.info

Connecticut
Yale Cancer Center*
Yale University School of Medicine
333 Cedar St.
P.O. Box 208028
New Haven CT 06520   (203) 785-4095
Website: www.info.med.yale.edu/ycc

Delaware
Robert and Eolyne Tunnell Cancer Center
Beebe Medical Center
424 Savannah Rd.
Lewes DE 19958   (302) 645-3770
Website: www.beebemed.org

District of Columbia
Lombardi Cancer Center*
Georgetown University Medical Center
3800 Reservoir Rd. NW
Washington DC 20007   (202) 784-4000
Website: http://lombardi.georgetown.edu

Florida
H. Lee Moffitt Cancer Center and Research Institute*
University of South Florida
12902 Magnolia Dr.
Tampa FL 33612   (813) 972-HOPE (813-972-4673)
Website: www.moffitt.usf.edu

M.D. Anderson Cancer Center Orlando (affiliated with M.D. Anderson Cancer Center in Houston)
1400 Orange Ave.
Orlando FL 32806   (407) 648-3800
Website: www.mdandersonorlando.org

Georgia
Winship Cancer Institute of Emory University
1365-C Clifton Rd. NE
Atlanta GA 30322   (888) 946-7447
Website: www.winshipcancerinstitute.org

Hawaii
Cancer Research Center of Hawaii**
1236 Lauhala St.
Honolulu HI 96813   (808) 586-3010
Website: www.crch.org

Idaho
Mountain States Tumor Institute
St. Luke's Regional Medical Center
100 East Idaho St.
Boise ID 83712   (208) 381-2711
Website: www.stlukesonline.org

Illinois
The Robert H. Lurie Comprehensive Cancer Center*
Northwestern University
Olson Pavilion 8250
710 North Fairbanks Ct.
Chicago IL 60611   (312) 908-5250
Website: www.lurie.nwu.edu

University of Chicago Cancer Research Center*
5758 South Maryland Ave.
Chicago IL 60637   (888) 824-0200
(773) 702-9200
Website: www-uccrc.uchicago.edu

Indiana
Indiana University Cancer Center**
535 Barnhill Dr.

Indianapolis IN 46202   (888) 600-4822
(317) 278-4822
Website: http://iucc.iu.edu

Iowa
Holden Comprehensive Cancer Center*
University of Iowa
200 Hawkins Dr.
Iowa City IA 52242
(800) 777-8442 (patient referral)
(800) 237-1225 (general information)
Website: www.uihealthcare.com

Kansas
Cancer Center
Via Christi Cancer Center
929 N. St. Francis St.
Wichita KS 67214   (316) 268-5784
Website: www.via-christi.org

University of Kansas Hospital
Cancer Center and Breast Center
3901 Rainbow Blvd.
Kansas City KS 66160   (913) 588-5000
Website: www.kumc.edu

Kentucky
Markey Cancer Center
University of Kentucky
800 Rose St.
Lexington KY 40536   (859) 257-4488
Website: www.mc.uky.edu/markey

Louisiana
Tulane Cancer Center
Tulane University
1430 Tulane Ave.
New Orleans LA 70112   (504) 988-6060
Website: www.som.tulane.edu/cancer

Maine
Maine Medical Center, a Member of Maine Health Family

Cancer Care
22 Bramhall St.
Portland ME 04102   (207) 871-0111
Website: www.mmc.org

Maryland
Sidney Kimmel Comprehensive Cancer Center*
The Johns Hopkins University
North Wolfe St.
Baltimore MD 21231   (410) 955-8822 (new patients)
Website: www.hopkinskimmelcancercenter.org

Massachusetts
Dana-Farber Cancer Institute*
Harvard University
44 Binney St.
Boston MA 02115   (617) 632-3000
Website: www.dana-farber.net

Cancer Center
Tufts-New England Medical Center
750 Washington St.
Boston MA 02111   (617) 636-2626
Website: http://cancercenter.nemc.org

Michigan
Barbara Ann Karmanos Cancer Institute*
Wayne State University
4100 John R St.
Detroit MI 48201-1379   (800) KARMANOS (800-527-6266)
Website: www.karmanos.org

University of Michigan Comprehensive Cancer Center*
University of Michigan Medical Center, Ann Arbor
1500 East Medical Center Dr.
Ann Arbor MI 48109   (800) 865-1125
Website: www.cancer.med.umich.edu

Minnesota
Mayo Clinic Cancer Center*
Mayo Foundation
200 First St., SW

Rochester MN 55905   (507) 284-3753
Website: http://mayoresearch.mayo.edu/mayo/research/cancercenter/

University of Minnesota Cancer Center*
420 Delaware St., SE
Minneapolis MN 55455   (612) 624-8484
Website: www.cancer.umn.edu

Mississippi
Cancer Services
Mississippi Baptist Medical Center
1225 N. State St.
Jackson MS 39202   (601) 968-1000
Website: www.mbmc.org

Missouri
Siteman Cancer Center**
Washington University School of Medicine
P.O. Box 8100
660 South Euclid Ave.
St. Louis MO 63110   (800) 600-3606
(314) 747-7222
Website: www.siteman.wustl.edu

Montana
Montana Cancer Center
St. Patrick Hospital and Health Sciences Center
500 West Broadway
Missoula MT 59802   (406) 543-7271
Website: www.saintpatrick.org

Nebraska
Eppley Cancer Center**
University of Nebraska Medical Center
Nebraska Medical Center
Omaha NE 68198   (402) 559-4238
Website: www.unmc.edu/cancercenter

Nevada
University Medical Center of Southern Nevada, Las Vegas
Cancer Center
1800 W. Charleston Blvd.

Las Vegas NV 89102   (702) 383-2000
Website: www.umc-cares.org/med_serv/cancer

New Hampshire
Norris Cotton Cancer Center*
Dartmouth-Hitchcock Medical Center
One Medical Center Dr.
Lebanon NH 03756   (603) 650-6300
(800) 639-6918 (cancer help line)
Website: www.cancer.dartmouth.edu

New Jersey
The Cancer Institute of New Jersey*
Robert Wood Johnson Medical School
195 Little Albany St.
New Brunswick NJ 08901
(732) 235-CINJ (732-235-2465)
Website: www.cinj.org

New Mexico
Cancer Research and Treatment Center
The University of New Mexico Health Sciences Center
2211 Lomas Blvd. NE
Albuquerque NM 87106   (505) 272-2111
Website: http://hsc.unm.edu/crtc

New York
Memorial Sloan-Kettering Cancer Center*
1275 York Ave.
New York NY 10021   (800) 525-2225
Website: www.mskcc.org

Roswell Park Cancer Institute*
Elm and Carlton Streets
Buffalo NY 14263-0001   (877) ASK-RPCI (877-275-7724)
Website: www.roswellpark.org

NYU Cancer Institute*
New York University
550 First Ave.
New York NY 10016   (212) 263-6485
Website: www.med.nyu.edu/nyuci

Herbert Irving Comprehensive Cancer Center*
New York Presbyterian/Columbia University
The University Hospital of Columbia and Cornell
622 West 168th St.
New York NY 10032   (212) 305-9327
Website: www.ccc.columbia.edu

Albert Einstein Comprehensive Cancer Center**
Albert Einstein College of Medicine
1300 Morris Park Ave.
Bronx NY 10461   (718) 430-2302
Website: www.aecom.yu.edu/cancer

North Carolina
Duke Comprehensive Cancer Center*
Duke University Medical Center
Durham NC 27710   (919) 684-3377
Website: www.cancer.duke.edu

University of North Carolina School of Medicine*
Lineberger Comprehensive Cancer Center
University of North Carolina at Chapel Hill
Campus Box 7295
Chapel Hill NC 27599   (919) 966-3036
Website: http://cancer.med.unc.edu

Comprehensive Cancer Center at Wake Forest University*
Wake Forest University Baptist Medical Center
Medical Center Blvd.
Winston-Salem NC 27157
(336) 716-4464
Website: www.bgsm.edu/cancer

North Dakota
Cancer Center
Altru Health System
1200 South Columbia Rd.
P.O. Box 6002
Grand Forks ND 58206   (701) 780-5000
Website: www.altru.org

Ohio
The Ohio State University Comprehensive Cancer Center*
The Arthur G. James Cancer Hospital and Richard J. Solove Research
Institute
300 West 10th Ave.
Columbus OH 43210   (800) 293-5066
Website: www.jamesline.com

Ireland Cancer Center*
Case Western Reserve and University Hospitals of Cleveland
11100 Euclid Ave.
Cleveland OH 44106   (800) 641-2422
(216) 844-5432
Website: www.irelandcancercenter.org

Oklahoma
Comprehensive Cancer Center
Oklahoma University Medical Center
1200 Everett Dr.
Oklahoma City OK 73104
(405) 271-4700
Website: www.oumedcenter.com

Oregon
The OHSU Cancer Institute**
Oregon Health Sciences University
3181 Southwest Sam Jackson Park Rd.
Portland OR 97201   (503) 494-1617
Website: www.ohsucancer.com

Pennsylvania
Fox Chase Cancer Center*
7701 Burholme Ave.
Philadelphia PA 19111   (888) FOX-CHASE (888-369-2427)
(215) 728-2570
Website: www.fccc.edu

University of Pennsylvania Cancer Center*
15th Floor, Penn Tower
3400 Spruce St.
Philadelphia PA 19104   (800) 789-PENN (800-789-7366)

(215) 662-4000
Website: www.pennhealth.com

University of Pittsburgh Cancer Institute*
Iroquois Building, Suite 206
3600 Forbes Ave.
Pittsburgh PA 15213   (800) 237-4PCI (800-237-4724)
Website: www.upci.upmc.edu

Kimmel Cancer Center
Thomas Jefferson University
233 South 10th St.
Philadelphia PA 19107
(800) JEFF-NOW (800-533-3669, Jefferson Cancer Network)
(800) 654-5984 (for deaf and hearing-impaired callers)
(215) 503-4500
Website: www.kcc.tju.edu

Rhode Island
Rhode Island Hospital
Comprehensive Cancer Center/Dept. of Medical Oncology
593 Eddy St.
Providence RI 02903   (401) 444-4000
Website: www.lifespan.org

South Carolina
Hollings Cancer Center
Medical University of South Carolina Hospital
86 Jonathan Lucas St.
Charleston SC 29425
(800) 424-MUSC (800-424-6872)
(843) 792-9300 (established patients and self-referrals)
(843) 792-1414 (information and physician referral)
Website: http://hcc.musc.edu

South Dakota
The Cancer Center
Sioux Valley Hospital
University of South Dakota Medical Center
1305 West 18th St.
P.O. Box 5039

Sioux Falls SD 57105   (605) 333-1000
Website: www.siouxvalley.org

Tennessee
The Vanderbilt-Ingram Cancer Center*
Vanderbilt University
649 The Preston Building
Nashville TN 37232
(800) 811-8480 (clinical trial or treatment-option information)
(888) 488-4089 (all other calls)
(615) 936-1782 or (615) 936-5847
Website: www.vicc.org

Texas
The University of Texas M.D. Anderson Cancer Center*
1515 Holcombe Blvd.
Houston TX 77030   (800) 392-1611
(713) 792-6161
Website: www.mdanderson.org

San Antonio Cancer Institute
8122 Datapoint Dr.
San Antonio TX 78229   (210) 616-5590
Website: www.ccc.saci.org

Utah
Huntsman Cancer Institute*
University of Utah
2000 Circle of Hope
Salt Lake City UT 84112
(877) 585-0303
(801) 585-0303
Website: www.hci.utah.edu

Vermont
Vermont Cancer Center
University of Vermont
Medical Alumni Building
Burlington VT 05401   (802) 656-4414
Website: www.vermontcancer.org

Virginia

Massey Cancer Center
Virginia Commonwealth University
401 College St.
P.O. Box 980037
Richmond VA 23298   (804) 828-0450
Website: www.vcu.edu/mcc

The Cancer Center at the University of Virginia**
University of Virginia Health System
P.O. Box 800334
Charlottesville VA 22908
(800) 223-9173
(804) 924-9333
Website: www.med.virginia.edu/cancer

Washington

Fred Hutchinson Cancer Research Center*
1100 Fairview Ave. North
P.O. Box 19024
Seattle WA 98109   (206) 667-5000
E-mail: hutchdoc@seattlecca.org (patient information)
Website: www.fhcrc.org

West Virginia

Mary Babb Randolph Cancer Center
West Virginia University Hospitals
P.O. Box 9300
Morgantown WV 26506   (304) 293-4500 (clinic)
(304) 293-3528 (administration)
Website: www.hsc.wvu.edu/mbrcc
*The center houses the National Cancer Institute's national information
and education network and operates the network's toll-free hotline,
(800) 4-CANCER (800-422-6237).*

Wisconsin

University of Wisconsin*
Comprehensive Cancer Center
600 Highland Ave.
Madison WI 53792   (608) 263-8600
Website: www.cancer.wisc.edu

Breast-Care Centers: What to Look For

This section contains an abbreviated list of breast-care centers, most of which are affiliated with major cancer centers. These specialized centers, whose sole specialty is breast cancer and sometimes other breast abnormalities, are increasingly important in the treatment of the disease. Oncologists, surgeons, nurses, and other staff at these centers help to better educate patients about treatment options. Additionally, specialists in these centers, which offer a multidisciplinary approach toward patient care, pride themselves on addressing patients' emotional needs as well as their medical ones. Information is made readily available to help patients develop a better understanding of breast cancer, which includes making informed decisions about treatment choices and playing an active role in overall treatment strategies.

To find a breast center near you, log on to the National Consortium of Breast Centers (NCBC) at www.breastcare.org. The consortium has an interactive feature on its website that allows you to search for a center. The consortium points out that there are different types of breast centers and that it is important to understand the differences in services that centers offer. Some breast-care centers provide mammography services only, while others are full-treatment cancer facilities affiliated with major cancer centers. You'll want to take note of those differences.

Many breast centers are named for advocates and breast cancer survivors, others for well-known corporations. Even if none of the centers listed are located near you, it may be a good idea to log on to one or more of the sites to get a sense of the kinds of services these facilities offer. In addition to cancer diagnosis and treatment, some programs are augmented with optional alternative and complementary medical services such as art and music therapy, guided imagery, and acupuncture.

Arizona
The Laura Dreier Breast Center
Banner Good Samaritan Medical Center
1111 E. McDowell Rd.
Phoenix AZ 85006   (602) 239-6300
Website: www.bannerhealth.com

California
Saul and Joyce Brandman Breast Center
Cedars-Sinai Medical Center
8700 Beverly Blvd.
Los Angeles CA 90048   (310) 4-CEDARS (310-423-3277)
Website: www.csmc.edu/651.html

The Joyce Eisenberg Keefer Breast Center
John Wayne Cancer Institute
St. John's Health Center
4th Fl., West Wing
1328 22nd St.
Santa Monica CA 90404   (310) 829-8089
Website: www.careforthebreast.com

Revlon/UCLA Breast Center
Jonsson Comprehensive Cancer Center
University of California, Los Angeles (UCLA)
8684 Factor Building UCLA Box 951781
Los Angeles CA 90095   (310) 825-2144
Website: www.jccf.mednet.ucla.edu/revlon.html

The Carol Franc Buck Breast Care Center
University of California, San Francisco
Comprehensive Cancer Center
1600 Divisadero St.
San Francisco CA 94115   (415) 353-3074
Website: http://breastcarecenter.ucsfmedicalcenter.org

Florida
Breast Care Program
H. Lee Moffitt Cancer Center and Research Institute
University of South Florida
12902 Magnolia Dr.
Tampa FL 33612   (813) 972-HOPE (813-972-4673)
Website: www.moffitt.usf.edu

Illinois
Breast Cancer Center
Rush University Medical Center
Rush Professional Office Building

1725 W. Harrison St., Suite 863
Chicago IL 60612   (312) 563-2325
Website: www.rush.edu

Massachusetts

Gillette Centers for Women's Cancers
Dana-Farber Partners CancerCare
44 Binney St.
Boston MA 02115   (800) 320-0022
Website: www.cancercare.harvard.edu
This center and all of the related institutions are major teaching centers of Harvard Medical School.

Michigan

Breast Care Center
University of Michigan
Comprehensive Cancer Center
1500 E. Medical Center Dr.
Ann Arbor MI 48109   (800) 865-1125
Website: www.cancer.med.umich.edu

Missouri

The Breast Cancer Program
St. John's Regional Health Center
1235 E. Cherokee
Springfield MO 65804   (417) 820-2000
Website: www.stjohns.com

New Jersey

The Jacqueline M. Wilentz Comprehensive Breast Center
St. Barnabas Health Care System
Monmouth Medical Center
300 Second Ave.
Long Branch NJ 07740   (732) 923-7700
Website: www.sbhcs.com/hospitals/monmouth_medical/breast_center

New York

The Carol M. Baldwin Breast Care Center
Stony Brook University Hospital
37 Research Way
East Setauket NY 11733   (631) 444-4550
Website: www.stonybrookhospital.com/BALDWIN

The Evelyn Lauder Breast Center and Iris Cantor Diagnostic Center
Memorial Sloan-Kettering Cancer Center
205 E. 64th St.
New York NY 10021   (212) 639-5200
Website: www.mskcc.org

North Carolina
The Breast Cancer Program
Duke Comprehensive Cancer Center
301 MSRB
DUMC Box 3843
Durham NC 27710   (919) 684-3377
Website: http://cancer.duke.edu

Pennsylvania
The Comprehensive Breast Program
Magee-Women's Hospital at the University of Pittsburgh Cancer Institute
300 Halket St.
Pittsburgh PA 15213
Website: www.fightingspirit.org/resources/comprehensive-cancer
-care.html

South Dakota
Breast Health
Women's Resource Center
Sioux Valley Hospital and Health System
Sioux Valley Campus
Medical Building 1, Suite 204
Sioux Falls SD 57117   (605) 328-7155
Website: www.siouxvalley.org/CentersofExcellence/Womens/Services/
BreastHealthServices

Tennessee
Thompson Comprehensive Breast Center
Covenant Health
1915 White Ave.
Knoxville TN 37916   (865) 541-1624
Website: www.covenanthealth.com

The Vanderbilt Breast Center
Vanderbilt-Ingram Cancer Center

Vanderbilt University Medical Center, Suite 2500
Villages at Vanderbilt
Nashville TN 37212   (615) 322-2064
Website: www.mc.vanderbilt.edu

Texas
The Nellie B. Connally Breast Center
University of Texas M.D. Anderson Cancer Center
1515 Holcombe Blvd.
Houston TX 77030
(800) 392-1611
(713) 797-6161
Website: www.mdanderson.org/Care_Centers/BreastCenter

Washington
Breast Cancer Specialty Center
University of Washington Medical Center
1959 NE Pacific St.
Seattle WA 98195   (206) 598-4628
Website: www.uwmedicine.org

Complementary and Alternative Care

Treatments that veer from conventional paths are becoming increasingly popular, but doctors warn that patients should fully investigate such strategies before taking part in them. Indeed, the reason the term *complementary* has been stressed by clinicians is simple: These methods are designed to augment, not replace, conventional therapies.

That said, the National Institutes of Health (NIH) has been investigating various alternative and complementary techniques that can be incorporated into conventional cancer treatment. Through its National Center for Complementary and Alternative Medicine, the NIH conducts a range of clinical studies in this burgeoning area. Many complementary treatments involve helping cancer patients with relaxing, becoming less anxious, or coping with depression. Mind/body medicine is one area being explored as a way to help patients cope with the harsh side effects of cancer treatment.

Many breast-care and cancer centers now offer some complementary and alternative techniques as optional aspects of care. However, if you decide to investigate alternative treatment strategies outside of a major treatment center, be aware that few of them have been fully investigated by medical scientists. The following list provides a few options to help you begin your research.

Cancer Treatment Centers of America
(800) 615-3055
Website: www.cancercenter.com
This network offers cancer treatment in four states as of this writing. According to the group's website, the centers, which advertise nationally on television, augment traditional cancer treatment with nutrition education, spiritual support, mind/body medicine, and naturopathic care. Representatives are available twenty-four hours a day to talk with prospective patients by phone.

National Center for Complementary and Alternative Medicine (part of the National Institutes of Health)
NCCAM Clearinghouse
P.O. Box 7923
Gaithersburg MD 20898
(888) 644-6226
(866) 464-3615 (TTY, for hearing-impaired callers)
Website: http://nccam.nih.gov
This center sponsors clinical trials in various complementary and alternative treatments. It also offers lectures and conferences.

The Wellness Web
http://groups.msn.com/TheWellnessWeb
Patients, clinicians, and caregivers provide information on this website. Participants exchange ideas about medications, clinical trials, mind/body medicine, and complementary care.

Quackwatch: Your Guide to Quackery, Health Fraud, and Intelligent Decisions
www.quackwatch.org
According to its website, Quackwatch is a "nonprofit corporation whose purpose is to combat health-related frauds, myths, fads, and fallacies. Its primary focus is on quackery-related information that is difficult or impossible to get elsewhere. It was founded in 1969 as the Lehigh Valley Committee Against Health Fraud and was incorporated in 1970. In 1997, it assumed its current name and began developing a worldwide network of volunteers and expert advisors." The bottom-line message of

Quackwatch is: Don't be fooled. Its website offers several noteworthy features, including "Quackery: How It Harms Cancer Patients" and "A Special Message for Cancer Patients Seeking Alternative Treatment."

Breast Cancer Organizations

Adelphi New York Statewide Breast Cancer Hotline and Support Program
School of Social Work
Adelphi University
Garden City NY 11530   (800) 877-8077
Website: www.adelphi.edu/nysbreastcancer

African American Breast Cancer Alliance
P.O. Box 8981
Minneapolis MN 55408   (612) 825-3675
E-mail: aabcainc@yahoo.com
Website: www.aabcainc.org

American Breast Cancer Foundation
1055 Taylor Ave.
Baltimore MD 21286   (877) 539-2543
Website: www.abcf.org

Breast Cancer Action
55 New Montgomery, Suite 323
San Francisco CA 94105   (415) 243-9301
Website: www.bcaction.org

The Breast Cancer Fund
1388 Sutter St., Suite 400
San Francisco CA 94109   (415) 346-8223
Website: www.breastcancerfund.org

The Breast Cancer Research Foundation
654 Madison Ave., Suite 1209
New York NY 10021   (646) 497-2600
Website: www.bcrfcure.org

The Breast Cancer Resource Committee
2005 Belmont St. NW
Washington DC 20009   (202) 463-8040
Website: www.bcresource.org

Breast Cancer Support and Reach to Recovery Discussion Group
(800) 227-2345
Website: www.cancer.org
An outgrowth of Reach to Recovery that formerly was a one-on-one support program but now sponsors group support meetings; contact your local or state chapter of the American Cancer Society.

Brides Against Breast Cancer: Making Memories Breast Cancer Foundation
12708 SE Stephens St.
Portland OR 97233   (503) 252-3955
Website: www.makingmemories.org/babc.html
Brides can help breast cancer patients by donating their wedding gowns. The gowns are then sold to raise money to aid patients with metastatic breast cancer.

Celebrating Life
P.O. Box 224076
Dallas TX 75222   (800) 207-0992
Website: www.celebratinglife.org
Resources and support for African American breast cancer patients.

Community Breast Health Project
545 Bryant St.
Palo Alto CA 94301   (650) 326-6686
Website: www.cbhp.org
Resources in the San Francisco Bay Area.

Fertile Hope
P.O. Box 624
New York NY 10014   (888) 994-HOPE (888-994-4673)
Website: www.fertilehope.org
Helps cancer survivors with fertility concerns.

The Inflammatory Breast Cancer Research Foundation, Inc.
(877) STOP-IBC (877-786-7422)
Website: www.ibcsupport.org
An online support organization.

Living Beyond Breast Cancer
10 East Athens Ave., Suite 204
Ardmore PA 19003   (610) 645-4567
Website: www.lbbc.org

Mary-Helen Mautner Project: The National Lesbian Health Organization
1707 St. NW, Suite 230
Washington DC 20036   (202) 332-5536
Website: www.mautnerproject.org

Men Against Breast Cancer: Caring about the Women We Love
P.O. Box 150
Adamstown MD 21710   (866) 547-MABC (866-547-6222)
Website: www.menagainstbreastcancer.org

Mothers Supporting Daughters with Breast Cancer
21710 Bayshore Rd.
Chestertown MD 21620   (410) 778-1982
Website: www.mothersdaughters.org

National Asian Women's Health Organization
250 Montgomery St., Suite 1500
San Francisco CA 94104   (415) 989-9747
Website: www.nawho.org

National Breast Cancer Coalition
1101 17th St. NW, Suite 1300
Washington DC 20036   (202) 296-7477
Website: www.natlbcc.org

National Native American Breast Cancer Survivors' Network
3022 S. Nova Rd.
Pine CO 80470   (303) 838-9359
Website: www.natamcancer.org
In association with the Native American Cancer Initiatives.

OBGYN.Latina.net
Website: http://latina.obgyn.net/espanol
An online organization that offers health information for women of Hispanic heritage; information is available in English or Spanish.

Pregnant with Cancer Network
P.O. Box 1234
Buffalo NY 14220   (800) 743-6724, ext. 308
Website: www.pregnantwithcancer.org

SHARE: Self-Help for Women with Breast or Ovarian Cancer
1501 Broadway, Suite 704A

New York NY 10036
(866) 891-2392
(212) 719-0364
Website: www.sharecancersupport.org

Susan G. Komen Breast Cancer Foundation
5005 LBJ Freeway, Suite 250
Dallas TX 75244
(800) I'M AWARE (800-462-9273) (help line)
(972) 855-1600
Website: www.komen.org

SusanLoveMD.Com
P.O. Box 846
Pacific Palisades CA 90272
(310) 230-1712
Website: www.susanlovemd.com

Women's Information Network Against Breast Cancer
536 S. Second Ave., Suite K
Covina CA 91723   (626) 332-2255
Website: www.winabc.org

Y-ME National Breast Cancer Organization
212 West Van Buren St., Suite 500
Chicago IL 60607
(312) 986-8338
(800) 221-2141 (twenty-four-hour hotline—English)
(800) 986-9505 (twenty-four hour hotline—Spanish)
Website: www.y-me.org
Y-Me volunteers speak 150 languages.

Young Survival Coalition
P.O. Box 528
52A Carmine St.
New York NY 10014   (212) 206-6610
Website: www.youngsurvival.com
For survivors under age forty.

General Cancer Information

American Cancer Society (ACS)
1599 Clifton Rd., NE

Atlanta GA 30329   (800) ACS-2345 (800-227-2345)
Website: www.cancer.org

American Society of Clinical Oncology (ASCO)
1900 Duke St., Suite 200
Alexandria VA 22314   (703) 299-0150
Website: www.asco.org

Association of Community Cancer Centers
11600 Nebel St., Suite 201
Rockville MD 20852   (301) 770-1949
Website: www.accc-cancer.org
The leading policy organization for community cancer centers; maintains a list of community cancer centers nationwide.

Association of Oncology Social Work
1211 Locust St.
Philadelphia PA 19107   (215) 545-8107
Website: www.aosw.org

Cancer Care, Inc.
275 7th Ave.
New York NY 10001
(212) 712-8080
(800) 813-4673
Website: www.cancercare.org
Support-group information, cancer education, counseling, etc.

Cancer Research Institute
681 Fifth Ave.
New York NY 10022   (800) 992-2623
Website: www.cancerresearch.org
Explores the immune system as a way to prevent, control, and cure cancer.

National Cancer Institute (NCI)
31 Center Dr.
Bethesda MD 20892
Website: www.cancer.gov

National Coalition for Cancer Survivorship
1010 Wayne Ave., Suite 770
Silver Spring MD 20910   (301) 650-9127
Website: www.canceradvocacy.org

National Comprehensive Cancer Network
500 Old York Rd., Suite 250
Jenkintown PA 19046   (215) 690-0300
Website: www.nccn.org

National Women's Health Network
514 10th St. NW
Washington DC 20004   (202) 347-1140
Website: www.womenshealthnetwork.org

Online Research Resources

Association for International Cancer Research
Website: www.aicr.org.uk
A British organization that supports basic cancer research into the causes, mechanisms, diagnosis, treatment, and prevention of cancer.

Breastcancer.org
Website: www.breastcancer.org
An online breast cancer resource that offers a wide range of information about breast cancer.

CANSearch
Website: www.canceradvocacy.org/resources/guide
A guide to cancer resources maintained by the National Coalition for Cancer Survivorship.

Cancer Information Network
Website: www.cancernetwork.com
Provides general information on cancer diagnosis, treatment, and prevention.

Cancer Survivors' Network
Website: www.cancersurvivorsnetwork.com
A resource developed by the American Cancer Society to aid cancer survivors; offers the opportunity, once you're registered with the site, to link your personal web page to the site.

CenterWatch
Website: www.centerwatch.com
A database of thousands of clinical trials for cancer as well as other medical conditions.

ClinicalTrials.gov
Website: www.clinicaltrials.gov
Provides information on a wide array of clinical trials; developed by the National Library of Medicine.

InteliHealth
Website: www.intelihealth.com
Features information from Harvard Medical School's Consumer Health Guide.

International Cancer Alliance
Website: www.icare.org
Offers a wide range of cancer information for patients with all forms of cancer, including breast cancer.

Mayo Clinic Health Oasis
Website: www.mayohealth.org
A vast resource of information from the famed clinic in Minnesota.

Office of Minority Health Resource Center
Website: www.omhrc.gov
Provides information on all forms of cancer for ethnic minorities; a division of the National Institutes of Health.

OncoLink
Website: www.oncolink.upenn.edu
Provides a broad range of data on clinical trials, coping with cancer, cancer treatments, etc. Operated by the University of Pennsylvania, this was the Internet's first major cancer resource.

PubMed
Website: www.ncbi.nlm.nih.gov/entrez
Physician's Data Query. The National Library of Medicine's database of scientific studies.

Women's Cancer Network
www.wcn.org
An online information resource funded by a grant from Bristol-Myers Squibb.

Listservs: Chatting on the Internet

Association of Cancer Online Resources
Website: http://acor.org

As of this writing, Acor.org sponsors twelve listservs for people with breast cancer. The listservs provide online "support groups" for people with a range of breast cancer diagnoses, including lists that focus on new treatments, inflammatory breast cancer, male breast cancer, metastatic disease, and partners of breast cancer patients, etc.

Friends in Need
Website: www.friendsinneed.com
Forums for online support for those being treated for breast cancer and survivors of the disease. The group's website notes that the listserv is for support and discussion. Medical advice should be sought from patients' physicians.

Breast-Cancer
Website: www.bcforum.org/list.html
Subscription address: ListServ@morgan.ucs.mun.ca
This is a discussion list that you can subscribe by sending an e-mail. To subscribe leave the subject area in your e-mail blank. In the body of your message write: subscribe Breast-Cancer. Add your first and last names. The website also has links to a chatroom for the Internet Breast Cancer Support Group as well as to a room for men who are in the life of a woman with breast cancer.

Symptom and Postsurgical Concerns

American Pain Society
Website: www.ampainsoc.org
Posts on its website a vast amount of information about pain, the use of pain medications, and the responsibilities of health-care professionals in prescribing potent painkilling drugs.

CancerSymptoms.org
Website: www.cancersymptoms.org
Sponsored by the Oncology Nursing Society and aimed at helping patients manage cancer symptoms, the site provides information on cancer-related fatigue, pain, depression, low white-blood-cell count, cognitive dysfunction, etc.

Chemocare.com
Website: www.chemocare.com
An excellent resource for patients on chemotherapy, this website has answers to many of the questions patients may ask about chemotherapy,

managing side effects, eating well during chemo, complementary ther-
apy, and survivors' experiences.

National Lymphedema Network
1611 Telegraph Ave.
Oakland CA 94612(800) 541-3259
(510) 208-3200
Website: www.lymphnet.org
Provides educational materials about a condition that is caused by the
surgical removal of lymph nodes. The organization offers information on
prevention and treatment.

Cosmetic Issues

American Cancer Society
Website: www.cancer.org www.cancer.org (keywords: *breast prostheses*
and *hair loss*)
The ACS maintains a web page with an extensive list of companies that
sell hats, wigs, and breast prostheses.

Bosom Buddy Breast Forms
Website: www.bosombuddy.com
Soft-fabric breast forms that fit in a bra.

Headcovers Unlimited
Website: www.headcovers.com
An online company aimed at chemotherapy patients as well as people
who have lost their hair due to other causes. The company sells hats,
turbans, caps, and other attractive headwear in an array of fashionable
choices.

Liberator Medical Supply
Website: www.liberatormedical.com
An online service that sells breast forms, mastectomy bras, mastectomy
swimwear, etc.

Look Good… Feel Better
Website: www.lookgoodfeelbetter.org
A national service to help with concerns about makeup, wigs, and other
cosmetic issues during chemotherapy and radiation. The site also provides
information to help men coping with cancer treatment. The American
Cancer Society and the National Cosmetology Association have collabo-
rated to bring this vital service to cancer patients around the country.

Dealing with Issues of Treatment Costs, Insurance, and Employment

Breast cancer treatment is not inexpensive. Most people will probably have a major portion of their expenses covered by health-care insurance. As a first step, you will want to review your policy to determine which costs are covered and which you may have to pay out-of-pocket. In addition to the organizations listed in Chapter 2 that can help with insurance-related issues, this section lists several more resources.

Online resources are available to help you understand insurance policies and to point you in the right direction when there is a dispute. Also bear in mind that insurance plans are not created equal. Some provide prescription drug coverage while others do not. You will want to know where you stand as far as prescription costs are concerned.

Health-insurance issues aside, an increasing number of reports in the medical and lay literature drive home a chilling fact: Cancer care is becoming so expensive that some patients must decide which among their prescribed medications they will buy. Exorbitant drug costs prohibit them from purchasing all that are required. An even more frightening scenario for some is facing cancer care without any medical coverage at all. An estimated forty-five million people in the United States are without health-care insurance.

Assistance with Insurance and Workplace Issues

The following sources provide information on insurance, workplace issues, and where to turn when you are unable to afford care.

American Association of Retired Persons (AARP)
601 E St. NW
Washington DC 20049   (888) OUR-AARP (888-687-2277)
Website: www.aarp.org
Initiated the Breast Cancer and Mammography Awareness campaign and is a strong advocate in the halls of Congress to reduce the cost of prescription drugs. AARP was among the first to note that the cost of prescription medications was outpacing inflation. The organization offers Medicare supplementary insurance.

Association of Community Cancer Centers
11600 Nebel St., Suite 201

Rockville MD 20852   (301) 984-9496

Website: www.accc-cancer.org

Offers a mother lode of information on a variety of cancer-related issues, including health insurance. The website includes a lengthy guide that can be downloaded, titled "Cancer Treatments Your Insurance Should Cover." In it, the authors address the following:

1. *Why some insurance companies are denying payment for effective cancer treatments*
2. *What can be done if payment is denied*
3. *How to ensure that your plan provides adequate coverage for cancer treatments*

The website also offers information about making treatment choices when diagnosed with early-stage breast cancer.

CancerCare
275 7th Ave.
New York NY 10001   (800) 813-4673
(212) 712-8080
Website: www.cancercare.org

Offers a broad range of information on financial assistance in its Helping Hand Resource Database. The database lists services that offer help through very small grants for specific cancers in some locations of the United States. The center does not provide grants for basic living expenses, such as food, rent, or mortgage payments. Through its Avon-Cares program, the organization offers small grants for breast cancer patients nationwide. On its website you'll find information about health-insurance and resources that provide information on assistance with medications.

Centers for Medicare and Medicaid Services (formerly the Health Care Financing Administration)
7500 Security Blvd.
Baltimore MD 21244   (877) 267-2323
Website: www.cms.hhs.gov

This is the federal agency that oversees Medicare and Medicaid. Medicare is the national health-insurance program that provides coverage for an estimated forty million U.S. citizens who are sixty-five or older, as well as for people under that age who have disabilities. Medicaid provides medical assistance for certain individuals and families with low incomes and few resources.

The Civilian Health and Medical Program of the Department of Veterans Affairs (CHAMPVA)
Website: www1.va.gov/health_benefits
This is the medical-benefits program for dependents of U.S. veterans. The Veterans Administration pays for certain medical services. The website is complex and lists more than a dozen telephone numbers at division headquarters. Two suggestions here: Visit the website, and call the regional Veterans Administration nearest you. A map is posted on the site.

The Civilian Health and Medical Programs of the Uniformed Services (CHAMPUS)
Website: www.ndw.navy.mil/Newcomers/Medical/champus.html
A federal agency that helps pay for civilian medical care for spouses and children of enlisted, active-duty military personnel, as well as retired uniformed-services personnel and their spouses and children. The agency also provides medical assistance to spouses of active or retired military personnel who have died. The CHAMPUS website has a pricing feature that allows you to obtain information on prevailing fees for certain procedures within a given area.

America's Health Insurance Plans (AHIP)
601 Pennsylvania Ave. NW
South Building, Suite 500
Washington DC 20004   (202) 778-3200
Website: www.ahip.org
This is a trade association that represents the nation's major insurance companies. HIAA offers consumer publications about health insurance.

HealthInsuranceInfo.Net
Website: www.healthinsuranceinfo.net
Do you have a problem with your health insurance? Are you being properly reimbursed? If not, perhaps this site can help. It contains information on how consumers should handle disputes with their insurers.

Hill-Burton Program
Website: http://ask.hrsa.gov/pc
In 1946, Congress passed the Hospital Survey and Construction Act, sponsored by Senators Lister Hill and Harold Burton. The legislation originally was designed as a way to infuse dollars into the modernization of hospitals. Over time the program has changed to contend with

another major need: patients who require care but who cannot afford it. Hundreds of hospitals, clinics, and other medical facilities that have received funding under the Hill-Burton Act offer free or reduced-cost services. But be aware: Not all communities have medical facilities that fall under the program's rules. You can find facilities closest to you by logging on to the program's website.

Medical Information Bureau, Inc.
P.O. Box 105
Essex Station
Boston MA 02112   (617) 426-3660
Website: www.mib.com
This company, which is a collaborative effort between U.S. and Canadian life-insurance firms, is aimed at preventing insurance fraud. Its website lists information to help you with credit repair, debt negotiation, and how to obtain your medical records.

Patient Advocate Foundation
700 Thimble Shoals Blvd., Suite 200
Newport News VA 23606
(800) 532-5274
Website: www.patientadvocate.org
A national nonprofit organization that acts as a liaison between patients and certain entities with whom there may be a dispute: an employer, an insurance company, creditors, etc. The aim is to help patients resolve employment, debt, and insurance issues. According to its literature, the foundation "seeks to safeguard patients through effective mediation assuring access to care, maintenance of employment and preservation of financial stability."

Assistance with Drug Costs

You can find medications at low or no cost through programs offered by many of the major pharmaceutical companies. Keep in mind that you must meet certain income requirements, usually at or below the federally assigned poverty threshold. To find information you may want to log on to the website of the company that produces the medication you need and plug in the keywords "patient assistance program." Alternatively, contact one or both of the following groups:

NeedyMeds, Inc.
P.O. Box 63716

Philadelphia PA 19147   (215) 625-9609
Website: www.NeedyMeds.com
An online organization that assists patients who meet certain income requirements to obtain no-cost prescription medications. The company does not want patients writing to them about financial problems.

Partnership for Prescription Assistance
1100 15th St. NW
Washington DC 20005
(800) 4PPA-NOW (800-477-2669)
(800) 762-4636
Website: www.pparx.org
A vital resource for patients who are having difficulty with the cost of prescription medications. The site has an interactive feature that allows searches for prescription-drug-assistance programs. Do not write to the Partnership for Prescription Assistance about your financial need.

Index

❧ ❧ ❧

WOMEN'S CANCERS: How to Prevent Them, How to Treat Them, How to Beat Them

by Kerry A. McGinn, R.N., and Pamela J. Haylock, R.N.

This guide gives women detailed information on treating and surviving the cancers that exclusively affect them: breast, cervical, ovarian, uterine, and vaginal cancer, as well as lung and colon cancer. The second edition covered the latest screening guidelines and diagnostic tests, and the discovery of the breast cancer gene. The third edition addresses the late and long-term effects of cancer, the new FDA approved and "smart" drugs, and possible environmental factors in cancer development.

544 pages ... 76 illus. ... Paperback $24.95 ... Third edition

LYMPHEDEMA: A Breast Cancer Patient's Guide to Prevention and Healing *by Jeannie Burt and Gwen White, P.T.*

This book emphasizes active self-help for lymphedema, the disfiguring and often painful swelling, particularly of the arm, that affects as many as 30 percent of breast cancer patients. It describes the many options women have for preventing and treating the condition, ranging from exercise to compression to massage. A second edition will be available in September 2005.

240 pages ... 44 illus. ... 2 photos ... Paperback $14.95 ... Second edition

RECOVERING FROM BREAST SURGERY: Exercises to Strengthen Your Body and Relieve Pain *by Diana Stumm, P.T.*

Speed your recovery from breast surgery, recover mobility, and eliminate pain. Physical therapist Diana Stumm shares what she has learned in her 30+ years of working with breast cancer patients. Using clear drawings, she describes a program of specific stretches, massage techniques, and exercises that form the crucial steps to a full and pain-free recovery from mastectomy, lumpectomy, radiation, reconstruction, and lymphedema.

128 pages ... 50 illus. ... Paperback $12.95

THE FEISTY WOMAN'S BREAST CANCER BOOK

by Elaine Ratner   Featured in The New York Times

This personal guide helps women navigate the emotional and psychological landscape surrounding breast cancer. Its positive message make this a perfect companion for every woman who wants not only to survive but also thrive after breast cancer.

"There are times when a woman needs a wise and level-headed friend, someone kind, savvy and caring... [This] book is just such a friend..." — **Rachel Naomi Remen, M.D.**

288 pages ... Paperback $14.95

To order books see last page or call (800) 266-5592

MEN'S CANCERS: How to Prevent Them, How to Treat Them, How to Beat Them ... *Pamela J. Haylock R.N., M.A., Editor*
This is a resource for men concerned about cancer, their family members, and caregivers. Each chapter is written by a specialized nurse or nurse practitioner and covers prevention, early detection, diagnosis, treatments, follow-up, and recurrence. Special chapters address sex changes related to cancer and future directions in scientific research and study. Includes an extensive resource section.

368 pages ... 9 illus. ... Paperback $19.95

THE PROSTATE HEALTH WORKBOOK: A Practical Guide for the Prostate Cancer Patient *by Newton Malerman*
Malerman, a prostate cancer survivor, attributes his recovery to a proactive approach. He encourages readers to understand their disease and get the best medical care possible. Based on his experience, extensive research, and discussions with doctors, nurses, and patients, he has written this hands-on book that includes 25 worksheets, from medical history checklists and treatment evaluation charts to test result records.

160 pages ... 6 illus. ... 35 worksheets ... Paperback $14.95

POSITIVE OPTIONS FOR COLORECTAL CANCER: Self-Help and Treatment *by Carol Ann Larson, Foreword by Kathleen Ogle, M.D.*
Colorectal cancer is treatable, even preventable. This practical book is a guide to warning signs, screening tests, treatment options, alternative healing methods, and life after colorectal cancer. The author, a survivor of colorectal cancer, explains how to cope with the disease and obtain the best treatments. The book includes contributions from cancer survivors, extensive input from medical experts, and a resource guide.

168 pages ... 6 illus. ... Paperback $12.95

CANCER DOESN'T HAVE TO HURT: How to Conquer the Pain Caused by Cancer and Cancer Treatment
by Pamela J. Haylock, R.N., and Carol P. Curtiss, R.N.
People with cancer often suffer pain needlessly. Research shows that cancer patients who have less pain do better. Readers learn how to describe pain in terms doctors understand and ask for the pain relief they need. The authors explain how to read prescriptions, administer medications, and adjust dosages if necessary. The book also includes information on proven non-drug methods of pain relief.

192 pages ... 17 illus. ... Paperback $14.95

MENOPAUSE WITHOUT MEDICINE *by Linda Ojeda, Ph.D.*

In this new edition of her bestselling book, Linda Ojeda discusses what the Women's Health Initiative study did and did not show about the dangers of HRT, the best options for peri- and postmenopausal women, the important differences between synthetic and bioidentical natural hormones, and hormone tests and nonhormonal remedies for correcting hormone imbalances. She gives natural remedies for depression, hot flashes, sexual changes, and skin and hair problems, and presents an updated, illustrated basic exercise program.

384 pages ... 37 illus. ... 45 tables ... Paperback $15.95 ... Fifth edition

THE *NATURAL* ESTROGEN DIET & RECIPE BOOK

by Dr. Lana Liew with Linda Ojeda, Ph.D.

From two top women's health and nutrition experts: almost 100 easy and delicious recipes that will naturally increase women's estrogen levels. Each recipe includes nutritional details including cholesterol and calcium contents. The authors discuss how estrogen can be derived from the food we eat, list foods that are the highest in estrogen content, and include meal plan ideas.

256 pages ... 25 illus. ... Paperback $14.95 ... Second edition

HER HEALTHY HEART: A Woman's Guide to Preventing and Reversing Heart Disease *Naturally* *by Linda Ojeda, Ph.D.*

Almost twice as many women die from heart disease and stroke as from all forms of cancer combined—in fact, heart disease is the #1 killer of American women ages 44 to 65. This book addresses the unique aspects of heart disease in women and the natural ways to prevent it, whether they take hormone replacement therapy (HRT) or not.

Ojeda also provides detailed information on how to reduce the risk of heart disease through nutrition and diet, physical activity, and stress management.

352 pages ... Paperback $14.95

HOW WOMEN CAN *FINALLY* STOP SMOKING

by Robert C. Klesges, Ph.D., and Margaret DeBon

Strategies for quitting are different for men and women. Women who quit smoking tend to gain more weight, menstrual cycles and menopause affect the likelihood of success, and their withdrawal symptoms are different. This program is based on the highly successful model at Memphis State University and is authored by pioneers in the field.

192 pages ... 4 illus. ... Paperback ... $11.95

CHRONIC FATIGUE SYNDROME, FIBROMYALGIA, AND OTHER INVISIBLE ILLNESSES: A Comprehensive and Compassionate Guide *by Katrina Berne, Ph.D.*

A new edition of the classic work *Running on Empty*, this greatly revised and expanded book has the latest findings on chronic fatigue syndrome and comprehensive information about fibromyalgia, a related condition. Overlapping diseases such as environmental illness, breast implant inflammatory syndrome, lupus, Sjögren's syndrome, and post-polio syndrome are also discussed. The book includes information on possible causes, symptoms, diagnostic processes, and options for treatment.

400 pages ... Paperback $15.95 ... Hardcover $25.95

THE ART OF GETTING WELL: A Five-Step Plan for Maximizing Health When You Have a Chronic Illness
by David Spero, R.N., Foreword by Martin L. Rossman, M.D.

David Spero brings together the medical, psychological, and spiritual aspects of getting well in a five-step approach: slow down and use your energy for things and people that matter — make small, progressive changes that build confidence — get help and nourish your social ties — value your body and treat it with affection and respect — take responsibility for getting the best care and health you can.

224 pages ... Paperback $16.95 ... Hardcover $25.95

CHINESE HERBAL MEDICINE MADE EASY: Natural and Effective Remedies for Common Illnesses
by Thomas Richard Joiner

Chinese herbal medicine is an ancient system for maintaining health and prolonging life. This book demystifies the subject, with clear explanations and alphabetical listings of 750 remedies for over 250 common illnesses ranging from acid reflux and AIDS to breast cancer, pain management, and weight loss.

432 pages ... Paperback $24.95 ... Hardcover $34.95

GET FIT WHILE YOU SIT: Easy Workouts from Your Chair
by Charlene Torkelson

Here is a total-body workout that can be done right from your chair, anywhere. Perfect for people with age-related movement limitations or special conditions, it includes the *One-Hour Chair Program*, a full-body, low-impact workout; the *5-Day Short Program* for those short on time; and *Ten-Minute Miracles*, exercises perfect for anyone on the go.

160 pages ... 212 photos ... Paperback $14.95

To order books see last page or call (800) 266-5592

POSITIVE OPTIONS FOR CROHN'S DISEASE
by Joan Gomez, M.D.

Crohn's disease is an inflammatory bowel condition that, while nonfatal, can be devastating. This book discusses who is at risk and why, and addresses what can be done, including self-care.

192 pages ... 1 illus. ... Paperback $12.95

POSITIVE OPTIONS FOR LIVING WITH YOUR OSTOMY
by Dr. Craig A. White

This book is a complete, supportive guide to dealing with the practical and emotional aspects of life after ostomy surgery.

144 pages ... 4 illus. ... Paperback $12.95

POSITIVE OPTIONS FOR HIATUS HERNIA
by Tom Smith, M.D.

A hiatus hernia is a common, potentially serious condition that occurs when the upper part of the stomach pushes through the diaphragm. This book describes tests, treatments, and self-help options.

128 pages ... 4 illus. ... 2 tables ... Paperback $12.95

POSITIVE OPTIONS FOR REFLEX SYMPATHETIC DYSTROPHY (RSD) *by Elena Juris*

RSD, also called Complex Regional Pain Syndrome, is characterized by severe nerve pain and extreme sensitivity to touch. This book covers medical information, practical advice, and holistic therapies.

224 pages ... 2 illus. ... Paperback $14.95

POSITIVE OPTIONS FOR ANTIPHOSPHOLIPID SYNDROME (APS) *by Triona Holden*

Also called Hughes syndrome and "sticky blood," APS is implicated in many serious health problems. This book identifies the symptoms and provides important information on diagnosis and treatment.

144 pages ... Paperback $12.95

POSITIVE OPTIONS FOR SEASONAL AFFECTIVE DISORDER (SAD) *by Fiona Marshall and Peter Cheevers*

About 10 million Americans suffer from SAD. This book helps distinguish the condition from classic depression and chronic fatigue, and suggests ways to alleviate the symptoms and live optimally.

144 pages ... Paperback $12.95

ORDER FORM

10% DISCOUNT on orders of $50 or more —
20% DISCOUNT on orders of $150 or more —
30% DISCOUNT on orders of $500 or more —
On cost of books for fully prepaid orders

NAME

ADDRESS

CITY/STATE   ZIP/POSTCODE

PHONE   COUNTRY (outside of U.S.)

TITLE	QTY	PRICE	TOTAL
Breast Cancer Basics and Beyond		@ $15.95	
Women's Cancers		@ $24.95	

Prices subject to change without notice

Please list other titles below:

		@ $	
		@ $	
		@ $	
		@ $	
		@ $	
		@ $	
		@ $	

Check here to receive our book catalog ☐   FREE

Shipping Costs

By Priority Mail: first book $4.50, each additional book $1.00
By UPS and to Canada: first book $5.50, each additional book $1.50
For rush orders and other countries call us at (510) 865-5282

TOTAL	_____
Less discount @____%	(_____)
TOTAL COST OF BOOKS	_____
Calif. residents add sales tax	_____
Shipping & handling	_____
TOTAL ENCLOSED	_____

Please pay in U.S. funds only

☐ Check ☐ Money Order ☐ Visa ☐ MasterCard ☐ Discover

Card # _____ Exp. date _____

Signature _____

Complete and mail to:
Hunter House Inc., Publishers
PO Box 2914, Alameda CA 94501-0914
Order at www.hunterhouse.com
call (800) 266-5592 or email: ordering@hunterhouse.com
Phone (510) 865-5282 Fax (510) 865-4295

BCB 07/2005